The Professional Medical Assistant: Clinical Practice

Bonnie J. Lindsey, CMA, CMT

and

Francis M. Rayburn, RN, CCRN

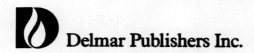

Delmar Publishers Inc.

NOTICE TO THE READER

Publisher does not warrant or guarantee any of the products described herein or perform any independent analysis in connection with any of the product information contained herein. Publisher does not assume, and expressly disclaims, any obligation to obtain and include information other than that provided to it by the manufacturer.

The reader is expressly warned to consider and adopt all safety precautions that might be indicated by the activities described herein and to avoid all potential hazards. By following the instructions contained herein, the reader willingly assumes all risks in connection with such instructions.

The publisher makes no representations or warranties of any kind, including but not limited to, the warranties of fitness for particular purpose or merchantability, nor are any such representations implied with respect to the material set forth herein, and the publisher takes no responsibility with respect to such material. The publisher shall not be liable for any special, consequential or exemplary damages resulting, in whole or in part, from the readers' use of, or reliance upon, this material.

Cover design by Bellone & Associates

Delmar Staff

Administrative Editor: Marion Waldman
Developmental Editor(s): Denise Black Gold and Helen Yackel
Project Editor: Andrea Edwards Myers
Production Coordinator: Mary Ellen Black
Art Supervisor: Judi Orozco
Design Coordinator: Karen Kunz Kemp
Senior Design Supervisor: Susan C. Mathews

For information, address Delmar Publishers Inc.
3 Columbia Circle, Box 15-015
Albany, New York 12212-5015

Printed in the United States of America
Published simultaneously in Canada
by Nelson Canada
a division of the Thomson Corporation

1 2 3 4 5 6 7 8 9 10 XXX 99 98 97 96 95 94 93

Library of Congress Cataloging-in-Publication Data

Lindsey, Bonnie Joan.
   The professional medical assistant : clinical practice / Bonnie J.
Lindsey and Francis M. Rayburn.
      p.   cm.
   Includes index.
   ISBN 0-8273-4150-4
   1. Medical assistants.   I. Rayburn, Francis M.   II. Title.
   [DNLM: 1. Allied Health Personnel.   2. Physicians' Assistants.
WA 21.5 L752p]
R728.8.L58   1993
610.69'53—dc20
DNLM/DLC
for Library of Congress   92-18589
                                                                CIP

The Professional
Medical Assistant

Contents

Preface

Purpose and Content

This text will introduce the medical assisting student to the duties and responsibilities of the professional medical assistant in clinical practice. In addition, we cover other aspects of professionalism—the professional organizations, interrelationships to other health-care professionals, and job-seeking information.

The authors have addressed the clinical competencies outlined in the 1990 DACUM update on the medical assisting profession to ensure that students will be able to achieve those basic entry-level skills necessary to the profession.

Information is also provided on the Clinical Laboratory Improvements Act of 1988 (CLIA). Students and instructors are admonished to be sure which laboratory tests may be performed by the medical assistant in the various states.

Organization

The nineteen chapters of the basic text are organized into a logical sequence presenting the information essential to the performance of the clinical competencies. This sequence is based on the teaching and on-job experience of the authors, but classroom presentation of the chapters may easily be rearranged to meet the needs of various programs and instructors. Following the main text is a chapter-by-chapter correlation of DACUM to the text (see appendix).

The intent of the authors is to introduce the student to the profession and its legal aspects. Then prior to covering the performance of the various procedures, we provide the student with the necessary information regarding the transmission of disease and preventive measures, medical asepsis, and data collection essential to diagnosis.

Where appropriate, more information than the essential theory has been provided in an attempt to assist the student in performing as a clinical medical assistant and in improving in the role of assisting the physician.

Examples and illustrations are provided where appropriate, as is patient education information. Vocabulary lists precede each chapter. Chapter review exercises conclude each chapter.

Information is provided on laboratory rules, Universal Precautions, patient education, AIDS, etc., along with information on arterial blood gases and pulmonary function studies, even though medical assistants will in all probability never be involved in the performance of these studies.

Recognizing that the duties of the clinical medical assistant vary from office to office and state to state, every attempt has been made to provide the student with the clinical and theoretical information essential to the profession.

Supplementary Materials

For the convenience of the instructor, an instructor reference manual is available with answer keys to the review questions, suggestions for presentation of material within the chapters, and answer keys to the objective materials presented in the student workbook, which contains additional testing and evaluation materials.

CHAPTER 1

Introduction to Clinical Medical Assisting

OBJECTIVES	On completion of this chapter, you will be able to:

- Demonstrate knowledge of the medical-assisting profession.
- Identify the relevant professional organizations and discuss the benefits derived from membership and active participation.
- Explain the legal aspects of a medical record and the need for documentation by the medical assistant.
- Define "clinical medical assisting."
- List the duties of a clinical medical assistant.
- Demonstrate correct charting technique and correction of charting errors.
- Differentiate among certification, license, and registration.
- Identify health-care associates.
- Define the chapter vocabulary terms.

Vocabulary— Glossary of Terms

Ancillary   Subordinate; controlled by authority. For example, an ancillary to the physician is the medical assistant, a registered nurse, or other licensed health-care professional.

Chart   Also called *medical record;* ongoing documentation of the care and treatment of a patient; also includes personal and financial information.

Concise   Free from elaboration or unnecessary detail.

Confidential   Containing information whose disclosure could be prejudicial to the person's interest.

Ethics   A code of conduct usually established by a profession through its professional organization.

Facet   Any definable aspect of a subject or object.

Law   A binding custom or practice enforced by a controlling authority.

Legible   Plain; readable.

Professional   One who conforms to the technical or ethical standards of a profession; conducting oneself in a manner fitting to a profession.

1

Statute	A law enacted by a legislative body of the government.
Subpoena	A command for a document or person to appear in court.
Technician	A specialist in the technical details of an occupation.
Vital Signs	Recordable data existing as a manifestation of life; e.g., temperature, pulse, respiration, and blood pressure.

Introduction

Welcome to the profession of medical assisting, a richly rewarding component of the national health-care delivery system. As a professional, you will be engaged in a field of endeavor with **ethical** and technical standards that you will be expected to uphold.

Medical assisting is a diverse field that includes a variety of tasks. As a clinical medical assistant, you will need to be patient oriented and will have direct patient contact.

Clinical medical assistants used to be called the "back office persons," meaning that they were not normally the first persons encountered by the patient in the medical office; their duties were performed directly with the patient or out of view of the waiting room. Since clinical duties require direct patient contact, the clinical person frequently wears a uniform and is occasionally inappropriately called, by the physician, the "nurse" or "my nurse," as opposed to "the medical assistant" or "my medical assistant." A name tag identifying you as a medical assistant will clearly reveal your professional status to patients and other health-care professionals.

Many of your duties as a clinical medical assistant are also duties performed by persons in other health occupations. These include taking and recording of vital signs, electrocardiograms, bandaging and dressing operative and postoperative sites and other wounds, assisting the physician with a variety of examinations and office surgeries, administering medications by a variety of modalities, and patient education; all duties generally associated with the nursing profession.

Patient education also will require that you develop good verbal skills so that patients will be able to understand you and your instructions to them. Good written communication skills also are required, since many directions you provide verbally must also be given in writing so the patient will have something to refer to at home.

You will also have responsibilities normally associated with the laboratory technology health occupations, such as specimen collection and handling and performing a variety of tests on body fluids such as blood and urine.

Your duties also will include disinfection and sterilization of equipment and supplies, and with the appropriate limited license, you may also perform certain types of radiologic examinations usually associated with the radiology **technician** profession. The procedures for performing these examinations are not covered in this text, but a variety of examinations and patient education related to radiologic examinations will be addressed.

You will also perform duties associated with the dietician and physical therapist as you counsel patients on diet and exercise. You will borrow from the home economist as you teach patients economical shopping techniques related to food purchasing and preparation and menu planning.

Relation to Other Health-Care Professionals

As a professional clinical medical assistant, you will continually interact with members of other health professions. You will interact with your physician employer, with other medical assistants, both administrative and clinical, and with other health professionals employed in the same office. You will also interact with health-care professionals in other offices, the hospital, medical laboratories, and so on.

Some of these individuals will be "licensed," such as physicians and nurses. *Licensed* means that they have been granted legal permission by state **statutes (laws)** to perform specific acts. Others will be *certified,* meaning that they have met certain requirements, normally documented by test, as set forth by their professional organization. The basic examination you will take to become a "certified medical assistant" covers both the administrative and clinical skills utilized in your profession and assures employers that you have met the competency levels of your profession.

A misconception held by some medical assistants is that they are certified upon graduation from their respective training program. ***This is not true.*** The diploma, certificate, or other documentation received upon completion of your training program certifies only that you have completed the requirements of the program with a passing grade (usually "C" or better).

Other health professionals will be *registered,* meaning that their name has been entered into an official record of those individuals who have met certain requirements. Individuals listed on a register may also be licensed or certified depending on the type of register. Some health professionals with whom you will interact are:

Physician: licensed by the state of practice, having met the requirements of the state licensing agency.

Registered Nurse (RN): licensed by the state of practice having met the requirements of the state licensing agency. They may be graduates of a two-year program, a three-year or diploma program, or a four-year program with a Bachelor's or higher degree in nursing. Included here are the *nurse practitioner* and *nurse midwife,* since they are registered nurses.

Practical Nurse (LPN), also Vocational Nurse (LVN): licensed by the state of practice having met the requirements of the state licensing agency. Training programs for practical/vocational nurses vary from six months to fifteen months or more, depending on the training school curriculum.

Laboratory Technician/Medical Technologist: licensed or certified.

Physician Assistant: certified. Graduate of an approved program; may be RN or LPN/LVN as well, and works under the license of a physician.

Radiology Technician/Technologist: usually licensed.

Medical Transcriptionist: certified/noncertified.

Other health-care professionals with whom you will interact include respiratory therapists, physical therapists, dieticians, emergency medical technicians, paramedics, electrocardiogram technicians, electroencephalogram technicians, medical secretaries, health information systems personnel, and others.

Professionalism

As a clinical medical assistant, you will be part of the medical assisting profession and as such will represent that profession in every **facet** of your employment and your relationships with other health-care professionals and with your patients. Whether you are certified or not, you will be expected to maintain your skills, upgrade your knowledge, and act in a professional manner that conforms to the ethical standards of your profession. You will represent your profession to the community by participating in one of the professional organizations and by educating the public and the patients who come into your care.

Professional Organizations

As a professional medical assistant you will want to become actively involved in one of the professional organizations. The American Association of Medical Assistants, Inc. (20 North Wacker Drive, Suite 1575, Chicago, IL 60606) was founded in 1956 and has local chapters throughout the United States. By writing to them directly, you can obtain the location of the chapter nearest to you and secure a membership application. As a member, you will receive *The Professional Medical Assistant,* the official journal of AAMA. This publication will help you keep abreast of developments in medical assisting and provide you with hints for increasing your efficiency, through original articles by experts in their field. AAMA offers national certification, continuing education and revalidation, and other benefits.

The American Medical Technologist was organized in 1930, and in 1976 introduced a component called "The Registered Medical Assistant" for the purpose of advancing the standards of the medical assisting professional and promoting educational and social advantages for those members. This organization also provides certification and continuing education programs and publishes quarterly educational publications and newsletters. Interested medical assistants should write directly to RMA/AMT, 710 Higgins Road, Park Ridge, IL 60068-5765, for information.

Active involvement in a professional organization at the student level will allow you to meet and interact with working professionals and increase your knowledge and understanding of the profession. This exposure certainly can be beneficial when you start seeking employment in the field.

Legal Aspects

As you are eliciting information from patients, assisting in their care and treatment, and educating them, you will learn much about them that is considered to be **confidential** information. This means that the information is *privileged;* that is, it cannot be revealed to anyone except those involved directly in the care and treatment of the patient, and only as it relates to that care and treatment. To reveal this information could result in a lawsuit based on *invasion of the patient's right to privacy.* Divulging financial, social, health, family, or treatment information is also an invasion of the patient's right to privacy.

Medical assisting is considered to be an **ancillary** health occupation. As such, under the law it falls under the legal doctrine of *respondeat superior,* literally meaning "let the master answer." This has been interpreted to mean that the physician must answer for everything that involves the treatment of the patient, even if that treatment was performed by someone other than the physician, such as a clinical medical assistant. As more professionals become involved in the care and treatment of the patient, and as more is expected of them in terms of professional preparation, education, and continuing education, medical assistants can expect to be held accountable, by law, for their own actions as they relate to the care and treatment of patients.

Chart/Medical Record

The **chart**/medical record is a legal document in which entries must be made in a thorough, clear, and **concise** fashion. This record provides a paper trail of everything done to and for the patient, when, by whom, and with what outcome. In some cases, it may also include statements about something not done and why. Every chart entry must be accompanied by a date and the name or initials of the charter. It is also recommended that entries include the time of day, particularly those involving procedures, such as venipuncture, capillary puncture, administration of medication, performance of laboratory tests, or obtaining specimens for testing.

Clear, concise, appropriate, well-documented chart entries may protect the entry maker from becoming implicated in a lawsuit for unlawful performance of a duty or action. Keep in mind, while making chart entries, that you may be held accountable for what you write today, right now, this minute, by a court of law years from now. The time from when a malpractice lawsuit is initiated until it actually goes to court may be several years.

The chart/medical record is considered a legal document and may be subpoenaed into court. A **subpoena** is a formal request by the court to review the chart/medical record and/or make it part of the formal court proceedings. As an entry maker into the document, you can be subpoenaed by the court as well.

Charting and Documentation

Just as the administrative medical assistant provides documentation consisting of day sheets, ledgers, statements, insurance forms, invoices, purchase orders, etc., for tracking and legal purposes, you also will have your own documentation called the chart/medical record. This record will include the patient's personal and financial information, medical, family, social, and personal history; from first to last entry it is ongoing documentation of the diagnosis and treatment of each patient. Entries will be made by the physician in handwritten or transcribed form, and by the medical assistant in handwritten form. In your charting entries you must express yourself clearly, concisely, accurately, and **legibly.**

You may write or print your entries, but they must be readable by anyone. You must write in blue or black ink, never in pencil or erasable ink pens. Fine- or medium-point ballpoint pens work very well. Think about what you want to say in your chart entry before you write it. This prevents many charting errors.

PROCEDURE FOR CHARTING

1. **Chart what was done.** Was this a laboratory test? If so, what was the name of the test? Did you administer a medication? What was the name of the medication, the dosage, and method of administration? If the medication was given by injection, you will need to include the site. (This will be discussed in further detail in the chapter on administration of medications.) Was this a procedure such as a dressing change? If you changed a dressing or removed sutures, what did the wound look like, how many sutures were removed, and what type of bandage or dressing materials were applied?
2. **Chart when it was done.** The date, and if a medication, laboratory test, or specimen collection, the time it was done.
3. **Chart the outcome, if any.** If this was a medication, was there a reaction, what kind of reaction, and when did the reaction occur? If this was a laboratory test, what was the result of the test? If there were **vital signs,** what were they? How were they taken?
4. **Initial (or sign your name) to the entry** (Figure 1.1).

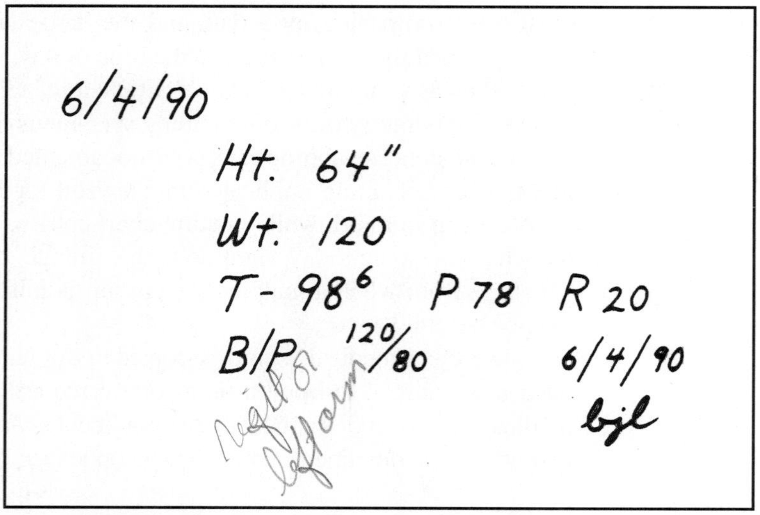

Figure 1.1 Example of correct charting

CORRECTING ERRORS

You are human, and humans do make mistakes. Therefore, it may occasionally be necessary for you to correct errors in your charting. When this happens, keep in mind that the error correction must be as clear and legible as the original charting and must include your initials. *Never erase the error. Never use a coverup such as Liquid Paper ("white-out").*

PROCEDURE FOR CORRECTING ERRORS

1. **Draw a single, clear line through the error.**
2. **Above the error, write your initials and the date and time the correction was made.**
3. **Chart the correct entry following correct procedure.** *Never,* make a correction to a chart entry after your office has received notification that a lawsuit is pending (Figure 1.2).

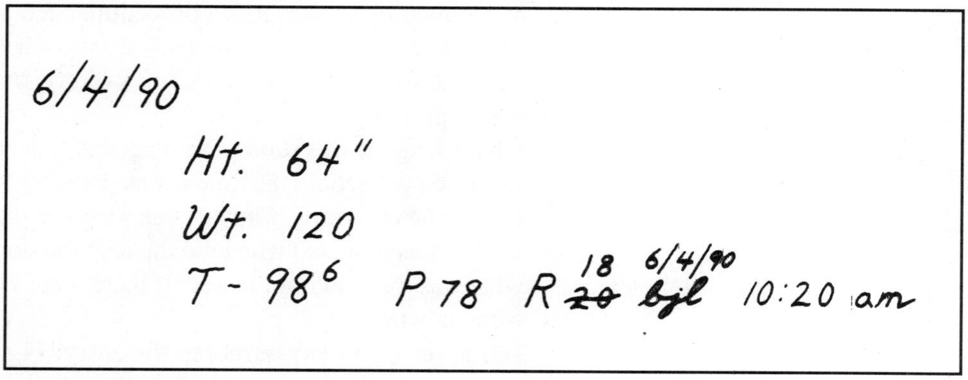

Figure 1.2 Example of chart error correction

**REVIEW/
SELF-EXAMINATION**

1. Differentiate between a patient chart and a patient medical record.
   are the same - legal document care + treatment

2. Can Liquid Paper or "white-out" be used to correct chart entries?
   Absolutely Not!

3. Why should a medical assistant not be referred to as a "nurse"?
   you don't have license

4. What is a medical record?
   legal document, care + treatment

5. Why is a medical record necessary?
   paper trail everything done, why, whom, instruction's

6. What is meant by confidential information? Give examples.
   disclosure in procedural that may cause harm

7. What is meant by *respondeat superior*?
   legal doctrine, Dr. must answer for treatment of patient

8. What information is needed in a chart entry?
   what when outcome +initals of person doing chart

9. What color ink should be used in making chart entries?
   black or blue

10. How can you invade someone's right to privacy?
    by telling someone treatment info. patient info.

11. Differentiate between licensed, certified, and registered.
    licenced-State certified - meet requirments registered-included in registary

12. How would you correct an error on a chart?
    drew line throw and initial, date, time *of people who have been*

13. Is it true that when you are notified that a lawsuit is pending, you should make whatever corrections are necessary to the patient's medical record? *no*

14. Must a professional possess a college degree? *No*

15. Licensed individuals must meet certain standards established by whom? *State*

16. Certification standards are established by whom? *professional orgazations*

17. What is meant by "privileged information"? *Confidential*

18. You are working with a physician assistant. Would you refer to him or her as "doctor"? *noo afo*

19. A patient calls you "nurse." How would you explain to them that you are a clinical medical assistant? *tell them you are not a nurse*

CHAPTER 2

Agents of Disease

On completion of this chapter, you will be able to:
- Identify common microbes.
- Identify vectors of disease in man.
- Identify at least ten diseases common to man.
- Identify the stages of the disease process.
- Identify the need for a universal blood and body fluid precaution system.
- Differentiate between normal and abnormal flora.
- Discuss various types of immunity.
- List the basic requirements for the growth of microorganisms.
- Explain the transmission process of HIV infections and AIDS.
- Differentiate between HIV, ARC, and AIDS.
- Demonstrate proper blood and body fluid precautions.

Vocabulary— Glossary of Terms

AIDS	Acquired immune deficiency syndrome.
Antigen	A substance capable of producing an immune response.
Bacterium	Any microorganism that multiplies by cell division and typically is contained within a cell wall.
Cilia	Hairlike processes projecting from the surface of a cell.
Coccoid	Resembling a coccus or globe.
Cytoplasm	The material outside the cell nucleus; the site of most of the chemical activities of the cell.
DNA	Deoxyribonucleic acid; a nucleic acid found in all living cells.
Flagellum	A whiplike projection from the surface of a cell that serves as a locomotion organ.
Flora	Bacteria normal to the body.
Fluke	Trematode worm.

Vector carrier

HIV	Human immunodeficiency virus.
Host	A plant or animal that harbors or nourishes another organism.
Immune	Resistant to disease.
Immunization	The process of producing immunity.
Impervious	Impenetrable; incapable of being damaged or harmed.
Indigenous	Native to a particular place.
Lumen	The cavity or channel of a tubelike structure.
Lymphocyte	Granulocytic leukocyte.
Microbe	A minute living organism.
Mollusks	Animals such as snails, slugs, mussels, oysters, clams, octopuses, and squids.
Nucleus	A small spheroid body contained within most cells.
Opportunistic	Used to refer to a microorganism that normally does not cause disease, but under certain conditions becomes pathogenic.
Optimum	Most favorable; e.g., *optimum* conditions.
Organelle	A specific particle of a cell whose functions involve locomotion or metabolism.
Parasite	A plant or animal living upon or within another living organism.
Pathogen	A disease-producing microorganism.
Prevalent	Dominant or powerful.
Refractile	Capable of deviation.
Retrovirus	A large group of RNA viruses including the viruses causing leukemia.
Toxin	A protein produced by certain pathogenic bacteria. A poison.
Vector	A carrier of an infective agent from one host to another.

Vectors of Disease in Humans

We live in a world of **parasitic microbial** agents, visible and not visible; normally we live in harmony with these agents. However, when our defense mechanisms are not functioning at **optimum** level, infection and disease can and frequently do occur, progressing through several stages:

1. *Incubation stage*—the time between the invasion of the **host** by the **pathogen** and the appearance of the symptoms of the disease.
2. *Prodrome stage*—onset of the initial symptoms, such as headache, malaise, runny nose, watery eyes, cough, chills, fever, etc., heralding the onset of illness.
3. *Acute stage*—occurs when the symptoms are fully developed and the disease is at its peak.

4. *Decline stage*—period during which the symptoms abate.
5. *Convalescence*—period between illness and return to health.

Health care personnel must be vigilant to protect both themselves and those under their care by controlling microbe activity in order to retard or prevent the spread of infection and disease. Host defenses against microbial attack include anatomic barriers such as intact skin and respiratory mucosa that is **ciliated** or lined with hair (e.g., the nose).

Immune factors, which include antibodies and various types of blood cells, play a tremendous role in maintaining health; physiologic barriers, such as gastric acid, also contribute to overall health maintenance.

Parasitic **vectors** commonly found in the diseases and infections that plague humans are classified as follows:

1. Bacteria
2. Fungi
3. Helminths
4. Protozoa
5. Rickettsiae
6. Viruses

BACTERIA

Bacteria are single-celled organisms that lack a true **nucleus** and other structures called **organelles,** which makes them different from all other organisms. Genetic material of bacteria consists of a single loop of double-stranded **DNA**. Reproduction is by cell division approximately every twenty minutes, giving them a high rate of population growth. Most bacteria possess a rigid cell wall outside of the cell membrane and may also possess certain external structures allowing for movement.

Bacteria are classified according to their shape or form and metabolic reactions. **Cocci** are spherical bacteria; diplococci do not always separate on mitosis or cell division, characteristically occur in pairs, and are responsible for such diseases as gonorrhea, meningitis, and pneumococcal pneumonia. Staphylococci occur in clusters resembling a bunch of grapes; streptococci appear as chains (Figure 2.1). Rod-shaped bacteria are referred to as bacilli: those with tapered ends are called fusiform bacilli, while those shaped like long threads are called filamentous bacilli. Bacilli that appear as spirals are called spirilla or spirochetes.

Bacteria are also classified according to their oxygen requirement: those that need oxygen are called aerobic, those that do not are called anaerobic. Anaerobic bacteria may be further subdivided into obligate anaerobes, which will grow only in

Figure 2.1 Examples of bacteria (Adapted with permission from Fong and Ferris, *Microbiology for Health Careers*, 4th Ed., Delmar Publishers Inc., 1987)

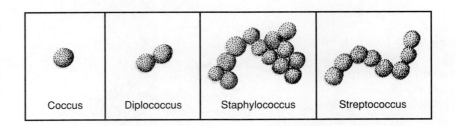

| Coccus | Diplococcus | Staphylococcus | Streptococcus |

the absence of oxygen, and facultative anaerobes, which possess the ability to adapt to an environment with or without oxygen.

Bacteria are also classified into two major groups called Gram-positive and Gram-negative, based on their reaction to the Gram stain. Gram-positive bacteria stain violet, while Gram-negative bacteria are decolorized and counterstain pink. Staphylococci and streptococci are both Gram-positive and are responsible for most bacterial infections occurring in humans. Staphylococci are responsible for a variety of infections, including boils, abscesses, and osteomyelitis. While they may produce systemic infections, their tendency is to produce localized infections with inflammation and pus. Staphylococci are particularly troublesome because of the ability of most strains to develop resistance to antibiotics. Streptococci, on the other hand, tend to resist localization and may spread throughout the bloodstream. They are responsible for such diseases as streptococcal throat infections, bacterial endocarditis, rheumatic fever, scarlet fever, and septicemia.

Some bacteria produce a **toxin** or poison; for example, *Corynebacterium diphtheriae,* which is responsible for the disease diphtheria or dysentery, is produced by various species of *Shigella*. A refractile, oval body called a *spore* may be formed within some bacteria and is highly resistant to environmental change; examples are *Bacillus* and *Clostridium,* which are responsible for such diseases as botulism, gas gangrene, Hansen's disease (leprosy), and tetanus. Other bacterial infections include cholera, pertussis (whooping cough), plague, syphilis, typhoid, and tuberculosis.

In the healthy individual, the skin, respiratory tract, and gastrointestinal tract are host to a variety of normal **flora** and parasitic bacteria that are harmless and occasionally helpful to their host by interfering with the growth of harmful bacteria. **Opportunistic** infections occur when organisms **indigenous** to one area of the body invade another part of the body where that bacillus is not native. An example would be the *Escherichia coli,* an intestinal bacillus, invading the urinary system.

FUNGI

Fungi are simple, plant-like organisms marked by the absence of chlorophyll and the presence of a rigid cell wall in some stages of their life cycle. Reproduction is by means of spores, which are oval bodies formed within the bacteria. Fungi are present in soil, air, and water and some species, such as the *Candida,* are part of the normal flora of the mouth, skin, intestinal tract, and vagina (Figure 2.2).

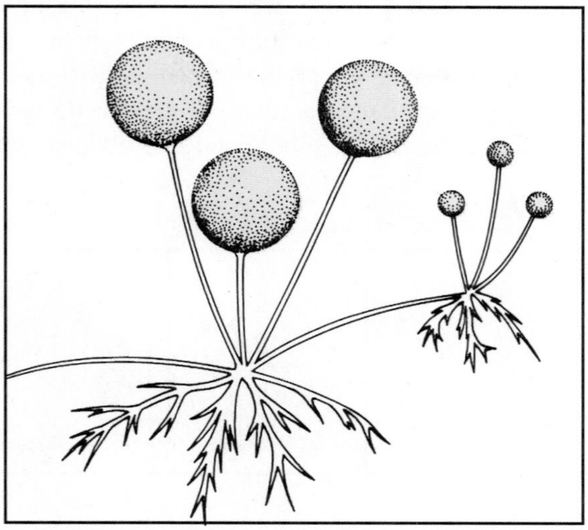

Figure 2.2 Example of a fungus: bread mold (Adapted with permission from Fong and Ferris, *Microbiology for Health Careers,* 4th Ed., Delmar Publishers Inc., 1987)

HELMINTHS

Helminths are parasitic worms—soft-bodied, elongated, naked invertebrates classified as nematodes or trematodes. Nematodes are roundworms characterized by longitudinally oriented muscles and an unusual esophagus. They occur as parasites in both humans and animals (Figure 2.3).

Trematodes are **flukes** and are also parasitic in both humans and animals. Since all flukes require a **mollusk** as their first host, primary infections generally result from the ingestion of uncooked or insufficiently cooked fish or shellfish, such as shrimp and lobster (Figure 2.4).

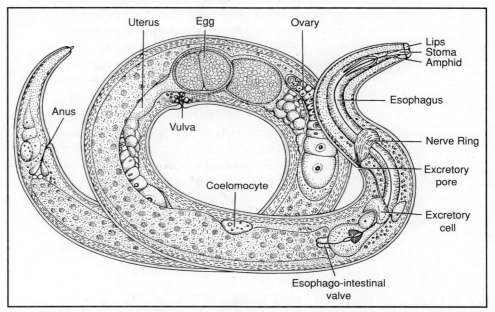

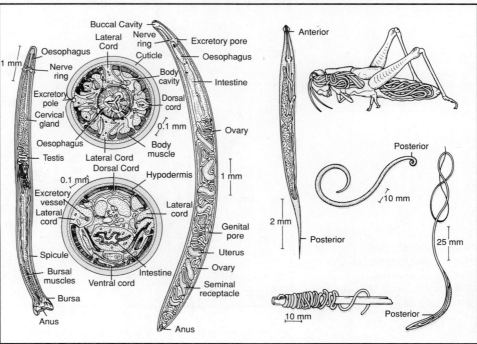

Figure 2.3 General nematode structure

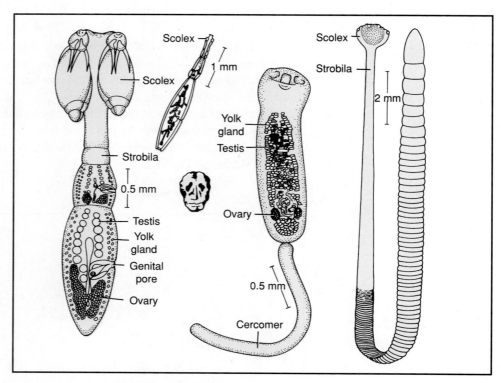

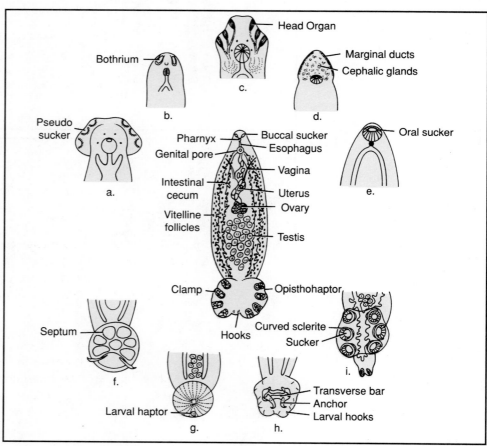

Figure 2.4 General trematode structure

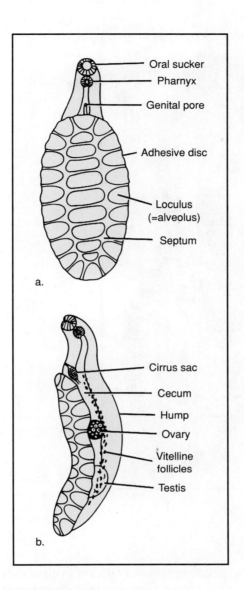

Figure 2.4 (continued)

PROTOZOA

Protozoa are the simplest organisms of the animal kingdom; they are single celled and range in size from submicroscopic (invisible under a standard microscope) to macroscopic (visible without the aid of a microscope). In various stages of their life cycle they possess **flagella** or cilia, which permit movement, but have no locomotor organs in the adult stage. Reproduction is by spore production. Parasitic infection of humans by protozoa is by means of contaminated food or water (Figure 2.5).

RICKETTSIA

Rickettsia are small, rod-shaped to globe-shaped bodies, often occurring in a variety of distinct forms within the **cytoplasm** or free in the **lumen** of the intestines in lice, fleas, ticks, and mites, by which they are transmitted to humans and other animals. Disease transmission is by bite from the infected host. Where good sanitary conditions and insect and rodent control are **prevalent**, rickettsial disease is not a major problem.

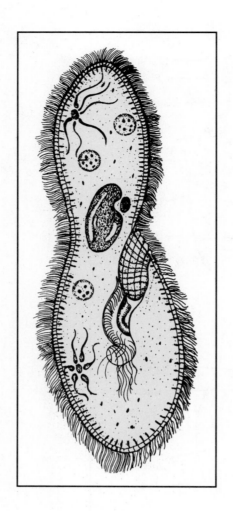

Figure 2.5 Example of protozoa: paramecium (Adapted with permission from Fong and Ferris, *Microbiology for Health Careers,* 4th Ed., Delmar Publishers Inc., 1987)

VIRUSES

Viruses are minute organisms ranging in size from 200–300 nm to 15 nm in size. They are composed of elements that do not possess uniform qualities and are able to replicate only within living host cells. They are frequently subgrouped according to host specificity, namely bacterial, animal, or plant. Classification is also made according to their origin, mode of transmission, or the manifestations they produce.

Viruses are responsible for many of the diseases that plague humans, from the common cold to hepatitis, herpetic infections, influenza, mumps, poliomyelitis, rabies, rubella (German measles), rubeola (measles), smallpox, and varicella (chickenpox) (Figure 2.6). Cytomegalovirus refers to host-specific herpes viruses that in humans produce cytomegalic inclusion disease with a syndrome that resembles infectious mononucleosis.

Virus reproduction is almost completely carried out within host cells, and chemotherapeutic agents have little or no effect on viral infections. Active **immunization** can be obtained by vaccination. Passive immunization is achieved with immune globulin. A class of antiviral drugs has been developed and is being utilized with some success in the treatment of some viral infections.

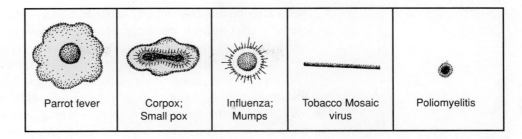

Figure 2.6 Examples of viruses (Adapted with permission from Fong and Ferris, *Microbiology for Health Careers,* 4th Ed., Delmar Publishers Inc., 1987)

| Parrot fever | Corpox; Small pox | Influenza; Mumps | Tobacco Mosaic virus | Poliomyelitis |

Microorganisms as Agents of Disease

Normal flora is a term used to describe microbes found normally in various parts of the body such as the mouth or intestines. When host defenses are not at optimum function, normal flora may increase and become manifest as the symptoms of infection or disease.

NORMAL VERSUS ABNORMAL FLORA

Humans are host to countless microscopic and macroscopic parasites. While the macroscopic parasites, the helminths, are of no benefit to man, they normally live in relative balance with their host, taking only enough nutrients to survive without destroying the health of the host.

On the other hand, microscopic organisms, in normal state, frequently contribute to normal system function in the area to which they are indigenous or native. *Escherichia coli,* as an example, is a species of Gram-positive bacteria, usually nonpathogenic, that constitutes the greater portion of the normal flora of the intestines in humans and other animals. *Candida,* an imperfect fungus with yeast-like characteristics, formerly called monilia, is another normally benign member of the parasitic flora of the skin, mouth, intestinal tract, and vagina.

FAVORABLE GROWTH CONDITIONS

When normal host defense mechanisms are not functioning at the optimum level, then normally benign parasites proliferate at abnormally high levels. The same situation occurs when an organism that is indigenous to one part of the body is introduced to a part of the body to which it is not indigenous.

Antibiotic therapy can, and frequently does, interfere with normal host defense mechanisms, a side effect of which frequently is the proliferation of certain types of normal flora. *Escherichia coli* often become the predominant bacteria in the flora of the mouth and throat.

Another side effect to some antibiotic therapy is candidiasis, formerly referred to as a yeast infection or moniliasis, occurring in the vagina and producing a number of extremely unpleasant symptoms.

VECTORS IN THE SPREAD OF DISEASE

Vectors are simply carriers in the spread of disease and include humans, animals, and insects that transfer a disease agent from one host to another.

Humans act as vectors in a variety of ways. One way is by transfer of normal flora of one part of the body to a part of the body to which it is not normal. *Escherichia coli,* for instance, are frequently transferred to the mouth or urinary tract via improper hygiene, such as failure to wash one's hands thoroughly with soap and water after elimination of body waste and then rubbing one's eye, putting a finger in one's mouth, or even handling food. In this fashion, humans are quite capable of self-inflicted vectoring of potentially infectious agents (Figure 2.7).

Direct contact with another human via kissing, touching, and sexual contact (via contact with body fluids and excretions) is another common source for the transmission of infectious agents (Figure 2.8). **HIV** infections and *Candida* can be transmitted in this fashion, as well as *Neisseria gonorrhoea*, the causative organism for gonorrhea. Transmission of the virus producing acquired immune deficiency syndrome (**AIDS**) via sexual contact or direct contact with the infected body fluids of an infected individual is now of worldwide concern.

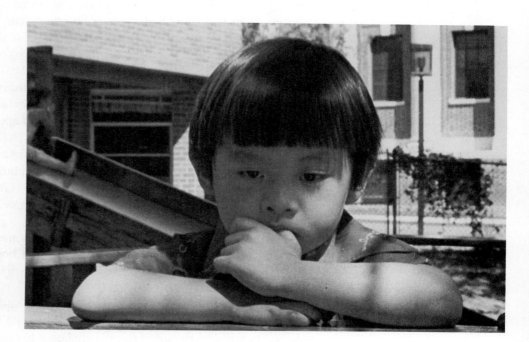

Figure 2.7 Sucking a thumb is one way in which a child might transfer a potentially infectious agent from one part of the body to another.

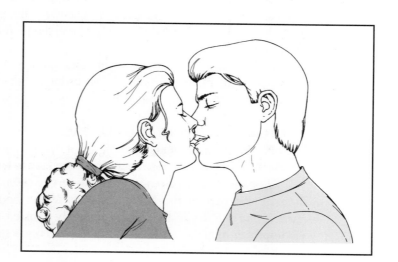

Figure 2.8 Kissing is a common way that infectious agents are transmitted from one person to another.

Nosocomial or hospital-borne infections are the result of direct contact with other patients, hospital personnel, or contaminated or improperly sterilized instruments and supplies; they account for hundreds of thousands of deaths each year, to say nothing of the millions of dollars in cost of increased hospitalizations. Common causative agents of nosocomial infections are *Escherichia coli, Proteus, Pseudomonas, Klebsiella* and *Staphylococcus.* The Joint Commission on the Accreditation of Hospitals is responsible for setting the standards for control of nosocomial infections.

Since physicians spend a great deal of time in the hospital environment (making rounds, in surgery, in the emergency room, etc.), they can act as vectors in the spread of nosocomial infections to the medical office environment. Medical assistants can also act as vectors in the spread of nosocomial infections since they also frequently interact with the hospital environment when they pick up or deliver X rays, laboratory specimens, or mail or just take lunch or coffee breaks in the hospital cafeteria, thereby interacting with hospital personnel and others.

Staphylococcal infections can be the result of proliferation of normal flora, may be transferred by direct contact, or may be nosocomial in origin. They are usually pyogenic or pus producing and are potentially fatal. *Staphylococcus aureus* is a common pathogenic form, producing conditions such as abscesses, boils, postoperative osteomyelitis, and some forms of bacterial endocarditis.

Excessive use and other misuses of antibiotic agents have resulted in the development of highly resistant strains of pathogens. Most hospitals monitor antibiotic usage closely to prevent and control abuse of antibiotics.

Indirect contact with an infected individual through intravenous transmission of body fluids such as blood or serum or simply via a contaminated needle or other instrument can transmit the AIDS virus, the viral agents producing hepatitis, and the *Treponema pallidum* spirochete producing syphilis, sometimes referred to as lues.

Droplet infections, which are the result of one host breathing in infectious agents from the sneeze or cough of an infected host, frequently account for the transmission of the viruses producing the common cold and influenza (Figure 2.9). The *Mycobacterium tuberculosis* and *Streptococcus pneumoniae*, the most common cause of lobar pneumonia, can also be transmitted by droplet infection.

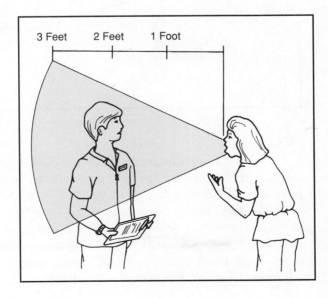

Figure 2.9 An example of a droplet infection: One person breathes in infectious agents from the cough or sneeze of an infected person (Reproduced with permission from Badasch and Chesebro, *Essentials for the Nursing Assistant in Long-Term Care,* Delmar Publishers Inc., 1990)

Earthborne fungi such as *Coccidioides immitis*, which produces coccidioidomycosis (also called desert rheumatism, San Joaquin Valley fever, or Valley Fever), are also transmitted in humans via the respiratory system through breathing and droplet contact with an infected host.

Humans, animals, and insects transmit infectious agents through the direct contact of biting. The bite of any warm-blooded animal, such as a bat, dog, or human can result in the transmission of the rabies virus, which produces an acute infectious disease of the central nervous system usually resulting in death (Figure 2.10).

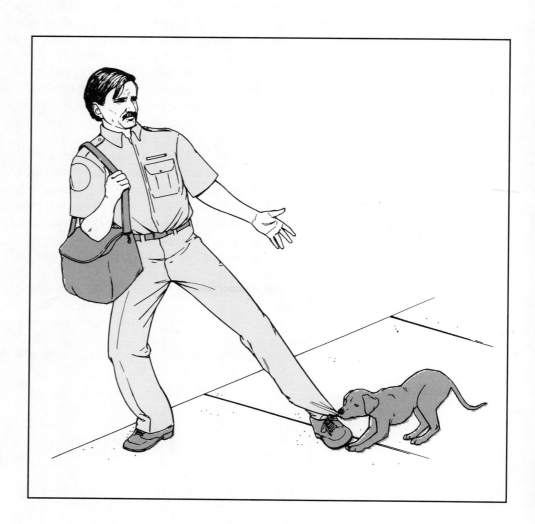

Figure 2.10 The rabies virus can be transmitted via a bite from an infected dog or other warm-blooded animal.

Malaria, an infectious febrile disease caused by protozoa of the genus *Plasmodium*, is transmitted by the bite of an infected mosquito. Yellow fever, an acute infectious viral disease, is also transmitted by the bite of the female of certain types of mosquitoes. Rocky Mountain spotted fever, caused by *Rickettsia rickettsiae,* is transmitted from rodent to man by the bite of various ticks. Of growing international concern is Lyme Disease, which is also transmitted by the bite of a tick. Plague, often called Black Death, is a fatal disease caused by the bacillus *Yersinia pestis,* transmitted from rodents to man by flea bites (Figure 2.11).

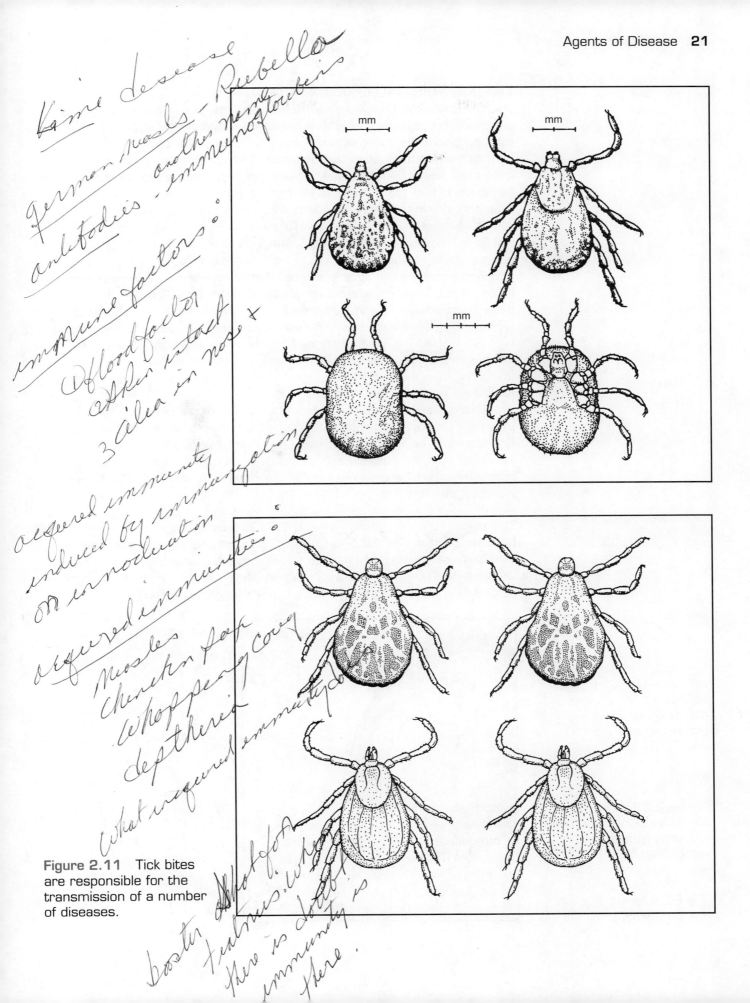

Figure 2.11 Tick bites are responsible for the transmission of a number of diseases.

DEFENSE MECHANISMS OF THE BODY

The defense of the host body against susceptibility to the invasive or pathogenic effects of microorganisms or to the toxic effects of **antigens** is referred to as **immunity** and is also described as *functional* or *protective*. Humoral and cell-mediated immunity are the heightened responses of the body to antigenic challenge that lead to more rapid binding or elimination of antigens than exists in the nonimmune state. Immunity is also the capacity to distinguish antigenic material from *self* and to neutralize, eliminate, or metabolize that which is foreign or *not self*.

Acquired immunity is the result of exposure to an infectious agent or its antigens and the subsequent development of the antigenic response. This is the type of immunity we develop as the result of having a disease such as rubella or German measles. Acquired immunity can also be induced through inoculation with preformed antibodies or specifically sensitized lymphoid cells (Figure 2.12). Inoculation with a dilute concentration of a disease-causing agent to initiate the body's antigenic response can also produce acquired immunity. Acquired immunity through inoculation is commonly used in the prevention of childhood diseases such as rubella (German measles), varicella (chickenpox), and pertussis (whooping cough). While lifetime immunity is frequently conferred, when there is doubt (as with Tetanus), a booster inoculation is frequently administered.

Humoral and cell-mediated immunity are types of responses instigated by **lymphocytes.** Two kinds of lymphocytes important to the establishment of immunity are T-lymphocytes or T-cells and B-lymphocytes or B-cells. Humoral immunity, that associated with the body humors or fluids, is characterized by the production of antibodies called *immunoglobulins* that are capable of neutralizing and destroying particular antigens.

HIV, ARC, and AIDS

The human immunodeficiency virus (HIV) has been identified as a **retrovirus** and causative organism for AIDS (acquired immunodeficiency syndrome). The virus is most commonly transmitted through sexual contact as with other sexually transmitted diseases (STDs) or by direct contact with infected blood, e.g., through the sharing of needles by drug users or by transfusion with contaminated blood.

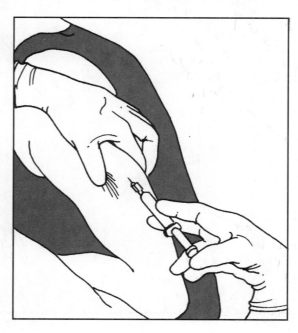

Figure 2.12 Inoculation often can induce acquired immunity (Adapted with permission from Keir, Wise, and Krebs-Shannon, *Medical Assisting*, 2nd Ed., Delmar Publishers Inc., 1989)

AIDS appears to be transmitted primarily through exposure to infected semen or blood, through vaginal or cervical secretions, and possibly via urine and feces. The virus has also been isolated in cerebrospinal fluid and amniotic fluid. Although the virus has been isolated in saliva and tears, there is no current evidence that AIDS is spread through these fluids during casual contact. There is, however, some real concern that saliva may be capable of transmitting the virus during intimate sexual contact.

The second most common way that AIDS is spread is through contaminated blood in blood-to-blood transmission, such as through blood transfusions or transfusions of blood products and the sharing of needles by intravenous drug users. Use of ELISA (enzyme-linked immunoabsorbent assay) and screening of potential donors for risk factors by commercial blood banks, plasma centers, and public health clinics have virtually eliminated the transmission of HIV through transfusions of blood and blood products. ELISA was approved for use by the Food and Drug Administration (FDA) in March, 1985.

AIDS can also be transmitted from mother to infant if the mother has the virus when she is pregnant or breast feeding.

So far in the United States the largest segments of the population with AIDS are homosexual and bisexual men, male and female drug users who share needles, and people who have received blood or blood products for medical reasons. There have been increasing numbers of people outside these groups who have contracted AIDS, including heterosexual sex partners of HIV carriers and children born to HIV-infected mothers.

It is possible that some people will develop antibodies to the virus, remain healthy, and show no symptoms of AIDS. However, the long-term effect of infection for this group of people is unknown. Because of the length of time it takes the body to develop HIV antibodies, tests to detect HIV may fail for as long as six months after an individual has been infected. Since HIV may be transmitted with or without symptoms, this period of latency is when the greatest danger of accidental transmission occurs.

Since there is, at present, no known cure for AIDS, it is currently believed that all those infected with HIV will eventually develop AIDS. Currently available evidence suggests that twenty to thirty percent of HIV-infected individuals will develop AIDS within the first five years of transmission; some authorities project eighty or more percent will develop AIDS within ten years following infection.

HIV-infected individuals normally experience a long incubation period, i.e., years of latency. During this time, they are frequently asymptomatic. Other HIV-infected individuals may have symptoms that last for months or that keep coming back and cannot be accounted for by the presence of another illness or infection. These symptoms frequently include rapid weight loss for no apparent reason, recurring fever or night sweats, profound and unexplained fatigue, swollen lymph glands in the axillae, groin, or neck, diarrhea that lasts for more than a week, leukoplakia or other lesions of the mouth and throat, memory loss, depression, and other neurological disorders. ARC (AIDS-related complex) is the term used for a combination of these symptoms.

Other HIV-infected individuals will develop more specific, life-threatening diseases, such as *Pneumocystis carnii pneumonia* (PCP) or Kaposi's sarcoma (KS), sure indicators of the development of AIDS. As new tests and treatment procedures are developed, it is hoped that this picture will improve.

There is no single, simple test for AIDS. AIDS is diagnosed by finding one or more life-threatening illnesses that would not appear in a person with a healthy immune system. These illnesses can only be diagnosed by a physician who performs certain types of tests based on the symptoms presented by the infected individuals.

PATIENT EDUCATION

Your patients need to know—this cannot be emphasized enough—that there is absolutely no evidence that AIDS is spread through casual contact. Activities such as working in a group setting, eating out in restaurants, swimming in public pools, shaking hands or hugging will not expose them to AIDS. There has not been a single case of AIDS among those living with persons who have AIDS, except for their sexual partners or children born to parents infected with the virus. Contact your local public health department for current pamphlets or handouts that you can put in your waiting room or pass out to patients needing or wanting HIV or AIDS information.

Patients experiencing any of the previously discussed symptoms over a period of weeks or months should get a complete medical examination, preferably from a physician who is familiar with AIDS.

Patients who are members of a high risk group for HIV infection should take the HTLV-III blood test, which detects antibodies to the virus that causes AIDS. A positive result does not mean that the patient has AIDS, but it does mean that they are infected with the virus that causes AIDS and should assume that they can infect others with whom they have sexual contact.

Patients need to be counseled on safe sex, which includes:

1. Do not have sexual contact with AIDS patients, with members of the at- risk groups, or with people who test positive for the AIDS virus.
2. Do not have sexual contact with multiple partners, including prostitutes (who may also be IV drug abusers).
3. Use a condom for all types of sex. Also use foam, cream, or jelly with nonoxynol-9 in it. This chemical may kill the AIDS virus.
4. Have sex with only one person. This lowers your chances of getting AIDS, but you should still use condoms to be safe.

Your patients who are drug users will also need to be counseled against sharing needles. For more or updated information, they can talk with their physician, or they can call the National AIDS Hotline; the toll-free number is 1–800–342–2437.

Patients and parents of female children need to be educated in the correct wiping techniques after elimination of body waste. Patients and parents of both male and female children also need to be educated in the necessity for washing their hands well with soap and water after the elimination of body waste.

Universal Precaution System

The Universal Precaution System is a blood and body fluid precaution measure system to be used with all patients in all situations in which the potential exists for coming into contact with blood or body fluids that are considered potentially dangerous. Strict adherence to the system results in greater protection from the risk of cross infection for the medical assistant, other health-care workers, and the patients. The rules are simple, but must be *strictly* adhered to:

1. **Gloves:** Must be worn any time there is potential for coming into contact with contaminated blood or body fluids, including the following situations:
   a. touching a patient with any type of lesion or break in the continuity of the skin;
   b. surgical or other invasive body procedures;
   c. dressing changes;

    d.   touching or handling a patient's blood or body fluids during examination, specimen collection, handling and processing of specimens, as well as cleaning, decontaminating, and disposal of blood or body fluids; this also includes cleaning and handling of contaminated instruments and supplies;

    e.   anytime there is danger of a procedure generating droplets of blood or body fluids, such as during various laboratory tests, body cavity examinations, etc.;

Dispose of gloves only when the danger of contamination has passed and always between patients.

2. **Gowns, masks, glasses, or goggles:** Cover gowns or disposable aprons must be worn in addition to gloves and for the same situations. Like gloves, these are to be disposed of only when the danger of contamination has passed and always between patients. Eyeglasses are considered an effective barrier, but if you do not wear eyeglasses, then reusable goggles should be available for use by the physician and the medical assistant and should be thoroughly cleaned between uses with warm, soapy water. Contact lenses are not considered adequate protection. Disposable masks should be worn to protect your oral and nasal mucous membranes from contamination. These masks can be properly discarded after each use.

3. **Hands and skin:** If you have any apparent lesions or other breaks in your skin, you should not perform any duty that will bring you into contact with the patient or blood or other body fluids. Hands should be thoroughly washed after:

    a.   removing gloves;

    b.   any contact with blood or body fluids;

    c.   collection, handling, or processing of specimens;

    d.   cleaning procedures or disposal involving contaminated instruments or supplies;

    e.   before leaving the office.

4. **Laboratory specimens:** All blood and other body fluid specimens collected from patients should be considered contaminated and require special handling:

    a.   Avoid contaminating the outside of the specimen container. If contamination does occur or doubt exists, disinfect the outside of the container with a 1:10 solution of household bleach and water or other germicide.

    b.   Place all specimens in well-constructed containers with secure lids, and then place them in a second container such as an **impervious** bag for transport. Be sure to check for breaks or leaks.

5. **Sharp instruments and needles:** Cleaning and disposal of needles and sharp instruments require special care to prevent injury. The following precautions should be adhered to:

    a.   Remove scalpel blades from their handles using a hemostat—not by hand.

    b.   Do not remove needles from syringes.

    c.   Do not bend, break, or otherwise manipulate needles or scalpel blades.

    d.   Do not recap used needles.

    e.   Dispose of needles, scalpel blades, and other sharp instruments immediately after use in a puncture-proof container, which should be placed as close as possible to the area where these items are used.

6. **Spills:** Accidents do happen and should blood or other body fluids spill, proceed as follows:

    a.   Put on protective gown, gloves, mask, and goggles.

    b.   Remove the visible material with disposable towels and immediately place the contaminated towels in an impervious bag at the spill site.

c. Decontaminate the area using a chemical germicide approved for use as a hospital disinfectant or with a 1:10 solution of household bleach and water.
d. Dispose of your protective gear, gloves, gown, etc., in an impervious bag.
e. Place all bagged items in a second impervious bag.
f. Clean your eyeglasses or goggles and wash your hands thoroughly.

7. **Other considerations:** These include nondisposable items and disposal of bulk blood and body fluids. Every office should have a written policy covering these items, but in general the following guidelines are acceptable:

a. Patient treatment areas such as examination tables should be cleaned on a regular basis and after each patient use.
b. General cleaning and soil removal should be done routinely.
c. Linens soiled with blood or body fluids should be bagged in an impervious bag for transport and then placed into a second impervious bag.
d. Bulk blood and body fluids may be poured carefully down a drain connected to a sanitary sewer. A septic tank is not acceptable.
e. All other waste should be decontaminated before being double bagged and disposed.

REVIEW/ SELF-EXAMINATION

1. How are parasitic vectors classified?
2. Give an example of an immune factor. *Celea in nose + lungs.*
3. Name the common parasitic vectors.
4. How are bacteria classified?
5. How do opportunistic infections occur?
6. Would fungi properly be described as animal or plant?
7. What are the two classifications of helminths parasitic to man?
8. Which is the simplest organism of the animal kingdom?
9. Do all viruses look exactly alike?
10. What is meant by normal flora?
11. How can normal flora produce disease symptoms?
12. How may a medical assistant be a vector in the spread of nosocomial infection?
13. Give examples of droplet infections.
14. List the stages of the disease process.
15. Give examples of diseases transmitted by insect and animal bites.
16. How can you acquire immunity?
17. Name at least seven bacterial infections.
18. How is AIDS transmitted?
19. What are some of the symptoms of HIV?
20. Name the specific indicators of the development of AIDS.
21. Is there a test for AIDS? If so, what is its name?
22. How would you counsel a patient on safe sex?
23. What are the common names for Hansen's Disease, pertussis, varicella, and rubella?
24. What are the basic requirements for the growth of microorganisms?
25. Does AIDS have an asymptomatic period? Can the disease be transmitted in the absence of symptoms?
26. Are the flea and mosquito the carriers of Lyme Disease?
27. Differentiate between rickettsiae and protozoa.
28. Give examples of diseases for which you may receive immunity through inoculation.

CHAPTER 3

Medical Asepsis

OBJECTIVES

On completion of this chapter, you will be able to:
- Define asepsis.
- Define disinfection.
- Define sterilization.
- Demonstrate correct handwashing technique.
- Prepare equipment and packs for sterilization.
- Demonstrate correct sterilization technique for prepared packs.
- Demonstrate proper disinfection technique for surgical instruments.
- Identify two common germicidal solutions.
- Differentiate among asepsis, disinfection, and sterilization.
- Identify the need for employing universal precautions while sanitizing equipment and supplies.

Vocabulary— Glossary of Terms

Asepsis	Condition of being free of infection.
Autoclave	A pressure chamber effecting sterilization using steam.
Contaminant	Microorganism.
Disinfection	Process of freeing from infection.
Germicide	Any agent that kills pathogenic organisms; common household germicides are soap and water and a 1:10 solution of household bleach and water.
Protein	Principal constituent of the protoplasm of all cells.
Sanitize	To clean.
Sterile	Free from living microorganisms.
Technique	The procedure and details of a mechanical process or surgical operation.

Introduction to Disinfection and Sterilization

To control the transmission of microbial infections it is imperative that all health-care personnel employ aseptic **techniques**. **Asepsis** helps prevent self-infection and nosocomial infecting of the patients under your care.

Since hands are a primary carrier of microbial infections, as a medical assistant you must employ conscientious and thorough hand washing to prevent the spread of disease from one patient to another and as a safeguard to your health and that of your family (Figure 3.1).

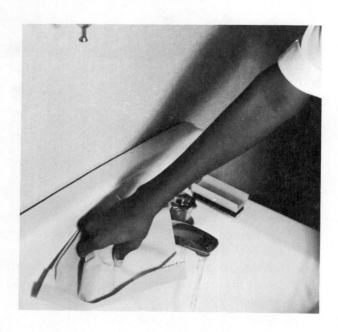

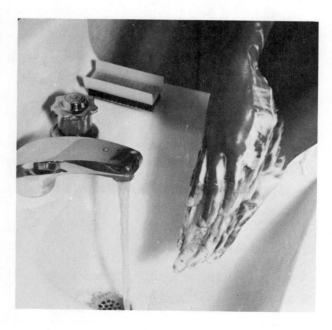

Figure 3.1 Steps in proper handwashing technique: (A) Use a dry paper towel to turn the faucet on and off. (B) Use the palm of one hand to clean the back of the other hand.

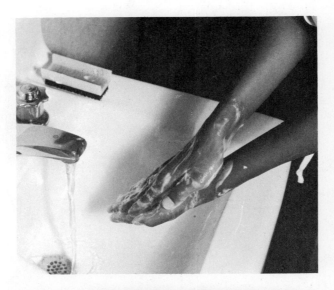

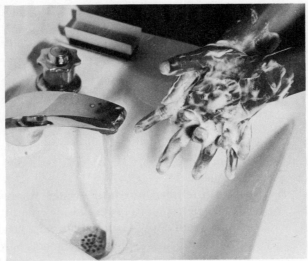

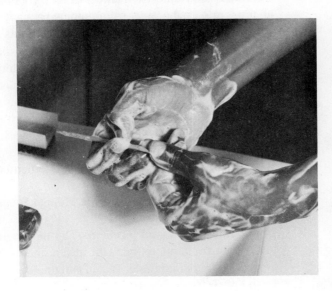

Figure 3.1 continued
Steps in proper hand
washing technique: (C)
Point fingertips down while
washing hands. (D) Inter-
lace the fingers to clean
between the fingers. Use
the blunt of an orange
cuticle stick (E)

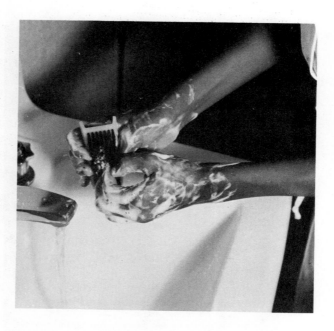

Figure 3.1 continued
Steps in proper hand washing technique: or a hand brush (F) to clean the nails. (Reproduced with permission from Simmers, *Diversified Health Occupations*, 3rd Ed., Delmar Publishers Inc., 1993)

PROCEDURE FOR HAND WASHING

1. **Remove all rings.** The grooves and crevices in jewelry provide excellent hiding places for microbes. The only ring that you may leave on is a plain gold wedding band.

2. **Stand up to the sink.** Be extremely careful that your clothing does not come into contact with the sink, as the sink is considered contaminated.

3. **Adjust the temperature of the water.** Warm water is preferred over hot or cold and will result in a better sudsing effect.

4. **Wet hands and apply soap.** Holding your hands down toward the sink, wet them generously and apply liberal amounts of soap (preferably liquid soap) to work up a good lather. Remember to keep your hands lower than your elbows at all times to keep the water from running back toward you.

5. **Wash hands using strong rubbing movements and rotary motions.** Wash the palms and the back of each hand using circular motions. Interlace your fingers and wash them thoroughly using plenty of friction.

6. **Rinse well.** Since your hands are the most contaminated, they are washed first, before wrists and forearms. Be sure to hold your hands lower than your elbows while rinsing.

7. **Relather and wash wrists and forearms.** Wash wrists and forearms using circular motions and friction.

8. **Rinse well.** Rinse arms and hands well, remembering to drain water toward the fingertips and away from the elbows.

9. **Inspect knuckles and fingernails. Repeat Steps 4 through 7.** Use a brush and orange stick as needed.

10. **Dry hands, wrists, and forearms.** Dry thoroughly, preferably using a paper towel. Be careful not to touch the area around your elbows or to come into contact with your clothing. Wipe from the forearms toward the fingertips using fresh towels for each wipe.

11. **Turn off the running water.** Use your paper towel to turn off the water. Wipe around the sink and then discard the towel.
12. **Apply lotion.** If desired, apply lotion to keep your skin soft and to prevent chapping.

Sanitization

Sanitization is a cleaning method for preparing instruments and equipment for **disinfection** or **sterilization**. This process lowers the microbe count and reduces contamination. Before beginning the sanitization process, be sure to follow the universal precautions (Chapter 2) and wear appropriate protective clothing.

Contaminated instruments should be removed to a separate work area away from patients as soon as possible after use. If they cannot be sanitized immediately, they should be put to soak in cold water to prevent blood or other **protein** matter from drying out and hardening. Hinged instruments should always be in open position while soaking. Reusable syringes should be put to soak with the barrel and plunger separated.

PROCEDURE FOR SANITIZING INSTRUMENTS

1. **Wash thoroughly** using a low-sudsing detergent, warm water, and a small, stiff brush to clean grooves, crevices, and serrations where **contaminants** such as blood, urine, feces, pus, tissue, and lubricants may have accumulated. Hinged instruments should always be separated and attention paid to the area of the hinge.
2. **Check the instrument carefully** to be sure it is in proper working condition—operating smoothly, free from damage and rust.
3. **Discard immediately damaged or rusted instruments.**
4. **Rinse each instrument thoroughly with hot water and dry the instrument thoroughly to prevent rusting.** All hinged instruments must be left in the open position.
5. **Place on a clean, dry surface** until they can be disinfected or sterilized.

PROCEDURE FOR SANITIZING REUSABLE SYRINGES

1. **Separate the barrel and plunger and wash thoroughly** in warm water with a low-sudsing, nonetching detergent that will not erode the glass surface of the syringe. A test tube brush works well for scrubbing inside the barrel of the syringe.
2. **Thoroughly brush** outside the syringe barrel and plunger and force detergent through the tip of the syringe with the plunger.
3. **Inspect syringes** for damage, chips, or cracks and discard immediately if any are found.
4. **Rinse thoroughly with tap water** to remove detergent.
5. **Rinse again using distilled water.**
6. **Place on a clean, dry surface** until they can be wrapped and sterilized.

PROCEDURE FOR SANITIZING REUSABLE NEEDLES

1. **Wash thoroughly** with low-sudsing detergent and warm water.
2. **Insert a stylet** through the lumen of the needle at the hub to remove any contaminated matter that is present and to prevent clogging of the lumen.
3. **Clean inside the hub** of the needle with a detergent-soaked cotton applicator.
4. **Use a syringe to force detergent solution through the lumen.**
5. **Rinse thoroughly with tap water.**
6. **Use a syringe to force distilled water** through the lumen.
7. **Inspect the needle carefully** for dullness or damage. If dull or damaged, discard immediately.
8. **Place needles on a clean, dry surface** until they can be wrapped and sterilized.

PROCEDURE FOR SANITIZING RUBBER GOODS

1. **Wash all rubber goods thoroughly** with a low-sudsing detergent and warm water.
2. **Rinse thoroughly.**
3. **Fill hot water bottles, etc., with water** and inspect for punctures or protein matter that has not been removed.
4. **Discard damaged rubber goods immediately.**
5. **Dry thoroughly** and place on a clean, dry surface until they can be wrapped and sterilized.

Preparation of Equipment for Sterilization

After the equipment has been properly sanitized and thoroughly dried, it is ready to be put into packages for sterilization, normally achieved by steam heating in an **autoclave** (Figure 3.2). While there are some routine guidelines for the preparation of packs for autoclaving, when it comes to the supplies and instruments to be included in the various packs, your physician employer may have some preferences. It is always a good idea to find out the physician's preferences and to make up "pack or tray" cards listing the contents of the various packages; these will save valuable time in the future when you are preparing equipment for sterilization (Figure 3.3). It is also a wise idea to encase these cards in cellophane or plastic to prevent water damage. Copies should be included in the office procedures manual for future reference and should be updated whenever changes are made.

Many offices prefer to use presterilized and disposable packs and trays for various frequently used items. The cost of the disposables is often far less than the cost of maintaining and preparing the instruments and supplies needed to package your own. It is essential when using disposable packs that they be checked for punctures or other damage prior to use. Damaged disposable packs should *always* be considered contaminated and discarded. Disposable packs are usually date-stamped with the date when the pack should be considered no longer sterile. If a pack is out of date, it should be discarded (Figure 3.4).

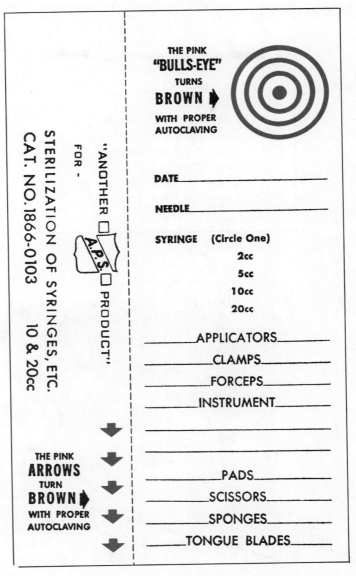

THE PINK
"BULLS-EYE"
TURNS
BROWN ▶
WITH PROPER
AUTOCLAVING

DATE_____

NEEDLE_____

SYRINGE (Circle One)

2cc

5cc

10cc

20cc

_____APPLICATORS_____

_____CLAMPS_____

_____FORCEPS_____

_____INSTRUMENT_____

_____

_____

_____PADS_____

_____SCISSORS_____

_____SPONGES_____

_____TONGUE BLADES_____

STERILIZATION OF SYRINGES, ETC.
CAT. NO.1866-0103   10 & 20cc

"ANOTHER ☐ PRODUCT"

FOR -

A.P.S.

THE PINK
ARROWS
TURN
BROWN ▶
WITH PROPER
AUTOCLAVING

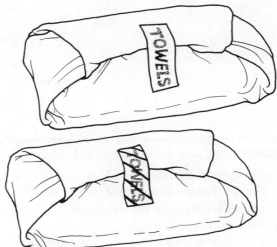

TOWELS

Figure 3.2 Examples of proper packaging for autoclaving: (A) Envelope-type packaging. (B) Package of towels before (top) and after (bottom) autoclaving; note that the sterilized package has diagonal lines on the tape, a positive sign that autoclaving has been done correctly. (Reproduced with permission from Keir, Wise, and Krebs-Shannon, *Medical Assisting*, 2nd Ed., Delmar Publishers Inc., 1989)

SAMPLE "PACK/TRAY" CARD

URETHRAL CATHETERIZATION TRAY

1	Fenestrated drape
1	CSR wrap
1	pair precuffed vinyl gloves
1	poly lined underpad
1	120 ml. specimen contained
5	rayon balls
1	vinyl catheter
2.7 gm.	lubricating jelly
2/3 oz.	PVP-1 solution

Figure 3.3 Sample "pack/tray" card

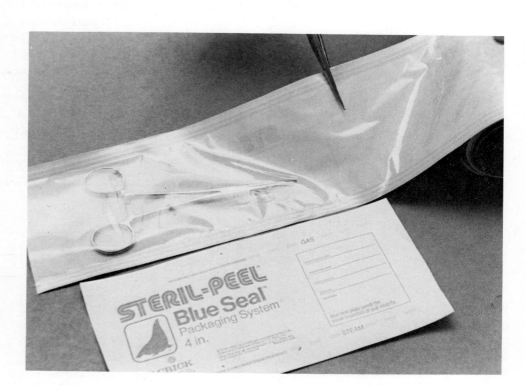

Figure 3.4 Sample disposable pack (Reproduced with permission from Simmers, *Diversified Health Occupations,* 3rd Ed., Delmar Publishers, Inc., 1993)

PROCEDURE FOR PREPARING GLASSWARE

1. **Wrap each piece separately** in 4 × 4 gauze for protection against breakage.
2. **Slip into disposable paper bags** that are available for sterilization or double wrap in two separate fabric wrappers and seal with sterile indicator tape.
3. **Correctly label the package or indicator tape.**

Sterile indicator tape, also called autoclave tape, contains a chemical agent that changes color after exposure to steam. The tape is available in a variety of colors and can be written on. Materials prepared for sterilization should have the date of sterilization and the package contents written on the indicator tape.

PROCEDURE FOR PREPARING RUBBER GLOVES

1. **Sanitize following the procedure for rubber goods.**
2. **Powder the gloves.**
3. **Using paper or gauze** to separate the surfaces from contact, fold the cuffs over toward the thumb of the glove.
4. **Insert paper or gauze into the inside palm of the glove** to prevent contact of the surfaces and allow for free circulation of steam.
5. **Place the gloves palm side up** with the thumb sides facing each other and the thumbs pointing away from center on a paper or fabric wrapper.
6. **Fold the bottom of the wrapper** up toward the fingers and the top of the wrapper over the previous fold toward the cuffs. Folding from left to right, fold the wrapper over the left glove and then fold again over the right glove.
7. **Place in a disposable bag** or wrap in a fabric wrapper and seal with sterile indicator tape for sterilization (Figure 3.5).

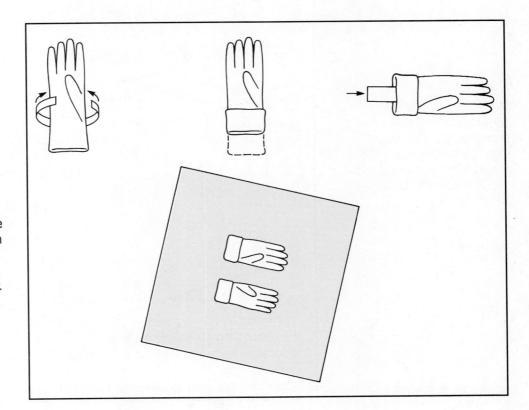

Figure 3.5 To sanitize rubber gloves, cleanse the outside of the gloves; then turn them inside out and repeat the cleansing process. Rinse thoroughly. Fill the gloves with water to ensure organic matter has been removed and punctures are not present. Dry gloves completely and wrap them.

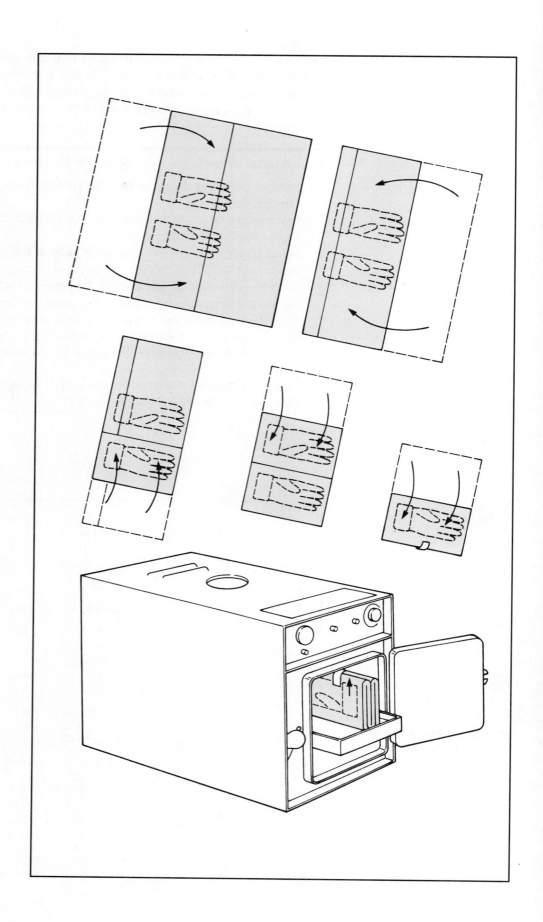

Figure 3.5 continued

PROCEDURE FOR PREPARING INSTRUMENTS

1. **Leave hinged instruments unhinged or in the open position.** They may be individually bagged in disposable bags designed for sterilization of instruments, or they may be double wrapped in fabric wrappers and sealed with sterile indicator tape.
2. **Correctly label the package or indicator tape.**

When wrapping instruments, place the instruments in the center of the wrapping fabric and fold the fabric first from the bottom toward the top, doubling back a small portion. Then fold the right side toward the left, doubling back a small portion. Then fold the left side toward the right, doubling back a small portion. Your package should now resemble an envelope ready for sealing. Fold the top of the envelope down. Double wrap identically and seal with a strip of sterile indicator tape (Figure 3.6).

PACKS

Packs or trays may be set up according to the needs of the office or the preference of the physician. They consist of the supplies and equipment needed for performing various procedures such as catheterization, lumbar puncture, suturing, suture removal, and office surgeries.

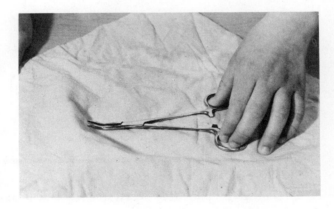

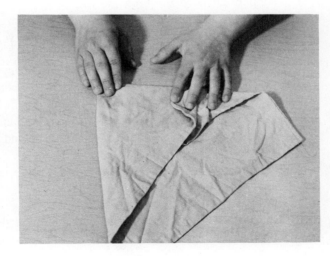

Figure 3.6 Procedure for preparing instruments for sterilization (Reproduced with permission from Simmers, *Diversified Health Occupations,* 3rd Ed., Delmar Publishers Inc., 1993)

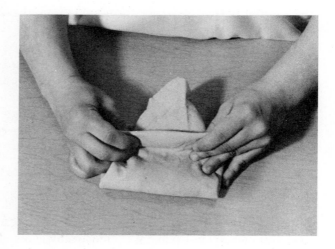

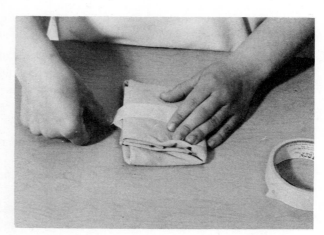

Figure 3.6 continued

PROCEDURE FOR PREPARING PACKS

1. **Pull your "pack/tray" card** so that you will know what instruments and supplies are needed.
2. **Take an autoclavable plastic or metal tray** large enough to hold the necessary equipment and supplies and of a size that will fit into the autoclave while leaving room for circulation of steam.
3. **Cover the surface of the tray with a clean, dry towel.**
4. **Place your instruments on the towel.** Instruments will stay put if you slip one of the finger holes of each of the hinged instruments over the tip of a hemostat.
5. **Place your necessary supplies** such as 2 × 2 and 4 × 4 gauze squares, medicine cup, gauze-wrapped syringe barrel and plunger, etc., in a convenient place on the tray.
6. **Next place prefolded towels and drape materials.** These may be placed on top of the instruments and other supplies.
7. **Place a sterile indicator on the tray.**
8. **Place the prepared tray in the center of a large piece of paper** or fabric wrap material.

9. **Fold from the bottom to the top edge of the tray**, doubling back a small portion.
10. **Fold the left side just past center**, doubling back a small portion.
11. **Fold the right side over the left**, doubling back a small portion.
12. **Fold the top portion down toward the bottom**, doubling back a small portion.
13. **Place this prepared pack in the center of another large wrapper** and wrap again in the same way.
14. **Seal the pack with sterile indicator tape.**
15. **Label and date the indicator tape.**

In some medical offices, such as a surgery specialty office, it may be desirable to have sterile packs of drapes, towels, and other materials already prepared. If this is applicable, prepare as indicated above.

Sterilization

The individuals who work in a medical office, like those employed in a hospital, must be constantly aware of the danger of microbial contamination. Sterilization is the complete elimination of microbial viability. This can be accomplished by:

1. Intense heat, such as boiling
2. Intense cold, such as freezing
3. Chemicals
4. Steam under pressure, such as autoclaving

The most commonly used and most efficient method of sterilization today is autoclaving with steam under pressure. There are times, however, when the other methods can be used to advantage, particularly in emergency situations.

When sterilizing by boiling, the tank or other container should be about one-third full of cold water. Sanitized instruments or glassware can then be placed in the container and one teaspoon of baking soda or special antirust agent added according to directions. The water is then brought to an active boil, and boiling is continued for a minimum of twenty minutes. This method of sterilization can be used for all dull instruments, syringes, glassware, porcelain, or enamelware.

In an emergency, dry-heat or hot-air sterilization can be most easily accomplished using an oven. It is less effective than moist heat, and higher temperatures and longer times must be employed. The following times and temperatures are suggested when dry heat is employed as a sterilization method: 250 degrees Fahrenheit for six hours, 320 degrees Fahrenheit for two hours, or 340 degrees Fahrenheit for one hour.

Intense cold such as freezing will destroy or retard some microbe activity, but with the exception of vaccines and food storage, this is no longer a viable method of sterilization. It is imperative that the expiration dates on vaccines be checked carefully prior to administration. Do not use vaccines once they have expired. When ordering supplies, be sure to check vaccines for forthcoming expiration dates.

With the chemical method of sterilization, a **germicidal** solution is poured into an airtight container with a stainless-steel top. Instruments sterilized by this method must be left to soak in the solution for a minimum of twenty minutes. This method is preferred over boiling for sharp instruments since boiling tends to dull the edges of sharp instruments, such as blades and scissors. Transfer or pick-up forceps are frequently sterilized in this fashion and are used in the opening and arranging of sterile packs or trays and for transferring sterile articles to a sterile field.

As previously indicated, today the most commonly used and most efficient method of sterilization of equipment and supplies is by steam heat autoclaving. An autoclave consists of a sterilizing chamber surrounded by pipes, valves, a pressure gauge, a safety valve, and a thermometer. The basic principle is the same as that employed in a pressure cooker. Packages to be autoclaved should always be sealed with sterile indicator tape and labeled with the contents of the package and the date and possibly time of autoclaving.

Autoclaves are distributed by a variety of manufacturers, whose directions for loading and operation should be followed explicitly (Figure 3.7). The loading and operation instructions should be sealed in plastic and placed near the autoclave for reference. Instructions provided with the autoclave will give the proper pressure and time for the types of articles you will be sterilizing. Most autoclaving is done at 15 pounds pressure, 250 degrees Fahrenheit, and usually for twenty to thirty minutes.

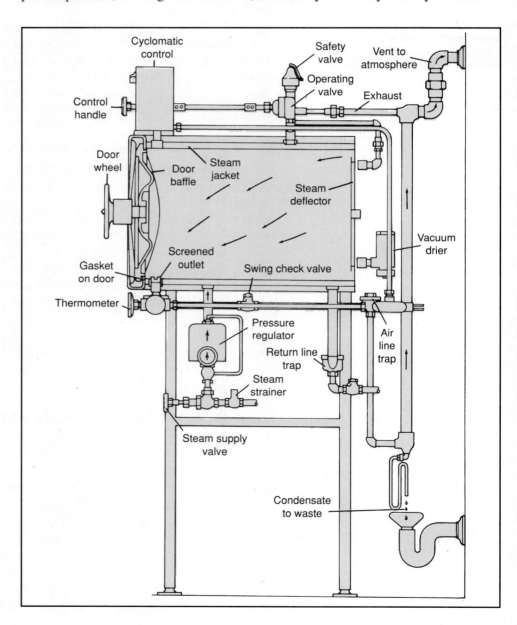

Figure 3.7 Diagram of an autoclave

PROCEDURE FOR AUTOCLAVING

1. **Following the manufacturer's directions, add distilled water to the water level in the reservoir**, if necessary.
2. **Adjust the control to fill.**
3. **Load the chamber**, following the manufacturer's directions, to allow for maximum circulation and penetration of steam.
4. **Close and seal the door.**
5. **Turn the control to the "on" position.**
6. When the temperature gauge reaches 250 degrees Fahrenheit and the pressure gauge reaches 15 pounds pressure, **set the timer** for the required time (usually twenty to thirty minutes).
7. When the timer signals completion of the timed cycle, **turn the control setting to "vent."**
8. When the pressure gauge reaches "0," leave the control set on "vent" and **open the chamber door slightly**, no more than a quarter of an inch.
9. **Allow complete drying of all articles**; then remove carefully, using heat-resistant gloves or hot pads.
10. **Place the sterile packages on dry, covered shelves** and turn the control knob to the "off" position, keeping the door slightly ajar.

The autoclave should be kept clean and in good repair. Commercial sterilization indicators contain a dye that changes color when the correct combination of time, temperature, and steam has been reached; an indicator should be placed in the center of each article prepared for sterilization.

Culture tests for determining the effectiveness of the sterilization process should be performed routinely. Strips of paper containing heat-resistant spores are placed in the center of two different wrapped articles and then loaded into the least accessible areas in the autoclave. Correct autoclaving procedure should be followed, and then the strips should be removed from their wrappers, dropped into culture tubes containing a broth, and incubated for the period suggested by the manufacturer. If the sterilization process has been done properly with regard to time, temperature, and steam, no growth should occur in the cultures. If growth occurs, repeat the process and if growth still occurs, the manufacturer should be contacted immediately for servicing of the autoclave.

After sterilization, articles should be stored in clean, dry, dustproof areas that are free from insect, animal, and other sources of contamination. Sterilized articles that are properly stored and damage free can be considered sterile for a period of one month. After that, they should be rewrapped and resterilized. Be sure to check sterilization date on the sterile indicator tape prior to using.

1. List the steps in correct hand washing procedure.
2. Differentiate between disinfection and sterilization.
3. Describe the procedure for sanitizing instruments.
4. Explain the procedure for inspecting rubber goods for punctures.
5. Describe "pack or tray" cards. What are they used for?
6. When should disposable packs or trays be considered no longer sterile?
7. Describe the procedure for preparing the following for sterilization:
   a. glassware
   b. rubber
   c. instruments
   d. packs
8. List the main parts of an autoclave.
9. Why should periodic culture tests be performed on an autoclave?
10. What is the correct time, pressure, and temperature for autoclaving?
11. List the procedural steps for autoclaving.
12. List two common household germicides.
13. Why should the autoclave directions be sealed in plastic?
14. Why are vaccines normally stored in a refrigerator?
15. What is an expiration date?

CHAPTER 4

Data Collection

OBJECTIVES

On completion of this chapter, you will be able to:

- Complete a patient history form demonstrating proper techniques for eliciting information.
- Establish an appropriate environment for history taking.
- Explain the need for a patient history and confidentiality.
- Identify the elements needed on a patient history form.
- Differentiate between "privilege" and "qualified privilege."
- Explain "review of systems."

Vocabulary— Glossary of Terms

Affect Feeling of pleasantness or unpleasantness produced by a stimulus.

Allergy A pathological reaction to a substance.

Anaphylaxis An unusual or exaggerated allergic reaction frequently accompanied by cardiac and respiratory arrest.

Authorization A document that empowers action. *Sign for record release.*

Confidential Private, secret; containing information whose disclosure could be prejudicial to a person's interest.

Data Information.

History A chronological record of significant events.

Privilege An advantage or favor granted by law.

Turgor Normal consistency of tissue.

Patient History

A complete patient **history** is essential to a patient's medical record (chart). When properly completed, the history provides personal, family, social, and medical information essential to the care of the patient and to the recordkeeping of the medical office. Although the information may be obtained in a variety of ways, it must be complete.

Confidentiality

The physician must keep **confidential** any communication, written or verbal, from the patient that is needed to provide treatment, unless required by law to divulge such information. The patient's right to privacy must be protected at all times. The medical assistant, acting as an agent of the physician and obtaining such confidential information through the scope of employment, is also bound by the patient's right to privacy not to reveal any information regarding the patient. When discussing a patient with another medical person who has some valid reason to know the information you are relaying, you must be careful not to be overheard by others.

The right of the patient to forbid physicians and other medical personnel from revealing confidential information is called **privilege** and is recognized by most states. There are times, however, when for the protection of the public, dissemination of certain information is required by code or statute. This information may include suspected abuse, gunshot and knife wounds, certain communicable diseases, and other similar information that must be reported to specified public agencies. This requirement is a complete defense to any action brought by the patient on the basis of defamation of character or invasion of privacy. *Qualified privilege* exists when information is revealed in court or is otherwise connected with legal or administrative proceedings.

An original, dated, and signed **authorization** by the patient or patient's parent or legal guardian requesting the release of medical information should always be obtained prior to releasing such information. An exception to this requirement is when medical information is subpoenaed for use in court. In this case, the court order completely bars any action by the patient against the professional or facility for releasing the information. Only the information requested in the subpoena or that has been explicitly authorized by the patient may be provided (Figure 4.1).

A properly completed authorization form signed by the patient or patient's parent or legal guardian is also required to release information to insurance companies, with the exception of worker's compensation cases, and to attorneys, even if they are representing the patient in a legal action.

Essential Information

There is a variety of preprinted forms available for obtaining and recording the information necessary for a patient history (Figure 4.2). Some medical offices have even designed and had printed history forms they feel are better suited to their needs than those already available. Other offices use computer-assisted **data** entry for information gathering. Information generally obtained includes the following:

1. *Patient's name*—last name, first name, and middle name or initial. If the patient does not have a middle name or initial you should insert NMI where the middle name or initial is called for. Be sure to include the correct title, i.e., Mr., Mrs., Miss, or Ms. This will help avoid confusion with names like Rusty that apply to either sex. For example: Jones, Rusty nmi (Miss).

2. *Vital statistics*—include date of birth, marital status, name of spouse (if married), parents' names or legal guardian's name if the patient is a minor, the name of the

C. R. Borup, M.D.
222 N. 2ND • Suite 201
Boise, Idaho 83702

**REQUEST FOR THE RELEASE
OF MEDICAL RECORDS**

To: _____

_____

_____

_____

I hereby request that any pertinent
information be sent to:

**Rex Borup, M.D.
222 North 2nd St., #201
Boise, ID 83702**

Signed:_____

Date:_____

Figure 4.1 Sample form authorizing the release of medical information

PATIENT HISTORY INFORMATION
(PLEASE PRINT)   Date......................................., 19.........

.... Phone ....
(Full Name Head of Household or Responsible Party)
Address ....
                (Street Number–City or Town)   Zip
Married ☐   Single ☐
Widowed ☐   Divorced ☐
No. of Children................   Give Name of Husband or Wife ....

Name .... Date of Birth .... Age ....
        (Full Name of Patient; Do Not Use Initials)

Employer ....
                (Employer of Patient or Husband, Wife, Etc.)   Department

Employer's Address ....

Spouse Employed by ....

Nearest Relative
and Address ....
                        (Relative Not Living at Same Address as Patient)

                                                                                            Patient's Social
Insurance Company ....Security No. ....

(If you have insurance, give details to secretary now)

Figure 4.2 Sample patient history form

financially responsible party, and in some cases the names and birth dates of any dependents. It is advisable to obtain the social security number and driver's license number.

3. *Addresses and telephone numbers*—in addition to the home address and telephone number, you should list the mailing address if different from the home address. The occupation of the patient should be listed, along with their business address and telephone number. If the patient is married or legally separated, you should obtain the occupation, business address, and telephone number of the spouse. If someone other than the patient is responsible for their financial arrangements, you will need that person's name, relationship to the patient, home address, telephone number, occupation, and business address and telephone number. *You should also have a written, dated, and signed third-party agreement.* In the case of minors, you will need complete information on both parents. If the case involves stepparents, you may find that the information you would normally obtain on the parents or guardian should also be obtained on the stepparents.

4. *Health insurance data*—the name and address of the insurance carrier(s) and group, code, or contract numbers. A photostat of their membership card or other identification should be attached to the medical record (chart). If there is more than one insurer, you should identify which one is primary, which is secondary, etc.

5. *Allergies*—to drugs or medications, foods, chemicals, and substances (such as iodine) used in various radiological procedures should be listed. It is essential to list the type of allergic response, such as nausea and vomiting, skin rash, etc. This is necessary since the administration of an allergen could result in serious consequences or death due to an anaphylactic reaction. Use a large lettered rubber stamp and red ink or a bold red ink marker to stamp or letter on the front of the medical record (chart) ALLERGIC TO: and then list the substances to which the patient has had an allergic response.

6. *Family history*—this section will include information about the patient's family, such as any history of diabetes, heart disease, kidney disease, etc., and condition and health status of parents and siblings.

7. *Social history*—this section will include information regarding the patient's personal habits, such as smoking, alcohol consumption, substance abuse, diet, exercise, etc.

8. *Medical history*—this section will include information about the patient's past and present medical problems, including information on previous operations and when performed, childhood and other diseases, and menstrual history for a female, with date of (or age during) menarche or last menstrual period. Included in this section are medications (prescription or over the counter) currently being taken and the dosages.

9. *Present medical problem*—includes the chief complaint and any symptoms.

See Figure 4.3 for a sample form used in gathering essential information about a patient.

IDENTIFICATION DATA Fill in the following information. PLEASE PRINT.

Date _____ # _____

Name _____ Date of birth _____ ___Male ___Female

Address _____ __Married __Separated __Divorced __Widowed __Single

_____ Education: ___years Elementary ___years High School

Home telephone _____ ___years College, Technical, Business, etc.
(area code)

Business telephone _____ Occupation _____
(area code)

FAMILY HISTORY Please follow the instructions given for each heading outlined below.

	YEAR OF BIRTH		
FAMILY	**HEALTH STATUS**	**ILLNESSES**	**DEATHS**

Print the names of your relatives, living or dead, in the list below. If there is not enough space, place an (x) here: ☐

Give the year of birth for all your relatives listed at the left and mark an (x) to indicate whether their health is good or poor.

Place an (x) in the appropriate column for any illnesses that you or the relatives listed at the left have now or have had.

If a relative you have listed has died, write the cause of death and the age at death in the columns below.

Illness column headers (diagonal): Good, Poor, Allergies or Asthma, Anemia, Bleeding Tendencies, Cancer or Tumor, Diabetes, Epilepsy, Glaucoma, Gout, Heart Trouble, High Blood Pressure, Kidney or Bladder Trouble, Nervous Breakdown, Rheumatism or Arthritis, Stomach or Duodenal Ulcer, Stroke, Tuberculosis

Columns: Year of Birth | (illnesses) | Cause of Death | Age

Rows:
Father:
Mother:
Brothers or Sisters:

Spouse:
Children:

Grandparents (Mark an (X) for illnesses only.)

YOUR ILLNESSES Start here ➤

Give your age at onset for any of the following illnesses you have now or have had.

Age	Age	Age	Age	Age
___eczema	___eye disease	___neuralgia neuritis	___measles	___rheumatic fever
___hives or rashes	___hemorrhoids	___pancreatitis	___mononucleosis	___venereal disease
___bronchitis	___hernia	___thyroid disease	___mumps	___yellow jaundice
___diverticulosis	___liver disease	___chicken pox	___nervous exhaustion	___other_____
___emphysema	___malaria	___German measles	___polio	

Have your ever been turned down for life insurance, military service or employment because of health problems? ...... ___Yes ___No

Have you been hospitalized more than three times? .... ___Yes ___No

Give the following information for the last three times you have been hospitalized starting with the most recent. (Women: Do not list normal pregnancies.)

	HOSPITALIZATION (1)	**HOSPITALIZATION (2)**	**HOSPITALIZATION (3)**
Type of operation or illness:............			
Month and year hospitalized:............			
Name of hospital:............................			
City and State:			

Place an (X) next to any of the following tests or immunizations you have had and if you can, give the year you last had them.

(X)	(Year)	**TESTS**	(X)	(Year)	**IMMUNIZATIONS**
_	_____	chest x-ray	_	_____	smallpox
_	_____	kidney x-ray	_	_____	tetanus
_	_____	G.I. series	_	_____	polio
_	_____	colon x-ray	_	_____	typhoid
_	_____	gallbladder x-ray	_	_____	flu
_	_____	electrocardiogram	_	_____	mumps
_	_____	T.B. test	_	_____	measles
_	_____	other x-rays	_	_____	other

Place an (X) in the appropriate column for any medicines you use or are allergic to.

(Use)	(Allergic to)	**MEDICINES**
_	_	aspirin
_	_	penicillin
_	_	sulfa
_	_	codeine
_	_	Demerol
_	_	antibiotics
_	_	laxatives or sedatives
_	_	other

Figure 4.3 Sample form used in gathering essential information about a patient

Please answer each of the following questions by placing an (X) in the "Yes" blank at the right if your answer to the question is yes, or by placing an (X) in the "No" blank at the right if your answer to the question is no. If you are unable to answer a question for any reason, place a solid circle (●) in the "Yes" blank.

1.	Are you troubled with stiff or painful muscles or joints?	1. Yes___ No___
2.	Are your joints ever swollen?	2. Yes___ No___
3.	Are you troubled by pains in the back or shoulder?	3. Yes___ No___
4.	Are your feet often painful?	4. Yes___ No___
5.	Are you handicapped in any way?	5. Yes___ No___
6.	Do you have any skin problems?	6. Yes___ No___
7.	Does your skin itch or burn?	7. Yes___ No___
8.	Do you have trouble stopping even a small cut from bleeding?	8. Yes___ No___
9.	Do you bruise easily?	9. Yes___ No___
10.	Do you ever faint or feel faint?	10. Yes___ No___
11.	Is any part of your body always numb?	11. Yes___ No___
12.	Have you ever had fits or convulsions?	12. Yes___ No___
13.	Has your handwriting changed lately?	13. Yes___ No___
14.	Do you have a tendency to shake or tremble?	14. Yes___ No___
15.	Are you very nervous around strangers?	15. Yes___ No___
16.	Do you find it hard to make decisions?	16. Yes___ No___
17.	Do you find it hard to concentrate or remember?	17. Yes___ No___
18.	Do you usually feel lonely or depressed?	18. Yes___ No___
19.	Do you often cry?	19. Yes___ No___
20.	Would you say you have a hopeless outlook?	20. Yes___ No___
21	Do you have difficulty relaxing?	21 Yes___ No___
22.	Do you have a tendency to worry a lot?	22. Yes___ No___
23.	Are you troubled by frightening dreams or thoughts?	23. Yes___ No___
24.	Do you have a tendency to be shy or sensitive?	24. Yes___ No___
25.	Do you have a strong dislike for criticism?	25. Yes___ No___
26.	Do you lose your temper often?	26. Yes___ No___
27.	Do little things often annoy you?	27. Yes___ No___
28.	Are you disturbed by any work or family problems?	28. Yes___ No___
29.	Are you having any sexual difficulties?	29. Yes___ No___
30.	Have you ever considered committing suicide?	30. Yes___ No___
31.	Have you ever desired or sought psychiatric help?	31. Yes___ No___
32.	Have you gained or lost much weight recently?	32. Yes___ No___
33.	Do you have a tendency to be too hot or too cold?	33. Yes___ No___
34.	Have you lost your interest in eating lately?	34. Yes___ No___
35.	Do you always seem to be hungry?	35. Yes___ No___
36.	Are there any swellings in your armpits or groin?	36. Yes___ No___
37.	Do you seem to feel exhausted or fatigued most of the time?	37. Yes___ No___
38.	Do you have difficulty either falling or staying asleep?	38. Yes___ No___
39.	Do you fail to get the exercise you should?	39. Yes___ No___
40.	Do you smoke?	40. Yes___ No___
41.	Do you take two or more alcoholic drinks a day?	41. Yes___ No___
42.	Do you drink more than six cups of coffee or tea a day?	42. Yes___ No___
43.	Have you ever used marijuana?	43. Yes___ No___
44.	Have you ever used heroin, LSD or similar drugs?	44. Yes___ No___
45.	Do you bite your nails?	45. Yes___ No___

Figure 4.3 continued

Methods of Eliciting Information

In many medical offices, the patient is asked to fill in the appropriate blanks on preprinted forms. Some medical offices have computer software that the patient can use in completing a form, which can then be printed out and included in the medical record (Figures 4.4 and 4.5).

Patient's Name _____ Date _____

Address: _____ Ins. _____

Home Phone: _____ Business Phone: _____

Occupation: _____

Referred By _____ Age_____ B.D._____ Sex_____ S M W D

Family History: Father_____ Mother_____

Brothers_____ Sisters_____ Cancer_____

Tuberculosis_____ Insanity_____ Diabetes _____

Heart Disease_____

Rheumatism_____ Gout _____ Goiter_____

Obesity_____ Nephritis_____ Epilepsy_____

Other_____

Past History: Diphtheria_____ Measles_____ Mumps_____

Chicken -Pox_____ Scarlet Fever_____ Smallpox_____ Thyroid_____

Infantile Paralysis_____ Malaria_____ Pneumonia_____

Dysentery_____ Jaundice_____ Boils_____ Rheumatic Fever_____

Tuberculosis_____ Asthma_____ Heart Disease_____

Hypertension_____ Diabetes_____ Infections_____

Gonorrhea_____ Syphillis_____ Tonsillitis_____

Nephritis_____ Operations_____

Menstrual: Onset_____ Frequency_____ Type_____

          Duration_____ Pain_____ L.M.P._____

Marital: Miscarriages_____ Abortions_____ Sterility_____

          Children_____

Habits: Alcohol_____ Tobacco_____ Drugs_____ Coffee_____

         Tea_____ Meals_____ Water_____ Sleep_____

         Bowel Movements_____ Exercise_____

         Amusements or Hobbies_____

Injuries:_____

Allergies:_____

Present Illness:_____

PHYSICAL EXAMINATION: Ht._____ Wt._____ Temp._____ B.P._____

Pulse_____ Respirations_____ General Appearance_____

Skin_____ Mucous Membranes_____

Eyes: Vision: O.D._____ O.S._____ O.U._____

Ishihara_____ Near Vision_____

Figure 4.4 Sample in-depth medical history form (Reproduced with permission from Keir, Wise, and Krebs-Shannon, *Medical Assisting,* 2nd Ed., Delmar Publishers Inc., 1989)

Pupil_____   Fundus_____

Ears_____   Nose_____

Chest_____   Breasts_____

Heart_____

Lungs_____

Abdomen_____

Genitalia_____

Rectum_____

Vagina_____

Extremities_____

Lymph Nodes: Neck_____   Axilla_____   Inguinal_____

              Abdominal_____   Reflexes_____

REMARKS:_____

_____

_____

_____

DIAGNOSIS:_____

_____

_____

TREATMENT:_____

_____

_____

Figure 4.4 continued

Generally, it is the medical assistant or the physician who elicits the information directly from the patient by asking the necessary questions and then writing down the patient's responses. In some offices, both the medical assistant and the physician elicit information, the medical assistant securing the information regarding the personal and financial aspects, the physician eliciting the family, social, and medical information.

It may seem somewhat redundant to question a patient repeatedly in an attempt to get answers to remarkably similar questions. But since patients are often unfamiliar with the terminology and embarrassed to ask for explanations, frequently they will change their response to a question when it is presented in a manner in which they are able to understand. Often this happens when questions are reduced to the simplest form, street language. There are many patients, for instance, who do not understand words like "void", "urinate", or "micturate"; but who can relate to "pass water" or "use the bathroom." When presented with a term that they do not understand, many patients to save embarrassment will just answer "No." This can often have a significant affect on a differential diagnosis.

NAME						AGE	SEX	S M D W
ADDRESS				PHONE		DATE		
SPONSOR			ADDRESS					
OCCUPATION			REF BY		ACKN			

COMPLAINTS

HISTORY

PRESENT CONDITION	PULSE	TEMP	RESP	B P	HEIGHT	WEIGHT

PHYSICAL FINDINGS

LAB TESTS

DIAGNOSIS

TREATMENT

REMARKS

Figure 4.5 Sample general medical history form (Reproduced with permission from Keir, Wise, and Krebs-Shannon, *Medical Assisting,* 2nd Ed., Delmar Publishers Inc., 1989)

Attempt to understand the patient. (This does not, however, condone being judgmental.) If you can relate to your patient and understand their situation, you will have completed the most difficult portion of your job. Once you are able to relate to the patient at their level, your efforts become more effective, and the patient and the practitioner benefit.

PROCEDURE FOR ELICITING INFORMATION

1. **Select a private, quiet environment.** You will be asking personal questions, so make sure that the patient's privacy will be guaranteed by ensuring your conversation cannot be overheard by others and that you will be free from interruption.
2. **Provide an interpreter or have the patient bring their own** if there is a language barrier.
3. **If the patient requests it, allow a family member or friend to accompany them.**
4. **Put the patient at ease.** You can usually do this with social conversation about topics like the weather, the patient's family, the patient's appearance, etc. Treat them like a social acquaintance who has stopped by your home; make them feel comfortable and at ease.
5. **Inform the patient about the need for the information you wish to obtain.**
6. **Take your time.** Do not make the patient feel hurried; allow the patient adequate time in which to respond.

Specialty-Specific Data

In all areas of specialization, there are items unique to that area. Peculiarities become evident to the medical assistant who has a genuine desire to learn and be effective. It is to your advantage to note those items of history upon which the physician repeatedly concentrates. Check with your employer to determine which items are considered particularly relevant.

In cardiology, the family history is most important. The most significant risk factor for myocardial infarction is not smoking, cholesterol levels, or stress, but the family history. Those patients who inherit a long line of cardiac disease are the most likely to succumb to cardiac-related illness. Family history is very important with many diseases that fall within the realm of internal medicine.

In obstetrics, problems in a previous pregnancy may be relevant in determining the risk factors applied to the current pregnancy. For example, if a woman has shown a tendency toward toxemia, diabetes, breech presentation, tubal pregnancy, or a variety of other difficulties throughout a previous pregnancy, there is significant risk that they may recur.

Those patients who have previously had postoperative difficulty from scarring or adhesions are of concern for the surgeon. Possible reactions to anesthesia are also significant in the patient's history.

An opportune time to obtain information needed in assessing the current complaint is during the initial physical assessment; it is usually done by the physician or physician assistant (PA). In order to cover all aspects of the patient's condition, the *body by systems* approach (frequently referred to as *review of systems*) is often used. As a clinical medical assistant you will assist the physician or PA with this review.

This technique separates the body into nine systems, each an assessment area. It may help to remember this technique as a *head-to-toe* assessment.

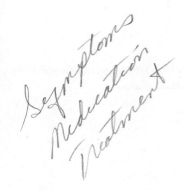

1. *Neurological:* Assesses level of consciousness (LOC), coordination, and pupillary response and compares strength on right and left hemispheres.
2. *Psychosocial:* Addresses the psychological well-being of the patient and **affect** and coping mechanisms.
3. *Cardiovascular:* Addresses circulation, quality and character of pulse, and heart tones.
4. *Respiratory:* Addresses skin color, quality and character of respiration, and respiratory effort.
5. *Gastrointestinal:* Addresses the character of the abdomen, quality and character of bowel sounds, tenderness to palpation, and bowel elimination history.
6. *Genitourinary:* Addresses patterns of elimination and problems with the reproductive system.
7. *Integument:* Addresses skin **turgor**, quality, temperature, and moisture and identifies any abnormalities.
8. *Bone:* Addresses abnormalities of the skeletal structure.
9. *Muscle:* Addresses general muscle tone and cites abnormalities if present.

See Figure 4.6.

Patient's Name _____ Birth Date_____

CC   HT._____ WT._____

PI

PH

    O
    A
    I
    HABITS

FH

P.E.   BP   T   P

Figure 4.6 POMR Assessment Form (Problem Oriented Medical Record)

<table>
<tr><td>

**REVIEW/
SELF-EXAMINATION**

</td></tr>
</table>

1. Who may authorize the release of medical information from a patient's medical record? *Patient Parent, legal guardian*

2. Who may authorize medical treatment of a minor?
   Parent Guardian or a court

3. What is meant by *privilege*?
   right of patient to hold confidential info

4. What is meant by *qualified privilege*?
   revealing info in court

5. List the personal information necessary on a patient information form.
   Name, Natural address, telephone No. Business phone

6. List the information needed about a spouse. *Spouses name occupation name, age, deps etc.*
   health & allergies

7. List the information needed about a stepparent or legal guardian.
   Same as spouse

8. What information is necessary when a third party is responsible for a patient's medical expenses? *insurance co who is 3rd party*

9. What health insurance information is necessary? *Primary, secondary name address, copy insurance card*

10. How would you identify a patient's allergies on their chart?

11. What information is included in a family history?

12. What information is included in a social history?

13. What information is included in a medical history?

14. Who is usually responsible for completing the patient history form?

15. How many body systems are there?

16. Who normally does the body systems assessment?

17. Cardiac and respiration arrest may indicate what type of reaction?

18. How would you assist a patient who is unable to read English and has poor understanding of the English language in completing the history form?

CHAPTER 5

Vital Signs

OBJECTIVES

On completion of this chapter, you will be able to:
- Accurately measure and record patient temperature.
- Accurately measure and record patient pulse rate.
- Accurately measure and record patient respiratory rate.
- Accurately measure and record patient blood pressure.
- Identify the normal parameters for patient vital signs.
- Identify the rationale for vital sign measurement.
- Define the vocabulary terms that appear in the chapter.

**Vocabulary—
Glossary of Terms**

Bradycardia	Adult heart rate less than sixty beats per minute.
Bradypnea	Adult respiratory rate less than twelve breaths per minute.
Bruit	An adventitious sound of vascular origin heard on auscultation.
Convection	One method of transference of heat.
Cyanosis	The bluish tinge that appears on the skin as a result of poor oxygenation.
Diastolic Pressure	The pressure exerted on the vasculature when the heart is at rest.
Dysrhythmia	Abnormal rhythm.
Eupnea	Normal respiratory pattern.
Fibrillation	Rapid, incomplete contractions of the heart, atria, or ventricles, resulting in irregular, rapid, and uncoordinated movement.
Gallop	A disorder of the heart rhythm.
Hg	Abbreviation for mercury.
Hypoxia	Condition of reduced oxygen supply to body tissue.
Metabolism	The sum of the physical and chemical processes essential to life.
Murmur	An ausculatory sound, usually of short duration, benign or pathological, of cardiac or vascular origin.

57

Rub	An ausculatory sound produced by friction from two surfaces rubbing together.
Sphygmomanometer	A blood pressure measuring device.
Systolic Pressure	The pressure exerted on the vasculature when the heart beats. Top
Tachycardia	Adult heart rate greater than 100 beats per minute.
Tachypnea	Adult respiratory rate greater than twenty breaths per minute.

Vital Signs

Vital signs are the group of parameters that function as an early warning system for the body against disease. Temperature, pulse, and respiration (TPR) along with blood pressure (BP) are the initial indicators that may signal the onset of illness. On each visit to a physician's office, the patient's vital signs are measured and recorded. By comparing the patient's readings to the established norm for each parameter, we are able to identify areas that may signal the presence of an early disease condition. By keeping a record of the patient's ongoing parameters, we are able to establish a baseline for that individual and thereby even more accurately detect a deviation from the norm for that individual patient. Accurate measurement of vital signs is essential to the patient's care and should never be taken lightly.

A variety of internal and external factors affect the patient's vital signs. Fear and stress may cause elevations of blood pressure, pulse, respiration, and even temperature by activating the autonomic nervous system ("fight or flight"). Smoking can affect the heart rate or blood pressure and, in some cases, the respiratory rate. Caffeine and some drugs affect the heart rate and blood pressure. Activity increases the respiratory and heart rates as well as blood pressure. Patients that regularly undertake vigorous physical activity (marathon runners, for example) may demonstrate exceptionally slow heart rates and low blood pressure.

Temperature

Regulation of body temperature is a function of the brain, specifically the hypothalamus. Heat is produced by voluntary and involuntary muscle movement and by the action of cellular **metabolism.** As heat builds in the body, it is lost through **convection,** conduction, radiation, perspiration, and elimination. Thermal regulation requires a delicate balance of these activities to keep the body temperature constant and allow the vital organs to function properly. Infection or metabolic imbalance can upset this function and cause temperatures to rise or fall dramatically.

A variety of measuring devices are available for taking a person's temperature. Clinical (glass) thermometers are used in some areas. Markings on the thermometer as well as the style of the bulb indicate the intended use. Oral thermometers have a longer narrow bulb and are color coded with a blue tip. Rectal thermometers have blunt bulbs and are color coded with a red tip. They can also be used for axillary temperatures (Figure 5.1). Clinical thermometers must be sterilized after each use (refer to Chapter 3 for information on cleaning and sterilizing equipment). To obtain an accurate measurement, a clinical thermometer should be left in place from three to five minutes when measuring an oral or rectal temperature and as long as ten minutes for an axillary temperature. These qualities make them undesirable for the busy doctor's office. It is also necessary to shake the mercury down before each use, which frequently accounts for breakage of the instrument, adding to their inconvenience.

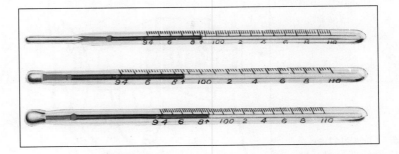

Figure 5.1 Clinical thermometers: oral (top), security (middle), rectal (bottom) (Reproduced with permission from Caldwell and Hegner, *Nursing Assistant,* 6th Ed., Delmar Publishers Inc., 1992)

PROCEDURE FOR USING A CLINICAL THERMOMETER

1. When lowering the column of mercury in a clinical thermometer, **grasp the thermometer by the barrel** near the distal end. Hold it firmly between the thumb and forefinger. With sharp motions of the wrist, **briskly shake the thermometer downward** until the column of mercury is approximately at the level of 93 degrees.

2. **Read the thermometer** by holding it at eye level and slowly rotating the barrel until the column of mercury and the scale of degrees are magnified and readable (Figure 5.2). The point where the column of mercury ends is the correct reading. If you neglect to shake the mercury column prior to taking a patient's temperature, then the thermometer will record only a reading that is equal to or higher than the level previously measured. The column of mercury will not travel backward to record a lower temperature.

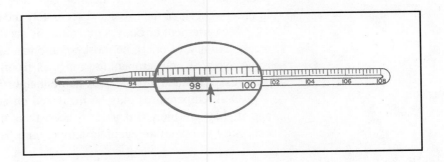

Figure 5.2 Reading a clinical thermometer (Reproduced with permission from Keir, Wise, and Krebs-Shannon, *Medical Assisting,* 2nd Ed., Delmar Publishers Inc., 1989)

Digital thermometers are much more common and efficient in today's medical setting (Figure 5.3). The digital thermometer has a disposable probe cover to allow for use with multiple patients; the probes are changeable and color coded for rectal and oral use. Digital thermometers have built-in timers and generally emit a tone when the measurement of the patient's temperature is completed. They are much

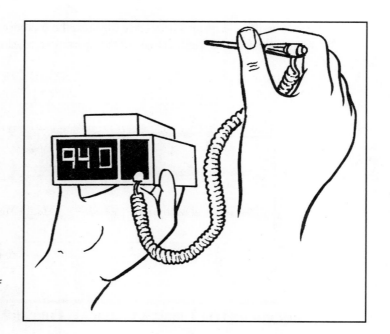

Figure 5.3 Digital thermometer (Reproduced with permission from Gomez and Hord, *Fundamentals of Clinical Nursing Skills,* John Wiley & Sons, Inc., 1988)

faster than clinical thermometers and can make an accurate measurement of the patient's temperature in as little as thirty seconds.

Disposable thermometers are also used. These thermometers are for a single use only and come individually wrapped. The person's temperature changes a series of colored dots on a plastic strip corresponding to temperature values (Figure 5.4). These systems are accurate and convenient for oral use but are not recommended for other uses.

Relatively new are otic thermometers, digital devices that take an accurate temperature in a matter of only a few seconds by means of a probe placed in the external auditory canal. Due to their speed and accuracy, these devices are particularly useful for small children and other patients who resist contact with medical personnel. The probe of the thermometer must be placed well into the auditory canal in order to occlude the canal and accurately measure the patient's core temperature.

Measurement of body temperature is accomplished by one of four routes: oral, rectal, axillary, or otic. The most common as well as the most convenient is the oral route. Normal oral temperature range is from 97 to 99 degrees Fahrenheit with a mean established at 98.6 degrees Fahrenheit or 37.0 degrees Celsius (centigrade).

Oral temperatures may be measured on adults and children over five years of age if they are alert and able to keep their mouth closed for the period of time necessary to obtain an accurate temperature. Unconscious patients, "mouth breath-

Figure 5.4 Disposable thermometer (Reproduced with permission from Keir, Wise, and Krebs-Shannon, *Medical Assisting,* 2nd Ed., Delmar Publishers Inc., 1989)

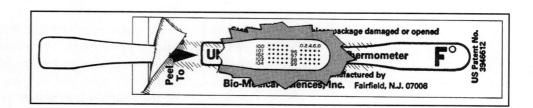

ers," patients with oral inflammation, and children younger than five years old or who are mentally impaired are inappropriate candidates for oral temperatures.

RATIONALE FOR PROCEDURE FOR TAKING ORAL TEMPERATURE

The medical assistant should wear gloves when taking a patient's temperature. Clinical oral thermometers should be placed beneath the tongue just to either side of the midline. Manufacturers of digital thermometers often recommend placing the thermometer farther back in the oral cavity between the molars and the lateral aspect of the tongue. This position places the probe in close proximity to the arterial blood supply and reportedly affords a more accurate temperature measurement. The patient should be instructed to close the mouth and to not bite down on the instrument (Figure 5.5). Record the temperature in the patient's medical record.

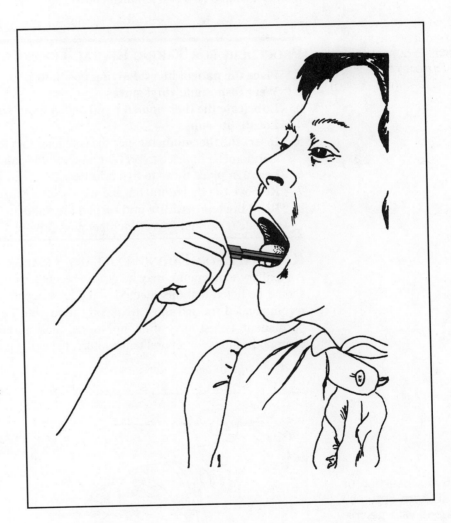

Figure 5.5 Placement of the oral thermometer (Reproduced with permission from Keir, Wise and Krebs-Shannon, *Medical Assisting,* 2nd Ed., Delmar Publishers Inc., 1989)

PRODECURE FOR TAKING ORAL TEMPERATURE

1. **Place the thermometer under the patient's tongue** and instruct the patient to keep the mouth closed.
2. **Leave in place three to five minutes** (clinical thermometer).

3. **Remove the thermometer** and wipe with a gauze pad to remove body fluids.
4. **Read the temperature and record the value** in the patient's chart. Be sure to include (o) to signify oral temperature.

RATIONALE FOR PROCEDURE FOR RECTAL TEMPERATURE

A rectal temperature is the most accurate due to the highly vascular composition of the rectal wall and the lack of air circulation to the cavity, but it is the least convenient. A rectal temperature is measured when an oral temperature is inappropriate. Normal range for rectal temperature is approximately one degree higher than for oral temperature. A lubricant should always be used when taking a rectal temperature to prevent injury to the delicate rectal mucosa. Gloves should be worn, and the thermometer should never be left unattended.

PROCEDURE FOR TAKING RECTAL TEMPERATURE

1. **Place the patient in a side-lying position.**
2. **Wear disposable vinyl gloves.**
3. **Lubricate the thermometer end** with a water-soluble lubricant.
4. **Locate the anus.**
5. **Insert the thermometer** past the sphincter into the rectal vault. Hold the thermometer in place to prevent injury to the patient.
6. **Leave in place three to five minutes.**
7. **Remove the thermometer** and wipe with a gauze pad to remove body fluids.
8. **Read the temperature and record the value** in the patient's chart. Be sure to include (r) to signify rectal temperature (Figure 5.6).

RATIONALE FOR TAKING AXILLARY TEMPERATURE

An axillary temperature may be used when other routes are inappropriate, though it should be noted that this method is the least accurate of the available choices. It is recommended for and most frequently used with infants. A patient who has had a permanent colostomy often no longer has a rectum, and if the patient has contraindications for an oral temperature, the axilla may be the only choice. Children

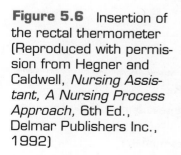

Figure 5.6 Insertion of the rectal thermometer (Reproduced with permission from Hegner and Caldwell, *Nursing Assistant, A Nursing Process Approach*, 6th Ed., Delmar Publishers Inc., 1992)

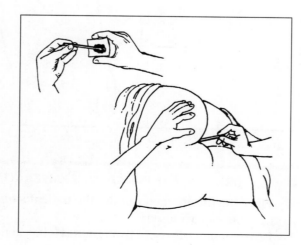

younger than five years old usually are unable to hold an oral thermometer correctly and may be candidates for an axillary temperature. Normal values for axillary temperature are one degree lower than those for oral temperatures. Gloves should be worn by the clinician.

PROCEDURE FOR TAKING AXILLARY TEMPERATURE

1. **Cleanse the axillary area** with an alcohol wipe and dry with a washcloth or gauze pad.
2. **Insert the thermometer under the patient's arm** and place the patient's arm at the patient's side.
3. **Leave in place three to five minutes.**
4. **Remove the thermometer** and wipe with a gauze pad to remove body fluids.
5. **Read the temperature and record the value** in the patient's chart. Be sure to include (ax) to signify axillary temperature (Figure 5.7).

Normal values for otic temperature are the same as for an oral temperature. The machines have disposable probe covers for each use. The probe is inserted gently into the external auditory meatus, a button is pressed, and the digital reading appears in three to five seconds.

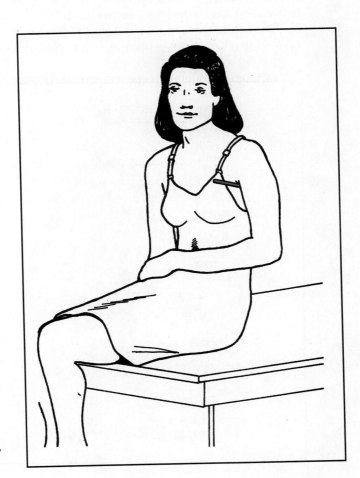

Figure 5.7 Technique for measuring axillary temperature (Reproduced with permission from Keir, Wise, and Krebs-Shannon, *Medical Assisting,* 2nd Ed., Delmar Publishers Inc., 1989)

Pulse

Measurement of pulse is accomplished by palpation of an artery against a firm base. The pulse is indicative of cardiac performance. Assessment of the pulse can tell the examiner a number of things about the patient's general condition.

PROCEDURE FOR TAKING THE PULSE

1. Using one or all of the first three fingers of the hand, **apply gentle but firm pressure** at the desired pulse site. (Never use the thumb. The thumb contains a strong pulse, and a pulse felt with the thumb is probably that of the examiner, not the patient.) By compressing the artery against a hard surface (generally a bone), the pulse can be felt.
2. **Count the pulse for one full minute.** If no abnormalities in rhythm are detected, it may be acceptable to count the pulse for fifteen seconds and multiply the result by four.
3. **Record the pulse** in the patient's medical record.

The most common site for obtaining a pulse is the radial artery, located at the anterior lateral aspect of the wrist. Other sites include the carotid artery, located on the neck inferior to the angle of the jaw; the brachial artery, located at the medial aspect of the arm just above the elbow; the femoral artery, located in the groin; the popliteal artery, located at the posterior aspect of the knee; the dorsalis pedis artery located just below the ankle on the dorsal surface of the foot; and the posterior tibial artery located on the posterior lateral aspect of the ankle (Figure 5.8). Once an accurate pulse rate has been obtained, record the information in the patient's medical record.

Figure 5.8 Pulse sites in the body (Adapted with permission from Hegner and Caldwell, *Nursing Assistant, A Nursing Process Approach*, 6th Ed., Delmar Publishers Inc., 1992)

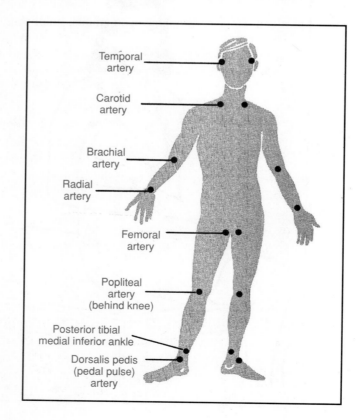

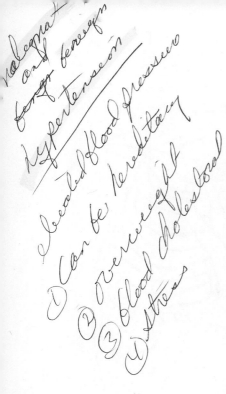

(handwritten margin notes)
inadequate and benign or ___
hypertension
1 Can be hereditary
2 Overweight
3 Elevated blood pressure
4 Elevated blood cholesterol
5 Stress

Normal pulse rates in adults range from 60 to 100 beats per minute. Below 60 the pulse is **bradycardic,** and above 100 the pulse is **tachycardic.**

There is more to assessing pulse than merely counting the beats and recording a number. Regularity of the rhythm is important, and taking the pulse can often be the first step in finding a cardiac **dysrhythmia.** Atrial **fibrillation** yields a pulse that is termed irregularly irregular; simply put, the pulse skips, but not in a definite pattern. Dropped beats may indicate premature ventricular contractions. (See Chapter 15, "Other Diagnostic Tests.")

Quality of the pulse is also significant. A pulse that can barely be felt is termed *thready.* A very strong pulse is termed *bounding.* Pulses are often rated as l+ to 4+. A pulse of l+ can be obliterated with minimal pressure and is also termed thready. A pulse of 2+ can be obliterated with firm pressure. A pulse of 3+ is strong and can only be obliterated with very firm pressure. A pulse of 4+ cannot be obliterated and is also termed bounding. Care should be taken to avoid putting pressure on the carotid arteries. Pressure on these arteries affects the carotid sinus and can cause dangerous slowing of the heart rate and potential injuries to the brain due to interruption of circulation.

PROCEDURE FOR PULSE AUSCULTATION

Another method of assessing pulse is by auscultation. The apical pulse is taken by placing a stethoscope over the point of maximum impulse (PMI), usually located just below the left nipple. This point may vary depending upon the orientation of the patient's heart in the thoracic cavity and the physical characteristics of the patient (Figure 5.9). Apical pulses are counted for a full minute, listening to the characteristic "lub-dub" sound and counting each "lub-dub" as one beat. Variations of the classic sound referred to as S^1 and S^2 can be the result of **murmurs, rubs,** or **gallops.** Apical pulses typically are taken on infants, small children, and patients who are to receive cardiotonic drugs, particularly digitalis preparations. Once the auscultated pulse rate has been obtained, record the information in the patient's medical record with a notation that this is an auscultated pulse rate.

Assessment of the quality of the heart tones is the responsibility of the physician, physician assistant, or a registered nurse. If an abnormality is detected by the medical assistant, it should be brought to the physician's attention.

In an emergency, the palpated pulse can be a rough indicator of **systolic blood pressure.** It is generally acceptable to assume that if a radial pulse can be palpated, the systolic blood pressure is at least 90 mm **Hg.** If a femoral pulse can be palpated, the systolic blood pressure is at least 70 mm **Hg.** If the carotid pulse can be palpated, systolic blood pressure is at least 40 mm **Hg.** These are no substitutes for a measured blood pressure, merely methods of estimating a blood pressure in cases of extreme emergency.

Respiration

PROCEDURE FOR OBTAINING THE RESPIRATORY RATE

Counting respiration is an art unto itself. Almost all patients either consciously or subconsciously will alter their respiratory pattern if they are aware that you are counting. In order to count respirations accurately, the method must be unobtrusive. An effective technique involves first taking the pulse for fifteen seconds and making

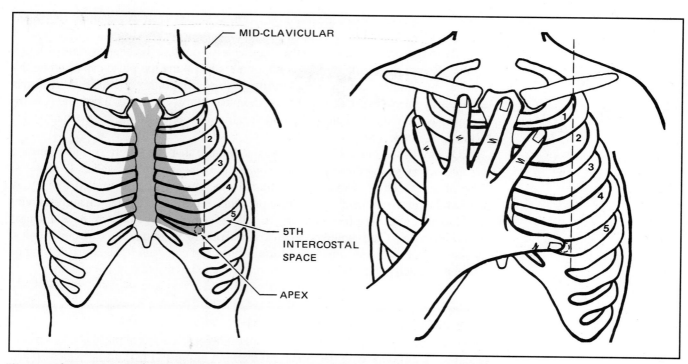

Figure 5.9 Location of the apical pulse (left); alternative method for locating the apex of the heart (right) (Reproduced with permission from Keir, Wise, and Krebs-Shannon, *Medical Assisting,* 2nd Ed., Delmar Publishers Inc., 1989)

mental note of the rate and quality. While continuing to hold the patient's wrist, count the rise and fall of the patient's chest for fifteen seconds and multiply the rate by four. Using this technique diverts the patient's attention and allows a more accurate assessment of the resting respiratory rate. If the patient is having respiratory problems, such as shortness of breath, the respiratory rate must be counted for one full minute. When an accurate measurement has been obtained, record the information in the patient's medical record. Any abnormalities observed in the patient's respiratory process should also be recorded.

The quality of the respiration is assessed best by using a stethoscope at strategic points anterior and posterior. This allows assessment of each of the lobes of the lung as well as the bronchials. However, a great deal of assessment can also be accomplished by carefully observing the patient.

Normal respiration, **eupnea,** is effortless and regular. An acceptable rate is twelve to twenty breaths per minute. An adult rate of fewer than twelve breaths per minute is called **bradypnea;** a rate of more than twenty is called **tachypnea.**

Most people breathe through the nose, and the diaphragm does the work. A patient, however, may be found to be using other muscles to assist their breathing. Observe the shoulders and the abdomen for exaggerated movement. If the patient is disrobed, note any obvious signs of movement between the ribs or at the sternum. Observe for marked nasal flaring with inspiration or pursed lips with exhalation. Is the patient "mouth breathing"? Consider the depth of respiration. Is it shallow and panting, or extraordinarily deep? Observe for regularity. If the respirations are irregular, try to observe a pattern. (See below for a discussion of abnormal respiratory patterns.)

While assessing the respiratory status of the patient, observe the patient's color. Look for signs of **hypoxia,** circumoral or nailbed **cyanosis** in a patient who has obvious difficulty ventilating. Note if the patient is pink, pale, or cyanotic. In darker-skinned patients the gums, oral mucosa, and nailbeds are indicative of oxygenation.

ABNORMAL RESPIRATORY PATTERNS (FIGURE 5.10)

Biot's Breathing

This respiratory pattern is characterized by a series of short, shallow respirations, followed by irregular periods of apnea. It is usually associated with increased intracranial pressure and head and spinal cord injuries.

Cheyne-Stokes Respirations

This is a cyclic pattern of shallow respiration, rapidly increasing to a crescendo, followed by irregular periods of apnea lasting ten to sixty seconds. It is thought usually to be an agonal respiratory pattern or precursor of death.

Kussmaul's Respirations

This is a pattern of rapid, gasping respiration, usually associated with diabetic ketoacidosis. Observe for sweet, fruity odor of patient's breath.

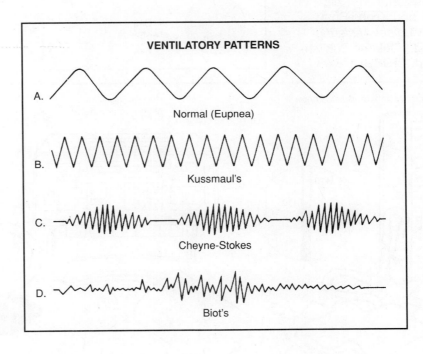

Figure 5.10 Respiratory patterns: (A) Normal (eupnea). (B) Kussmaul's. (C) Cheyne-Stokes. (D) Biot's. (Adapted with permission from White, *Basic Clinical Lab Competencies for Laboratory Care, An Integrated Approach*, Delmar Publishers Inc., 1988)

Blood Pressure

A **sphygmomanometer** and stethoscope are the instruments needed in obtaining a blood pressure reading (Figure 5.11). Sphygmomanometers come in several types (Figure 5.12). The mercury sphygmomanometer has a column of mercury with the scale printed on the sides of the glass tube. The aneroid sphygmomanometer has a clock-like dial with the values printed around the edge and a pointer (some home units print out digital values). There are also electronic sphygmomanometers. For our purposes we will deal with the mercury and aneroid units. In both cases, the technique is the same.

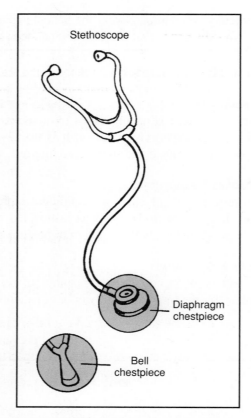

Figure 5.11 Stethoscope (Adapted with permission from Keir, Wise, and Krebs-Shannon, *Medical Assisting*, 2nd Ed., Delmar Publishers Inc., 1989)

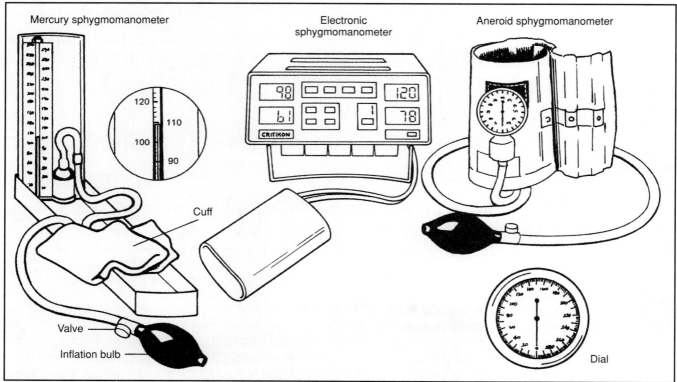

Figure 5.12 Three types of sphygmomanometer: mercury, aneroid, and electronic (mercury and aneroid illustrations adapted with permission from Keir, Wise, and Krebs-Shannon, *Medical Assisting,* 2nd Ed., Delmar Publishers Inc., 1989)

PROCEDURE FOR OBTAINING A BLOOD PRESSURE READING

1. After completely deflating the cuff, **place the cuff on the arm** securely and smoothly, approximately two inches above the elbow.
2. After palpating the anterior medial aspect of the arm at or above the antecubital space to locate the pulse, **place the diaphragm of the stethoscope** over the site where the pulse was palpated, being careful to keep the diaphragm out from under the margin of the cuff (Figure 5.13) Just as patients come in different sizes, so do blood pressure cuffs. There are adult sizes for adolescent and adult use, pediatric sizes for children and infants, and thigh cuffs that may be used on the arm for patients who are obese.
3. **Close the valve on the cuff** and gently inflate the cuff while listening for the **bruit** of the pulse.
4. As the pulse is auscultated, **continue inflation of the cuff until the sound disappears.**
5. At this point, **gently loosen the valve** by turning slightly counterclockwise and allow the air to escape slowly, indicated by the column of mercury or pointer on the dial descending slowly.
6. As the bruit of the pulse returns, **make note of the value** at the time the first pulsation is noted; this is the systolic blood pressure.
7. **Continue to slowly deflate the cuff,** listening to the pulsation in the artery. When the pulsation disappears, make note of the value; this is the **diastolic pressure.**
8. When an accurate blood pressure reading has been obtained, **record the information in the patient's** medical **record.**

In some patients you win hear the pulsation all the way down to the level of zero; this is often referred to as the "second diastolic" pressure. While measuring blood pressure, you first hear the pulsation for systole; the tone of the pulsation then becomes quiet or muffled—this is the true diastolic pressure. If the pulsation is still heard after a change in quality, some people prefer to record all values.

Example
You measure the patient's blood pressure and auscultate the first tone at 160 mm Hg; the tone changes in quality at 70 mm Hg and continues to 20 mm Hg. You would record the pressure as 160/70/20. Check with your physician employer to become familiar with preference in this matter.

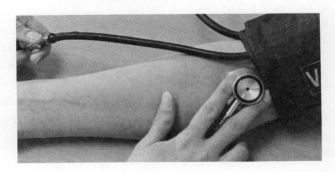

Figure 5.13 Proper cuff placement for blood pressure reading (Reproduced with permission from Simmers, *Diversified Health Occupations,* 2nd Ed., Delmar Publishers Inc., 1988)

If you are unable to hear the pulsation, check the placement of the stethoscope. Palpate the brachial pulse and place the head of the stethoscope directly over this point. If you are using a stethoscope with a bell and diaphragm, check that the diaphragm is in proper position.

If you are still unable to auscultate a pulse, it may be necessary to use a **doppler,** a special stethoscope that electronically magnifies the sound (Figure 5.14).

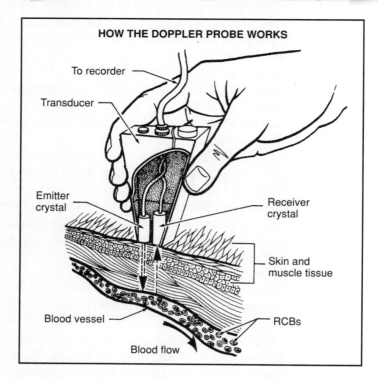

HOW THE DOPPLER PROBE WORKS

To recorder

Transducer

Emitter crystal

Receiver crystal

Skin and muscle tissue

Blood vessel

RCBs

Blood flow

Figure 5.14
Doppler probe (Reproduced with permission from Keir, Wise, and Krebs-Shannon, *Medical Assisting,* 2nd Ed., Delmar Publishers Inc., 1989)

PROCEDURE FOR OBTAINING A BLOOD PRESSURE USING A DOPPLER

1. **Apply conduction gel** to the skin surface where the brachial pulse was palpated.
2. **Place the head of the doppler directly in the conduction gel** and reposition until the pulse is heard.
3. **Inflate the cuff until the pulse disappears.**
4. **Slowly deflate the cuff until** the pulse is heard again and record this value as the systolic pressure.

The pressure is then recorded in the patient's medical record as systolic over doppler. No diastolic value is recorded with a doppler pressure.

Systolic pressure may also be palpated.

PROCEDURE FOR OBTAINING A SYSTOLIC BLOOD PRESSURE BY PALPATION

1. **Find the brachial pulse.**
2. **Inflate the cuff** while palpating the pulse until the pulse disappears.
3. **Slowly deflate the cuff** and when the pulse returns record the value as the systolic pressure.

As in the method of doppler pressures, the word "palpated" is substituted for the diastolic value. Record the blood pressure in the patient's medical record.

When taking blood pressures, you will note a slight fluctuation of the column of mercury or of the needle just prior to auscultating or palpating the systolic pressure. Never record this value as the systolic pressure. The true systolic pressure is auscultated. The visual fluctuation may occur as much as twenty millimeters of mercury higher than the true systolic pressure. Recording this value is erroneous, very misleading, and potentially harmful to the patient. Medications and treatments are often prescribed as a result of the values of the patient's vital signs.

Height and Weight

Measurements of the patient's height and weight should be made at the time of the first office visit and may also be made at subsequent office visits. There are several reasons for this. The most obvious has to do with the patient's general condition and how the patient compares to the norm for their age and sex (Figure 5.15). More important than whether a patient is over or under the norm is the fact that the dosage for certain prescription medications is determined by weight or body surface area.

The physician may prefer that patients be weighed with or without clothing and that their height be measured in their stocking feet. The important point is that whatever the method, it should be consistent in order to establish an accurate baseline and progression for each patient.

PROCEDURE FOR OBTAINING HEIGHT AND WEIGHT OF A PATIENT

1. Most offices use a standing medical scale. **Have the patient stand on the center of the platform of the scale,** wearing clothing consistent with your office procedure.
2. **Adjust the large counterweight** to the appropriate increment (usually in fifty-pound segments).
3. **Move the smaller counterweight** to the left or right until the pointer of the scale is balanced at the midline.
4. **Record the patient's weight** in the medical record as the total of the two values. For example, if the large counterweight is at the 150 mark and the small counterweight is at 26, the patient's weight is 176 pounds.
5. While the patient remains on the platform, preferably in their stocking feet, **extend the arm at the back of the scale to a level above the patient's head and lower the arm until firm contact with the patient's head is made.** Move the arm slowly to avoid injury to the patient. **Read the numerical scale at the back of the instrument and record the patient's height** in total inches in the medical record.

It is generally a good idea to occasionally check the accuracy of the scale by placing both counterweights in the zero position and verifying that the pointer is at the midline when nothing is on the scale. If the pointer varies, the scale should be recalibrated in accordance with your office maintenance procedure. Failure to have the scale recalibrated will result in inaccurate readings.

MEN			
Height	Small	Medium	Large
5' 2"	128–134	131–141	138–150
5' 3"	130–136	133–143	140–153
5' 4"	132–138	135–145	142–156
5' 5"	134–140	137–148	144–160
5' 6"	136–142	139–151	146–164
5' 7"	138–146	142–154	149–168
5' 8"	140–148	145–157	152–172
5' 9"	142–151	148–160	155–176
5'10"	144–154	151–163	158–180
5'11"	146–157	154–166	161–184
6' 0"	149–160	157–170	164–188
6' 1"	152–164	160–174	188–192
6' 2"	155–168	164–178	172–197
6' 3"	158–172	167–182	176–202
6' 4"	162–176	171–187	181-207

WOMEN			
Height	Small	Medium	Large
4'10"	102–111	109–121	118–131
4'11"	103–113	111–123	120–134
5' 0"	104–115	113–126	122–137
5' 1"	106–118	115–129	125–140
5' 2"	108–121	118–132	128–143
5' 3"	111–124	121–135	131–147
5' 4"	114–127	124–138	134–151
5' 5"	117–130	127–141	137–155
5' 6"	120–133	130–144	140–159
5' 7"	123–136	133–147	143–163
5' 8"	128–139	138–150	146–167
5' 9"	129–142	139–153	149–170
5'10"	132–146	142–156	152–173
5'11"	135–148	145–159	155–176
6' 0"	138–151	148–162	158–179

Figure 5.15 Chart of desirable weights for men and women (Reproduced with permission from Keir, Wise, and Krebs-Shannon, *Medical Assisting,* 2nd Ed., Delmar Publishers Inc., 1989)

**REVIEW/
SELF-EXAMINATION**

1. What is the purpose of recording vital signs?

2. Name three methods of measuring a patient's temperature.

3. What method would you use to take the temperature of a three-year-old child?

4. What factors affect temperature?

5. Why should you not use your thumb when taking a pulse?

6. What does the systolic blood pressure represent?

7. What is meant by diastolic blood pressure?

8. What should you do if you are unable to hear the pulsation when attempting to measure a blood pressure?

9. What is a palpated blood pressure?

10. What is an apical pulse? When is one required?

11. List two instances when a clinical thermometer should not be used for an oral temperature.

12. What is a doppler?

13. List four sites where pulses may be palpated.

14. What is meant by auscultation?

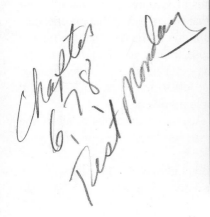

CHAPTER 6

Assisting with the Physical Examination

On completion of this chapter, you will be able to:
- Demonstrate proper procedure in assisting the physician with the physical examination.
- Demonstrate the proper methods of caring for the examination room and instruments after completion of the procedure.
- Identify the proper techniques in preparing the patient and the area for the physical examination with respect to the procedure being performed.
- Define the characteristic principles of the specialty examination.
- Demonstrate proper procedure in assisting the physician with specialty examinations.
- Define the vocabulary terms used in the chapter.

Vocabulary— Glossary of Terms

Anoscope	An instrument for examining the anus and lower rectum.
Anxiety	A feeling of uncertainty, apprehension, or fear.
Colonoscope	A fiber-optic instrument used to study the interior structure of the colon.
Culture	A specimen obtained during the exam and applied under sterile conditions to agar or a similar growth medium to elicit the growth of microorganisms.
Cystoscope	A fiber-optic instrument used to study the interior structure of the urinary bladder.
Cytology	The study of cells.
Ophthalmoscope	An instrument used to examine the eyes.
Otoscope	An instrument used to examine the ears.
Sigmoidoscope	An fiber-optic instrument used to examine the lower portion of the colon.
Stimulus	Any agent, act, or influence producing a reaction.
Trauma	Any wound, physical or psychic.

Assisting with the Physical Examination

E ach of us, at one time or another, has undergone an office exam by a physician or accompanied someone else during this procedure. Think back to that initial experience and review the feelings and **anxiety** that were a part of that experience.

If your experience was pleasant, it was no doubt due to the fact that the people with whom you were in contact placed you at ease, made you feel secure, and assisted you in understanding the procedure. On the other hand, if your experience was a source of **trauma,** than very likely you were left to the mercy of your own imagination without benefit of support from the people involved.

Carry those memories with you into practice. Adjust your actions to allow the patients with whom you come in contact to achieve maximum benefit from your own experience and education.

Some patients harbor an inherent fear of doctors and dentists. Fortunately they are in the minority. Those who are fearful are usually those who have had bad experiences or those for whom this is a first experience.

Most of us fear the unknown. Providing as detailed an explanation of the procedures to be conducted during the exam may help ease the patient's anxiety, thereby making the visit less stressful for both the patient and yourself.

Upon accepting employment in a medical office, the medical assistant should receive a period of orientation to the facility. During this period, the new employee should become familiar with the general routine of the office and some of the idiosyncracies of the physician.

Most offices have one or more examination rooms equipped with the items needed during the physical exam. These will include an examination table, an examination light source, equipment for collecting specimens, and the basic instruments for conducting the exam.

In specialty areas, some of the instruments may be included in trays or other containers and will need to be placed in the room prior to the beginning of the procedure. As you become familiar with the technique of the physician, you will learn to anticipate the physicians's needs. There are instances when a piece of equipment is needed and must be obtained from another area after the exam is in progress, but these should be kept to a minimum. One way to eliminate this problem is to ask the physician during the set-up phase if there will be any special equipment needed for the procedure.

PROCEDURE FOR GENERAL EXAMINATION PREPARATION

1. **The examination room should be neat and orderly,** with an ample supply of examination table covers and drapes available.
2. **There should be an area available for the patient to disrobe and hang up clothes.**
3. **Patient gowns should be available to the patient after disrobing.**
4. **A cover sheet should be made available to the patient,** particularly if the examination room is cool.
5. Once the patient is escorted to the room, introduce yourself and **obtain initial vital sign measurements** and any other information necessary for the patient's medical record.
6. **Briefly explain the procedure** to the patient. If the patient is a child, explain the procedure to the child's parent(s).

When explaining a procedure to the parent(s) of a child old enough to understand the procedure, be sure to include the child in the discussion. Children have anxieties like the rest of us and sometimes to a far greater degree than their adult counterparts. Do your best to reduce anxiety during your explanation of the procedure, choosing your words carefully. After the explanation is complete, ask if the patient has any questions. Answer them to the best of your ability or refer them to the physician, as appropriate.

If this is the patient's first visit to your office, the physician will probably want to do a systems review and talk with the patient prior to the examination. This may or may not be the case with subsequent examinations. When the physician enters the examination room, introduce the patient to the physician if the patient has not been seen by this examiner before.

PROCEDURE FOR PREPARING THE PATIENT FOR THE EXAMINATION

1. **Instruct the patient in disrobing** based on the examination to be performed. Be specific as to what clothing is to be removed and what may be left in place.
2. **Escort the patient to the area used for disrobing,** show them where they may hang clothing, and provide them with a patient gown. If the patient needs assistance with disrobing and gowning, provide whatever assistance is required.
3. **Give instructions on where the patient should go after they have completed disrobing.** For example, "After you are finished, please have a seat on the examination table." (Identify the table by gesture.)
4. **Leave the room, informing the patient that you will return in a few minutes, after they have finished.** You should remain in the room with anxious patients and unaccompanied pediatric patients. It may be preferable to remain with any patient you have concerns about leaving unattended.
5. **After allowing the patient sufficient time to disrobe, return to the examination room.** Remember to knock before entering.
6. **Assist the patient to the position necessary for the exam,** while explaining the rationale to the patient.
7. **Drape the patient to allow them maximum privacy.**
8. **Advise the physician that the patient is now ready for the examination.**

Assisting the Physician During the Examination

After preparing for the examination by collecting the necessary equipment and arranging it on a tray placed for the convenience of the physician, your next responsibility is to assist the physician. The medical assistant has two main duties during the examination. The first is to assist the physician in positioning the patient during the procedure, to handle equipment with care so as not to contaminate a sterile field, and to follow the physician's instructions during the exam. The second is to comfort and reassure the patient before, during, and after the examination.

There is a normal sequence to the complete physical examination that varies only with the examiner's preferences. In general, the sequence is as follows:

1. *Appearance*—overall appearance of the patient.
2. *Gait*—the manner or style of the patient's walking.
3. *Posture*—the way the patient stands and sits.
4. *Physical systems review*—this is normally the portion of the examination that requires the medical assistant to assist the physician. It is your responsibility to have the equipment necessary for the examination ready and at hand. As the physician requests instruments or other materials, hand them firmly to the physician handles first so that they are ready to be used. If the patient is an adult or male of puberty age, you will probably not assist with the examination of the rectal area or genitalia during a routine physical examination. If the patient is a female, you should always remain in attendance during this portion of the examination. (A female assistant should always be present during a complete physical examination of a female client by a male physician.) If specimens are taken, label them immediately.

AFTER THE EXAMINATION

Remember to review any instructions given to the patient with the patient and/or a family member. Explain each instruction separately in terms that the patient can understand easily, remembering to ask if there are any questions. Supply the patient with a written copy of the instructions, including a phone number to call if questions arise.

Once the physical examination has been completed, assist the patient off the examination table and, if necessary, help with dressing. Record any necessary information in the patient's medical record. Prepare any specimens for examination or transport. Clean table tops with disinfectant. Cover the examination table with clean paper or linen.

Equipment must be cleaned, and in some cases sterilized, after the completion of the procedure. Once the patient has left the area, proceed to clean and reorganize the examination room in preparation for the next patient. Clean the instruments and put them away in their proper place and take those instruments to be sterilized to the appropriate area for sterilization. Replace all supplies used during the examination to avoid a shortage during the next procedure.

Specialty Examinations

The role of the medical assistant in specialized examination procedures includes preparing the room by ensuring the presence of necessary equipment for the particular examination, assisting the patient in getting ready for the examination by instructing them in disrobing, assisting them to the appropriate position for the procedure, and draping them appropriately, and assisting the physician as necessary during the examination.

GYNECOLOGY AND OBSTRETRICS

The patient should completely disrobe and wear a gown. The most common position for the OB/GYN exam is the *lithotomy* position. The patient is placed on a specially designed table in the supine position, with feet placed in "stirrups" mounted on the end of the table. The knees are bent and the legs separated, with a drape placed over the lower portion of the body for privacy. A pillow is placed under the head for comfort. In some cases, elderly patients may find this position extremely uncomfortable, so the physician may elect to perform the exam with the patient in a lateral recumbent (side-lying) position.

Various sizes or types of specula and scopes may be used for the examinations. Lubricant, **culture** tubes, wooden cervical spatulas, sterile slides for smears, uterine dressings, and fixative sprays or **cytology** jars should be readily available (Figure 6.1). A supply of vinyl examination gloves and finger cots should be available for the physician's use.

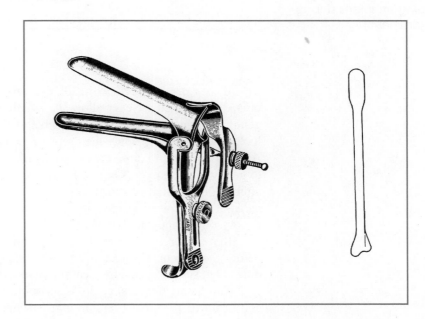

Figure 6.1 Instruments used in the OB/GYN examination: (A) Speculum. (B) Cervical spatula. (Reproduced with permission from Jarit Surgical Instruments Catalog, copyright 1991.)

PEDIATRICS

Positioning varies, depending on the age of the child and the examination to be performed. Usually placing the child on a standard examination table is sufficient. Disrobing varies, depending on the extent of the examination to be performed.

NEVER leave children or infants unattended on an examination table, due to the danger of injury from a fall. Infants and some younger children are often uncooperative during the exam and may need to be restrained by a "papoose wrap" to allow the physician to complete the exam (Figure 6.2). If so, place the youngster diagonally on a small blanket; bring the corner of the blanket at the feet up toward the abdomen, and wrap the right corner of the blanket laterally around the torso with the arm inside at the infant's side. Then wrap the left corner of the blanket laterally around the torso with the arm enclosed at the child's side and tuck under the torso. This wrap should be snug enough to prevent movement of the arms and legs during the exam, but loose enough to prevent discomfort to the child.

It is also acceptable to allow the parent to hold the child in arms during the examination procedure as long as the parent feels comfortable with this approach.

OPHTHALMOLOGY

In this exam the patient is placed in a specially designed chair with head and neck support. Often the physician will request that drops be instilled in the eye prior to the exam. In some cases this will be done by the medical assistant, in others by the physician.

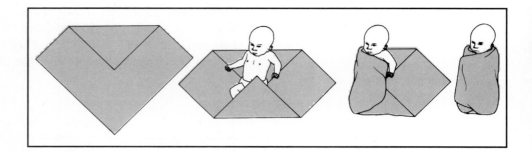

Figure 6.2 Use of a "papoose wrap" in restraining an infant during an examination

If you are required to instill eye drops, adhere to the following to do the procedure correctly. Never allow the solution to drop directly on the cornea. After gently applying traction to the cheek below the lower eyelid, request that the patient look upward. Gently apply the drops to the conjunctival sac near the inner canthus. Allow the patient to close the eye to distribute the medication; have tissues available to gently blot the excess liquid. It may be necessary to dim the lighting in the room after the instillation of drops. Be sure to record in the patient's medical record the name of the medication, the number of drops used in each eye, the date and time, and the outcome, anticipated or otherwise.

Remember to prepare the patient for any unusual side effects to the drops before they occur. For example, visual changes are common when the pupils are dilated but subside as the medication wears off.

The testing of visual acuity is accomplished by means of the Snellen Eye Chart, consisting of rows of letters arranged in lines of decreasing size. The test is conducted with one eye covered, then with the other eye covered, and finally with both eyes open. The medical assistant should ask the patient to read the smallest print that they are able to see. When the patient has completed a line of print correctly, ask them to read the next largest line above, as well, to ensure accuracy in the test. When testing the right and left eye singly, the medical assistant may choose to have the patient read a line from left to right with one eye and then from right to left with the other. The value listed adjacent to the line of print should then be recorded in the patient's medical record (e.g., 20/20, 20/30, 20/40, etc.).

When testing visual acuity of children who are unable to read, the Snellen "Big E" chart is used; this chart consists of various sizes of the capital letter "E" arranged in different directions. The child is asked to demonstrate the direction of the tines of the letter instead of reading a line of the alphabet (Figure 6.3).

Oτorhinolaryngology

Examinations of the ear, nose, and throat require a fully charged, operational **otoscope, ophthalmoscope,** and laryngoscope. Modern units combine all three into one instrument pack fitted with a variety of appropriate heads and a rechargeable battery. Units are usually placed in a charging unit when not in use, guaranteeing their readiness when needed. Also used are the nasal speculum, tuning forks, laryngeal mirror, and tongue blades (Figure 6.4).

Proctology

The patient should disrobe, at least from the waist down, and wear a hospital gown. Positions vary, depending on the procedure to be performed. The most common

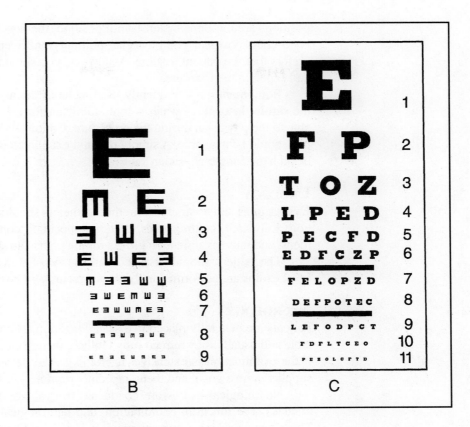

Figure 6.3 Eye charts

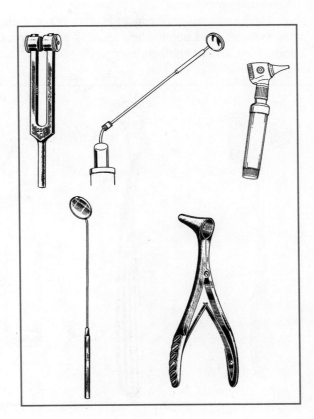

Figure 6.4 Instruments used during ear, nose, and throat examination: (A) Tuning fork. (B) Laryngoscope. (C) Otoscope. (D) Laryngeal mirror. (E) Nasal speculum. (Reproduced with permission from Jarit Surgical Instruments Catalog, copyright 1991)

positions are the Sims or left lateral position, the dorsal recumbent position, and the knee–chest position. The physician normally will identify which position he or she prefers that the patient assume. As always, you should drape the patient for privacy and explain the procedure.

Equipment most frequently used includes the **anoscope,** the **colonoscope,** and the **sigmoidoscope.** A water soluble lubricant for the scopes should be made available to the physician during the procedure. Cotton swabs, culture tubes, and cytology jars should be available. A supply of vinyl examination gloves and finger cots should be on hand for the physician's use.

UROLOGY

Cystoscopes and a variety of urethral catheters should be available for the examination. Lubricant, culture tubes, a sterile specimen container, glass slides for specimens, and vinyl examination gloves for the physician should also be available.

The patient should disrobe from the waist down and be draped for privacy. Most exams are performed in the dorsal recumbent position.

NEUROLOGY

Patients are generally placed in a seated position (High Fowler's) on an examination table and usually may remain fully clothed, though clothing may need to be removed if the examination is extensive. If clothing is to be removed, the patient should be supplied with a gown and then draped appropriately.

Neurological exams are conducted to evaluate deep tendon reflexes (DTRs), cranial nerve function, coordination, and neurological response to various **stimuli.** These exams seldom cause discomfort, but should be explained to the patient while preparations are made.

Equipment necessary includes (but is not limited to) a rubber percussion hammer, cotton-tipped applicators, a safety pin or Wartenberg neurological pin wheel, tuning fork, and an ophthalmoscope (Figure 6.5).

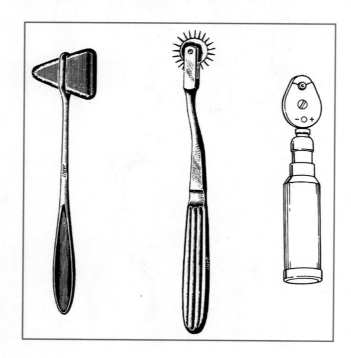

Figure 6.5 Instruments used in the neurological examination: (A) Rubber percussion hammer. (B) Wartenberg neurological pinwheel. (C) Ophthalmoscope. (Reproduced with permission from Jarit Surgical Instruments Catalog, copyright 1991.)

1. List the basic components included in a standard examination room.

2. What position is most common for OB/GYN examinations?

3. Describe the method of restraint for infants and small children during examination and procedures.

4. Describe the correct technique for placing drops in a patient's eye.

5. What is a Snellen chart?

6. What are the medical assistant's responsibilities during the examination? After the examination?

7. How should after-exam instructions be delivered to the patient?

8. List the specialty examinations.

9. Describe how you might allay a patient's fears about an examination.

10. What information needs to be recorded in a patient's medical record following a Snellen eye examination?

11. What information needs to be recorded in a patient's medical record following insertion of eye drops?

12. How should instruments be handed to the physician during an examination?

13. What care is necessary for the examination room following an examination?

14. If lithotomy position is uncomfortable or impossible for a patient having a gynecologic examination, what alternative position might be employed?

15. What information is anticipated from a neurological examination?

CHAPTER 7

Bandages and Dressings

OBJECTIVES

On completion of this chapter, you will be able to:
- Select appropriate bandages.
- Apply bandages correctly.
- Define the various types of dressings.
- List the various applications for bandages and dressings.
- Select appropriate dressings.
- Apply dressings correctly.
- Correctly record bandage/dressing change in patient medical record.

**Vocabulary—
Glossary of Terms**

Abrasion	Damage to the external layers of skin; a scrape.
Cravat	The technique of folding a triangular bandage to make a strip bandage.
Distal	Farthest.
Incision	A clean, straight cut made by a scalpel.
Infection	The body's response to invasion by a pathogenic organism.
Proximal	Nearest.
Sanguineous	Liquid having the appearance of blood; bloody.
Serous Fluid	Clear, yellow-tinged liquid drainage from a wound.
Wound	An interruption of skin integrity.

Introduction

T o avoid confusion in the following discussion of bandages and dressings, we begin by explaining the function of each and identifying their differences. The term *bandage* is applied to any material used to wrap or bind a body part.

Bandages include rolled gauze, woven elastic material, triangular cloth for slings, and prepared bindings for various areas of the body. *Dressing* applies to any material placed in direct contact with a **wound**. Bandages are clean; dressings are sterile.

Bandages are applied to extremities and other body parts, sometimes alone, sometimes in combination with a dressing. The principle of bandaging remains the same regardless of the body area involved or the function of the bandage.

GAUZE BANDAGES

Gauze bandaging/dressing materials are usually supplied in roll form and are identified by width, which varies from 1" to 8". The material varies from a nonstretch linen to highly absorbent elasticized material. A specialty gauze used for wrapping relatively straight body parts comes with a special applicator (tube gauze) and is ideal for fingers, arms, hands, and feet (Figure 7.1). Gauze is primarily used to cover a sterile dressing. Generally, the physician will order the specific type to be used.

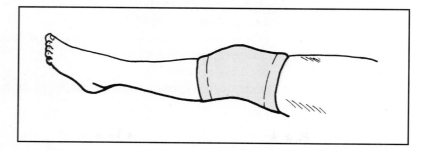

Figure 7.1 Tube gauze (Reproduced with permission from Keir, Wise, and Krebs-Shannon, *Medical Assisting,* 2nd Ed., Delmar Publishers Inc., 1989)

ELASTIC BANDAGES

Elastic bandages also come in roll form and vary in width from 2" to 8". They are most commonly used to support an injured joint or extremity, to increase venous return, or to hold dressings or splints in place. The size used varies with the application. Universally referred to as Ace bandages (a brand name), the elastic bandage is notorious for impeding circulation and causing swelling and loss of sensation when improperly applied. Careful application is imperative for the protection of the patient. Serious and possibly irreversible damage can result from an improperly applied elastic bandage.

"Padded elastic bandages" are frequently used for the treatment of severe sprains. This term refers to the use of cast padding or bunting wrapped around the body part prior to the application of the elastic wrap. The purpose is to provide more stability to the injured extremity.

TRIANGULAR BANDAGES

A common component of first-aid kits, this bandage is a large triangle of linen construction. In an emergency, it can fill any role. In common practice it is folded over to make a bandage of varying width (**cravat**) or fashioned into an arm sling (Figure 7.2).

Bandages and Their Applications

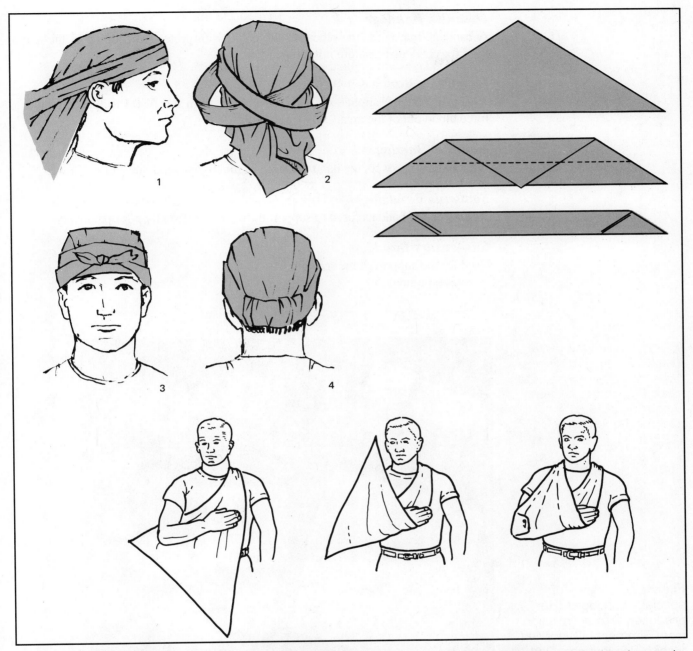

Figure 7.2 Examples of uses of a triangular bandage: (A) Applying a triangular bandage to the head or scalp. (B) Folding a cravat bandage from a triangular bandage. (C) Applying an arm sling. (Reproduced with permission from Simmers, *Diversified Health Occupations*, 2nd Ed., Delmar Publishers Inc., 1988 and Keir, Wise, and Krebs-Shannon, *Medical Assisting*, 2nd Ed., Delmar Publishers Inc., 1989)

SPECIALTY BANDAGES AND APPLICATIONS

Barton's Bandage
A double figure-eight bandage, used for fractures of the lower jaw.

Demigauntlet Bandage
A gauze bandage covering the hand but leaving the fingers exposed.

Desault's Bandage

A bandage that binds the elbow to the flank, with protective padding in the axilla, used for clavicular fracture immobilization.

Esmarch's Bandage

A rubber bandage applied around a body part from the **distal** to the **proximal** to force blood out of the area.

Gauntlet Bandage

A bandage that covers the hand and each of the fingers separately, like a glove.

Scultetus Bandage

A many-tailed bandage used to support the abdomen, usually postoperatively.

Suspensory Bandage

Used for the support of the scrotum.
(See Figure 7.3.)

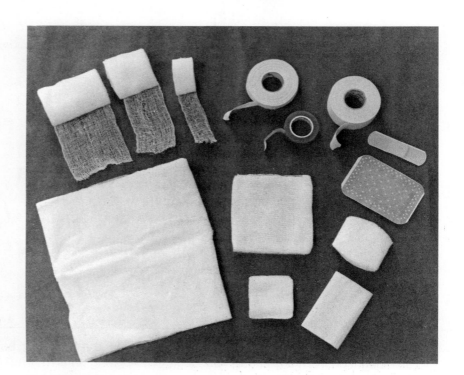

Figure 7.3 Types of specialty bandages (Reproduced with permission from Simmers, *Diversified Health Occupations,* 2nd Ed., 1988)

PROCEDURE FOR APPLYING BANDAGES

The part of the body requiring the bandage dictates the proper technique to use for bandaging. Often several bandaging styles may be incorporated to accommodate difficult areas.

Regardless of function the same rules apply:

1. **Wrap any body part from the distal end toward the proximal to improve circulation and aid the healing process.** When wrapping an arm/hand or leg/

foot, leave the fingers/toes exposed to aid in assessing circulation and sensation after the bandage has been applied. Wrap the body part securely, being careful that the bandage is not loosely applied.

2. **Never wrap tight enough to impair circulation.**
3. **Never wrap tight enough to impair sensation at the distal point of the bandage.**
4. Once the bandage has been applied, **verify circulation and sensation at the distal point of the bandage** and check the function of the bandage. *Document these findings in the patient's chart.*
5. During the procedure, **instruct the patient in the proper technique for applying the bandage.**

METHODS OF APPLICATION

Circular Wrap

Used as a start for most wrapping techniques or for small areas of an extremity (e.g., wrist). Start the bandage around the extremity and wrap on top of the previous turn. Continue for at least two turns to anchor a bandage or as necessary to cover a dressing adequately. Tape in place (Figure 7.4).

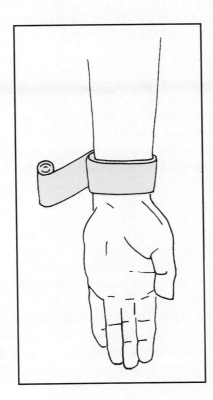

Figure 7.4 Circular wrap (Reproduced with permission from Narrow and Buschle, *Fundamentals of Nursing Practice*, 2nd Ed., John Wiley & Sons, Inc., 1982)

Figure-Eight Wrap

Used for joint areas that must be allowed to bend. Start with a circular wrap distal to the joint area. Continue to the proximal end of the joint area in the figure-eight pattern and conclude with two turns of circular wrap. Tape dressing in place or use metal clips as appropriate (Figure 7.5).

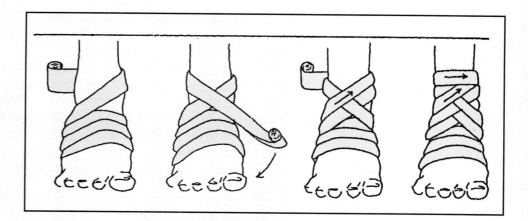

Figure 7.5 Figure-eight wrap (Reproduced with permission from Narrow and Buschle, *Fundamentals of Nursing Practice*, 2nd Ed., John Wiley & Sons, Inc., 1982)

Recurrent Wrap

Used for the top of the head and amputation stumps. Begin with two turns of circular wrap at the proximal point of the bandage for an anchor. Fold the bandage over itself making a 45-degree angle, then apply the dressing back and forth (anterior to posterior) over the end of the area being bandaged. Complete the procedure with two turns of circular wrap to anchor the recurrent turns of the bandage. This is one of the few times the bandage is not applied from distal to proximal aspect (Figure 7.6).

Reverse Spiral Wrap

Used to keep bandage in place in areas that rapidly change in diameter (e.g., forearm, calf). Start at the distal end of the area to be bandaged with two turns of circular wrap. Proceed one turn around the extremity in a spiral pattern, fold the dressing material over itself, and proceed in the opposite direction in a spiral pattern. Continue this procedure and end the dressing with two turns of circular wrap. The completed dressing yields a "herringbone" pattern. Tape or use metal clips, as appropriate (Figure 7.7).

Spiral Wrap

Used for long areas of extremities where there is no joint involvement. Frequently used for splinting procedures to hold the splint in place. Start at the distal point with two turns of circular wrap. Proceed toward the proximal in a spiral pattern. End with two turns of circular wrap. Tape or use metal clips, as appropriate (Figure 7.8).

On completion of the bandage, check the distal point of the bandaged area for changes in color, swelling, or decreased/absent pulse. If any of these symptoms occur, the bandage should be reapplied in a manner that does not impede circulation or sensation. Remember to document the check in the patient's chart and make note that pulses and color of the extremity distal to the bandage were normal.

Application of Splints and Casts

Casts and splints generally are applied by the physician. In some areas, office personnel may be trained as orthopedic technicians and assume this responsibility. In most cases, the medical assistant has the responsibility of gathering materials and assisting the physician in the application of the device.

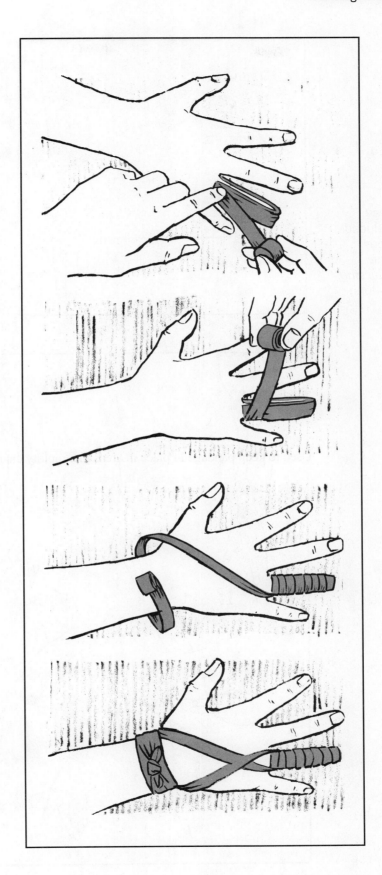

Figure 7.6 Recurrent wrap (Reproduced with permission from Simmers, *Diversified Health Occupations,* 2nd Ed., Delmar Publishers Inc., 1988)

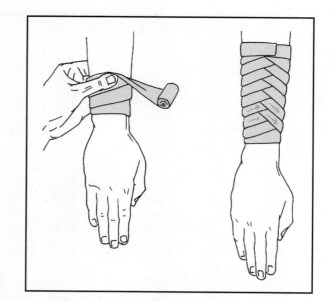

Figure 7.7 Reverse spiral wrap (Reproduced with permission from Narrow and Buschle, *Fundamentals of Nursing Practice*, 2nd Ed., John Wiley & Sons, Inc., 1982)

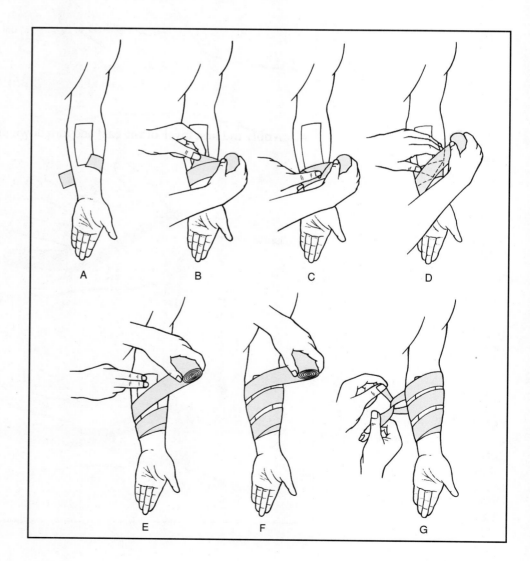

Figure 7.8 Spiral wrap

PROCEDURE FOR APPLYING SPLINTS AND CASTS

Splints are used for temporary immobilization of a fresh fracture, a severe sprain, or a muscle tear. Although a variety of preformed, commercial splints is available, expense and convenience make the plaster splint a favorite of many physicians.

The "sugar tong" splint is one of the most popular varieties. Strips of plaster are used to form a U-shaped brace around the affected area (usually an arm) and are held in place by elastic bandage or bias dressing. Posterior splints are often applied to leg and ankle injuries. Here the plaster strip is placed against the back of the affected area and again held in place by a bandage.

The advantage of a splint is that it allows for swelling in the few days immediately after an injury. The bandage may be adjusted to accommodate the changes in tissue and is generally replaced with a permanent cast in three to seven days.

Casts are a more permanent, long-term method for stabilizing fractures. Though splints are generally made of plaster, casts may be made either of plaster or synthetic material (fiberglass).

In application of both splints and casts materials are essentially the same. Casting materials are available in rolls or strips in widths ranging from two to six inches. Gloves should be worn when handling casting materials. If plaster is used, a bucket of warm water is needed. If fiberglass is used, cool water is needed. The procedure is as follows:

1. **Thoroughly cleanse the affected area.**
2. **Apply stockinette to the area**, allowing a generous margin to form a cuff.
3. **Wrap the area** with cast padding or bunting.
4. **Apply the first layer of the cast** and turn down the stockinette over the cast to form a finished edge.
5. **Apply successive layers of cast material** and allow the cast to cure.
   a. Take care to rest the cast on a soft surface (pillow, etc.). To prevent indentations from forming, do not hold the cast with the hands or rest on a firm surface.
   b. It is normal for the cast to become warm during the curing process due to the chemical reaction of the casting material.
6. **Instruct the patient or caregiver in the care and observation of the cast.**
   a. The distal extremity should be assessed for swelling, discoloration, or loss of sensation and circulation. If any of these occur, or if pain is unrelieved by the medications prescribed, the cast should be checked by a physician immediately.
   b. The cast should be kept dry at all times.
   c. The extremity should be kept elevated.
   d. Ice packs may be applied to the affected area directly over the cast to help reduce swelling.

DRESSING MATERIALS

Absorbent Dressing

Used for wounds with drains or large amounts of liquid drainage. Composed of layers of surgical sponges and gauze pads, usually covered with a gauze bandage taped in place.

Dry Dressing

Sterile gauze pads are applied to the wound directly from the package. No medications or solutions are used. The dressing may be taped in place or covered with a gauze bandage taped in place.

Fenestrated Dressing

A dressing with a hole or slot to allow an appliance or drain to protrude through the dressing. Often used to cover ostomy sites or to allow drains to deliver liquid to more absorbent material (Figure 7.9).

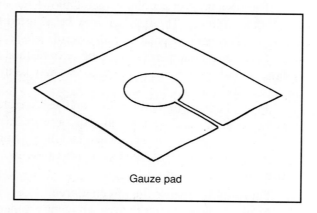

Gauze pad

Figure 7.9 Fenestrated dressing

Medicated Dressing

A dressing applied to a wound with a variety of solutions or ointments as ordered by the physician to promote healing or prevent infection. Some dressings are premedicated and packaged in bottles of strip gauze packing for use on deep wounds.

Occlusive Dressing

Applied to keep air and microorganisms out. Usually consists of gauze covered by plasticized tape or gauze saturated with a petroleum-based ointment (e.g., vaseline gauze, Xeroform gauze). The latter is commonly used to seal "sucking chest wounds."

Pressure Dressing

Applied to keep drainage from accumulating in tissues or to stop bleeding. Usually consists of a roll of sterile gauze or a collection of folded gauze pads placed directly against the area and taped tightly in place to provide pressure. Commonly used to stop bleeding at arterial puncture sites or any time hemostasis is difficult to achieve.

Wet to Dry Dressing

Dressings are applied to the wound and saturated with sterile water or sterile saline or other designated solution. They are covered and allowed to dry over a period of time. When removed they take some of the upper layers of tissue with them. Often used in burn debridement or in removing areas of necrotic tissue from a wound to promote healing.

Drains

Drains are often placed in surgical wounds to allow escape of fluids trapped deep within a surgical **incision**. The drainage of fluid from the wound lessens edema and minimizes the medium available for growth of bacteria, lessening the danger of

infection. Drains vary in configuration but share one quality: their premature removal will anger even the most pleasant physician.

Penrose drains are simply a small piece of soft rubber tubing protruding from the wound; they are usually not anchored with sutures. Penrose drain stock is frequently used as a tourniquet when drawing blood.

Other drains are composed of more rigid tubing extending from the wound and connected to a compressible, bulb-type suction to help syphon drainage (e.g., Jackson/Pratt, Hemovac). These drains are usually sutured in place but can be removed quite easily if need be (Figure 7.10).

Dressings

As mentioned at the beginning of the chapter, dressings are used to cover a wound. They are always applied using sterile technique to prevent contamination and infection of the wound. Gloves should always be worn during a dressing change to prevent contact with the drainage. Always document the presence or absence of drainage and the color and character of drainage when making a dressing change. The type of drainage can be an important factor in identifying the presence of infection or hemorrhage.

When performing a dressing change for the first time, carefully remove the old dressing layer by layer to avoid inadvertently removing drains from the wound and to determine the methods used to apply the original dressing. When changing a dressing, make every effort to dress the wound in the same manner used previously.

PROCEDURE FOR APPLYING/CHANGING A DRESSING

Assemble the following:

1. Sterile forceps for the dressing change.
2. Sterile gloves.
3. A sterile towel to create a sterile field.

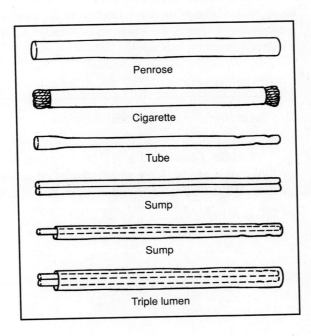

Figure 7.10 Commonly used drains

4. Irrigant or cleansing solution, as ordered.
5. Medication, as ordered.
6. Dressing and bandaging materials similar to that found in the previous dressing.

The equipment and supplies necessary for a dressing change should be assembled prior to starting, but if the medical assistant is unfamiliar with what lies under the cover of a dressing it may be necessary to remove the old dressing to find out what supplies are needed. If this is the case:

1. **Put on clean gloves and untape the dressing cover.**
2. Using sterile forceps, **carefully remove the dressing layer by layer** until the wound is exposed. Be careful to leave drains in place, unless the physician has ordered them removed.
3. If the wound has been packed, **remove the packing gently** using sterile forceps.
4. **Cover the wound with a sterile towel** while you assemble the necessary supplies.

When dressing a wound, sterile technique is a must (refer to Chapter 9 for a detailed description of maintaining a sterile field). Collecting the materials needed for the dressing change prior to starting will allow a smooth operation that gives the patient confidence in the medical assistant's ability and reduces the danger of contamination of the wound.

Often the physician will order that the wound be *cleansed* or *irrigated* during the dressing change; do not confuse these terms. When an area is to be cleansed, the physician will order the solution to be used (e.g., hydrogen peroxide [H_2O_2], normal saline, Betadine, etc.). The intent is to sponge the surface area with the solution using sterile gauze pads. If the physician orders *irrigation*, the intent is for the solution to be sprayed into the wound gently by means of a syringe or poured into the wound, then allowed to flow out of the wound.

If there are orders to irrigate or cleanse the wound, proceed as directed. If the wound has packing, verify whether the packing was plain or medicated and replace with the same type, using sterile forceps to gently fill the cavity of the wound, maintaining aseptic technique. Follow the directions for completing the dressing and bandage securely, as directed. Document the condition of the wound, the absence or presence of drainage, the color and character of any drainage found, and how the patient tolerated the procedure.

An example of correct documentation:

2-1-89

10:30 am Dressing change completed on R forearm incision. No redness or swelling noted at site. Very small amount of **sero-sanguineous** drainage noted on dressing. Wound irrigated with half-strength hydrogen peroxide. 4x4 gauze dressing applied with tape. Pt. tolerated procedure well.

Alice Smith, CMA.

**REVIEW/
SELF-EXAMINATION**

1. Explain the difference between bandages and dressings.

2. Why are bandages always applied from distal to proximal?

3. Name three types of bandages and list their functions.

4. Name three types of dressings and list their functions.

5. Name five types of wrapping technique and state when each application is appropriate.

6. Why should you wear gloves during a dressing change?

7. Define "sterile technique."

8. At the completion of the application of a bandage, what should be checked and documented in the patient's chart?

9. Explain the difference between cleansing and irrigating a wound.

10. What is the purpose of a drain in a wound?

11. What is the purpose of documenting the color and character of wound drainage?

12. What is the purpose of a wet to dry dressing?

13. What is the function of a pressure dressing?

14. What type of wrap is used for a knee?

15. What is a fenestrated dressing?

16. If after applying an elastic bandage, you are unable to palpate the patient's pulse distal to the dressing, what should you do?

17. If you are to perform a dressing change and you are unfamiliar with the site, what steps should you take?

18. What information must be recorded in the patient's medical record on completion of:

    a. bandaging

    b. dressing change

    c. first application of a dressing

19. What instructions should be given to a patient with a cast or splint?

20. What factor determines whether cold or warm water is used in the application of a cast or splint?

21. Why are splints used?

CHAPTER 8

Surgical Instruments and Supplies

Suture
Stitch
3 types of needle
straight
curved

OBJECTIVES

On completion of this chapter, you will be able to:
- Identify instruments commonly used in the medical office.
- Select the instruments needed for a physical examination.
- Select the instruments necessary for inserting and removing sutures.
- Classify commonly used instruments.
- Differentiate among various types of suture materials.
- Identify needle types.

Vocabulary— Glossary of Terms

Blunt	Dull; not having a sharp edge.
Cannula	A tube for insertion into a cavity.
Clamp	An instrument with parts that come together for holding or compressing.
Curette	A blade, scoop, loop, or ring used to scrape or cut.
Dilate	To enlarge or widen.
Drill	An instrument with an edged or pointed end for making holes.
Fenestrate	To make an opening.
Forceps	An instrument for grasping, holding, or exerting traction.
Grasp	To seize, hold, or control.
Hemostat	An instrument used to control bleeding by compressing vessels.
Probe	An instrument used to examine a cavity.
Punch	An instrument used to perforate or cut.
Puncture	To pierce with a pointed instrument.
Retract	To draw or hold back.
Scalpel	A thin-bladed knife used in surgery.

Scrape	To cut by repeated strokes of an edged instrument.
Sharp	Having a thin edge or fine point for cutting or piercing.
Speculum	An instrument for examining a body cavity.
Trocar	A sharp, pointed instrument fitted with a cannula.

Classification of Instruments

Medical and surgical instruments are costly precision tools that require careful handling. They are frequently named for the part of the body they are used to examine (e.g., the vaginal **speculum**) or for the designer (e.g., Mayo scissors, Silverman biopsy needle, Foley catheter, Taylor percussion hammer, and Schiotz tonometer).

Medical assistants should familiarize themselves as quickly as possible with the instruments they will be using and with any special care or handling instructions for those instruments. Many of the instruments will be utilized as part of the physical examination, treatment, diagnostic procedures, and office surgical procedures. The medical assistant will also be responsible for disinfecting and sterilizing the instruments, as well as selecting the appropriate instruments for a variety of sterile packs and trays.

Surgical instruments normally are classified according to their use and, for practical purposes, may be described as:

1. cutting and **scraping**
2. **clamping** and **grasping**
3. holding and **retracting**
4. **dilating** and **probing**
5. viewing

Surgical instruments normally are made of stainless steel and may have either a dull finish or a highly polished one. The parts of an instrument are clearly identifiable and allow for visual differentiation. Every instrument consists of a handle and the part that comes in contact with the patient. In addition, many instruments have a closing mechanism. Instrument handles may be ring-style, such as scissors and **hemostats**, or spring-type such as tissue **forceps** and tweezers. The closing mechanism of an instrument is called a rachet; it resembles gears and is located below the ring handles, as in hemostats and needle holders. For convenience in use with materials of varying thicknesses, rachets can be normally locked in one of three positions.

Instruments used for grasping and holding have a variety of inner surfaces. Some have serrations, which may be horizontal or longitudinal, or crisscross as with hemostats. Other instruments may have plain inner surfaces or, if used for grasping and holding, may have one or more teeth, such as the Allis tissue forceps.

There are also instruments for the visual inspection of body cavities and organs and the measurement of a site or organ or of its pressure; examples are the Graves vaginal speculum, Hirschman anoscope, and Schiotz tonometer.

Instrument Identification

Cutting and scraping instruments are used to cut, scrape, and **puncture**. They include **curettes**, **drills**, needles, **punches**, **scalpels**, and scissors. These instruments will have a **sharp** blade or surface and, like the scalpel, may be disposable or have disposable blades or cutting surfaces.

Drills are utilized in orthopedic surgery as well as dental surgery and consist of a hand-held or power drill and drill bits in assorted sizes.

Punches are used to indent, perforate, or excise and are frequently used in orthopedics, dermatology, dentistry, and other specialties.

Curettes are scraping instruments used to smooth surfaces, remove material or growths from cavities, or remove growths from the interiors or surfaces of organs (Figure 8.1).

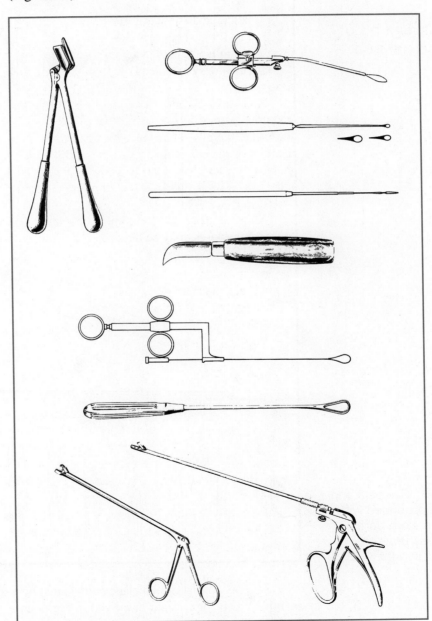

Figure 8.1 Examples of cutting instruments (Reproduced with permission from Jarit Surgical Instruments Catalog, copyright 1991)

Scalpels consist of a handle and a blade and are used to make incisions (cut into) or to remove tissue. Most are disposable or have disposable blades. The standard handles are the No. 3, No. 3 long, and the No. 7. Blades come in a variety of shapes and sizes. For medical office use, the most common blade is the No. 11, with Nos. 10, 12, and 15 also being used frequently (Figure 8.2).

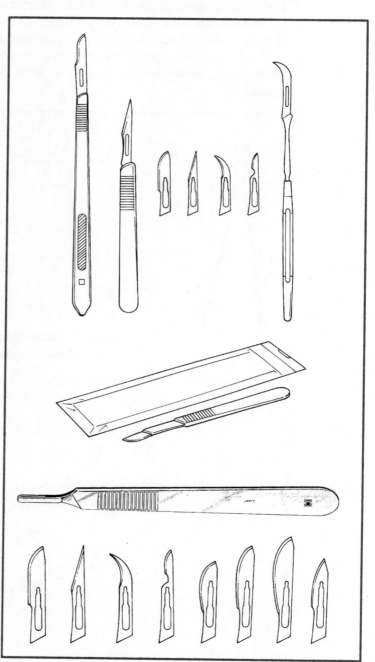

Figure 8.2 Scalpels and blades (Reproduced with permission from Jarit Surgical Instruments Catalog, copyright 1991)

Scissors consist of two blade parts joined by a screw and a screw joint. They are identified as being straight or curved in accordance with their appearance and sharp or **blunt** by their blade points. A pair of scissors may be described as sharp–sharp (s/s), sharp–blunt (s/b), or blunt–blunt (b/b). They are used to incise or excise tissue as well as to remove sutures and dressings or bandages (Figure 8.3).

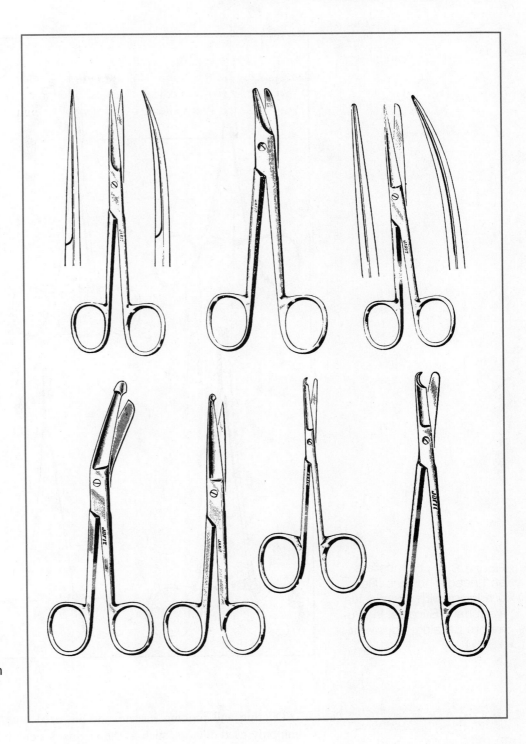

Figure 8.3 Surgical scissors (Reproduced with permission from Jarit Surgical Instruments Catalog, copyright 1991)

Clamping and grasping instruments are used in a variety of tasks, such as hemostasis, blunt dissection, and holding and manipulating tissue. Examples of these instruments are Allis tissue forceps and Kelly hemostats. (Figures 8.4 and 8.5).

Holding and retracting instruments are used to hold tissues and organs away from an operative site. Many of the clamping and grasping instruments are frequently used as holding and retracting instruments in office surgery.

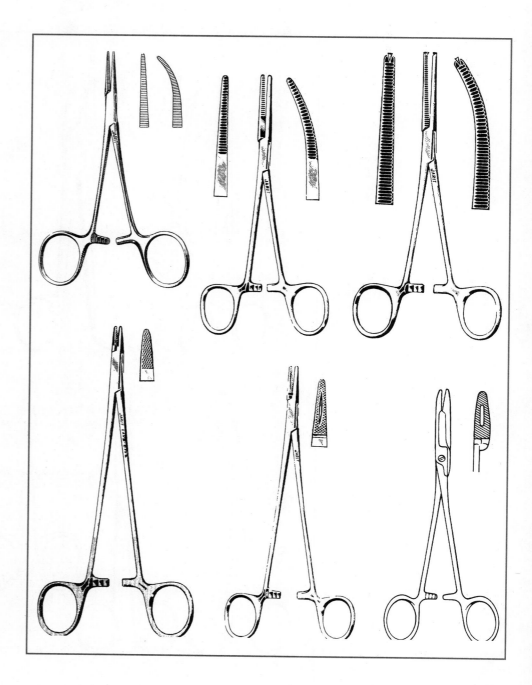

Figure 8.4 Hemostats and needle holders (Reproduced with permission from Jarit Surgical Instruments Catalog, copyright 1991)

Dilating and probing instruments are used both in examination and surgery. Commonly used dilators, such as the vaginal speculum, are available as disposables (Figures 8.6 and 8.7).

Basic Tray Setups

The following are some basic trays found in most medical offices. Every physician, surgeon, or specialist has preferences for certain instruments (such as scalpels), and you may want to modify the basic tray setup to include those preferences. If you are working for a specialist, you will need to find out what special trays you will need to prepare and then make up a tray card for each.

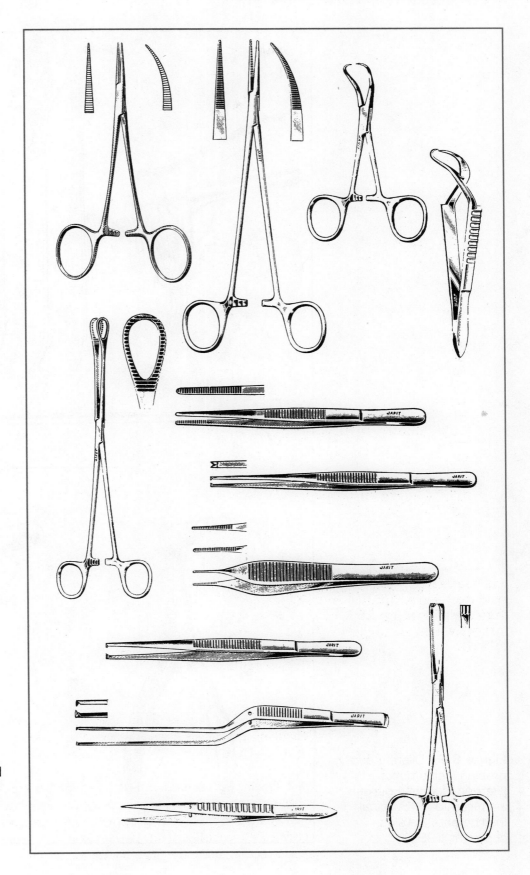

Figure 8.5 Grasping and holding instruments (Reproduced with permission from Jarit Surgical Instruments Catalog, copyright 1991)

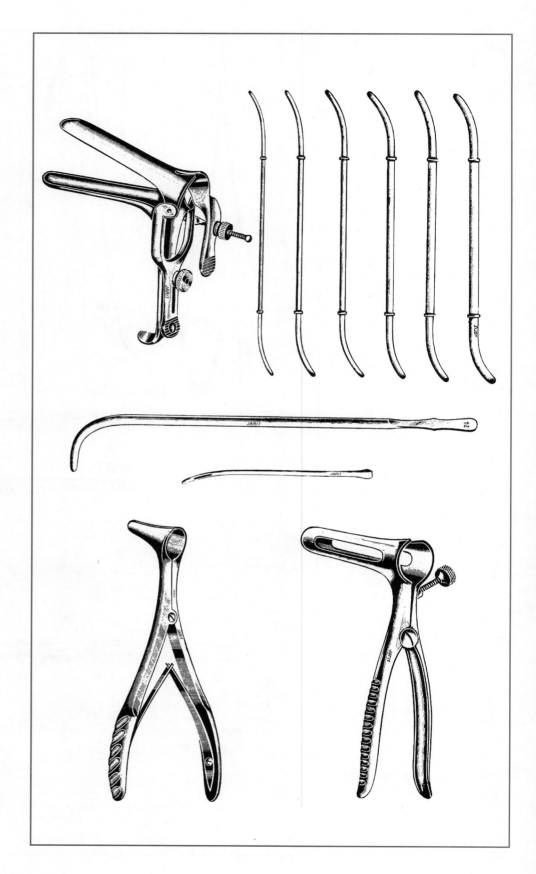

Figure 8.6 Dilating and probing instruments (Reproduced with permission from Jarit Surgical Instruments Catalog, copyright 1991)

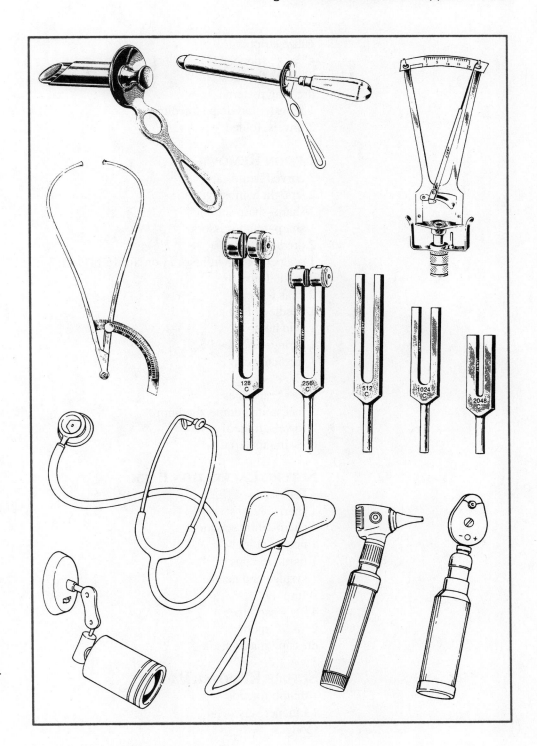

Figure 8.7 Diagnostic and other instruments (Reproduced with permission from Jarit Surgical Instruments Catalog, copyright 1991)

INCISION AND DRAINAGE

2 hemostats
1 scalpel No. 3 with No. 15 blade
2 dressing forceps
1 tissue forceps
drain

gauze stripping
4" × 4" sponges
2" × 2" sponges
dressing material
1 **fenestrated** drape, medium
2 towels, folded

LESION REMOVAL

2 curved hemostats
2 straight hemostats
1 sharp–sharp scissors
1 sharp–blunt scissors
2 dressing forceps
1 scalpel No. 3 with No. 11 or No. 15 blade
2 tissue forceps
2 Allis forceps
1 needle holder
1 skin hook
1 syringe and needle
1 medicine cup
4" × 4" sponges
2" × 2" sponges
1 fenestrated drape, medium
2 towels, folded
dressing material

SUTURE/LACERATION PACK

3 hemostats
1 sharp–sharp scissors
1 sharp–blunt scissors
1 needle holder
1 tissue forceps
1 syringe and needle
suture
4" × 4" sponges
2" × 2" sponges
dressing materials

SUTURE REMOVAL PACK

1 thumb forceps
1 Littauer scissors 4"
sponges

Suture Materials

The term *suture* refers both to the act of surgically stitching and to the material used in the process. Suture is sometimes referred to as *ligature* since it may also be used to ligate or tie off a vessel or tissue.

Absorbable suture is called surgical gut, plain catgut, or chromic gut or catgut. Plain catgut or surgical gut is made from sheep or beef intestine and is generally absorbed by the body in five to forty days. Chromic gut or catgut is treated with chromic salts in a type of tanning process that decreases its absorption rate in the tissues. Thus treated, chromic catgut can last approximately a month before absorption.

Nonabsorbable suture materials include silk, which is easy to tie yet strong; it is frequently treated with a coating that prevents snagging of the tissues. Cotton is tough and resilient, but not as strong as silk. Nylon and other synthetic materials, such as polyester, are strong with a high degree of elasticity and are relatively nonirritating to the tissues. Stainless steel is the strongest of all suture materials, but difficult to work with. Surgical staples are made of stainless steel .

Sizing of suture material is standardized and is set by the United States Pharmacopeia. Size is determined by the diameter of the strand and range from 11–0 (the smallest) to 1–0 (the largest); the higher the number, the smaller the diameter. In the medical office, 2–0 to 6–0 are the most commonly used.

Needles

Needles may be straight, half-curved, curved, atraumatic (or eyeless), or traumatic (having an eye). Their points are described as cutting, **trocar**, and taper. They are chosen according to the area in which they will be used and the depth and width of stitch desired. The atraumatic needle is the one most commonly used in the medical

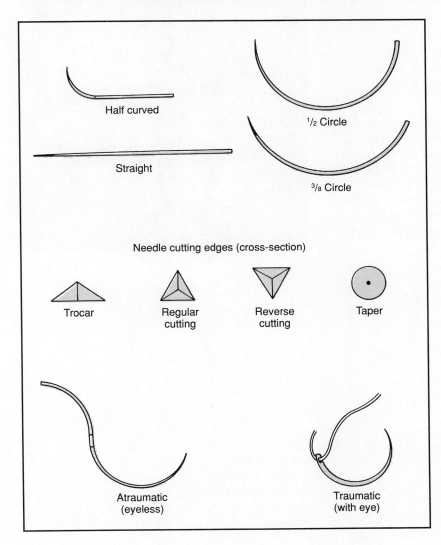

Figure 8.8 Needles

office; it is supplied in peel-apart packages with suture attached or in separate needle packages and continuous reels of suture (Figure 8.8).

Disposables

Disposables are a boon to the busy medical practice; they are convenient and eliminate the need for the medical assistant spending time checking, disinfecting, and sterilizing instruments, packs, etc. Disposables include dressing materials, drapes, wraps, gloves, syringes, needles, instruments, and a wide variety of packs; it must be remembered that their containers must be checked for damage, and the discard date must be checked carefully for sterile disposables (Figure 8.9). While many medical offices use disposables routinely, they normally will keep at least one back-up set of instruments, trays, etc., that are not disposable and can be used if disposable supplies are exhausted.

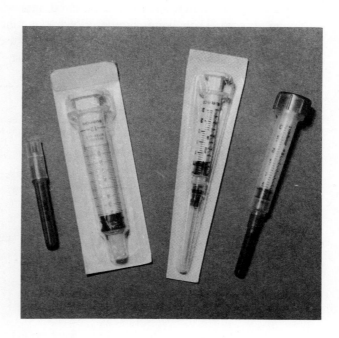

Figure 8.9 Sample disposables: needles and syringes (Reproduced with permission from Simmers, *Diversified Health Occupations,* 2nd Ed., Delmar Publishers Inc., 1988)

1.   Instruments are classified in what manner?

2.   Name at least four cutting and scraping instruments.

3.   Give an example of the use of a punch.

4.   Give an example of the use of a curette.

5.   What is meant by s/s, s/b, and b/b? To what instrument do the terms apply?

6.   Give two uses for clamping and grasping instruments.

7.   Name a commonly used dilator.

8.   What instruments would be needed for a suture removal pack?

9.   Give two examples of absorbable suture.

10.   Give three examples of nonabsorbable suture.

11.   How is suture material sized?

12.   What is meant by an atraumatic needle?

13.   List five examples of disposable materials.

14.   Define the following:

   a.   dilate

   b.   speculum

15.   What suture sizes are most commonly used in the medical office?

CHAPTER 9

Office Surgery

OBJECTIVES

On completion of this chapter, you will be able to:
- Deliver postoperative instructions to the patient.
- Position and drape a patient for a procedure.
- Establish and maintain a sterile field.
- Open sterile packs and place materials on the sterile field without contamination.
- Demonstrate the proper technique for preparing equipment and supplies for the office surgery.
- Demonstrate the method of preparing the room for office surgery.
- Role play giving a patient emotional support.
- Demonstrate proper technique for pouring sterile liquids.
- Demonstrate the proper method of hand washing prior to a procedure.
- Demonstrate proper technique in gowning and gloving both self and physician prior to procedure.
- Demonstrate proper technique for handling sterile specimens.
- Demonstrate proper care of equipment and room after completion of the procedure.

Vocabulary— Glossary of Terms

Contamination	Any contact of a sterile item with a nonsterile surface or item.
Depilatory	Describes a solution that has the ability to remove hair.
Epistaxis	Severe bleeding from the nose.
Hemostasis	The cessation of bleeding.
Mole	A pigmented growth of tissue.
Wart	A tumor of the epidermis, usually caused by a virus.

Preparation

Prior to beginning a procedure, the medical assistant must prepare the area for the procedure for the physician. The medical assistant should refer to procedure or tray cards for the procedure in question and assemble the sterile and nonsterile supplies in the procedure room.

The room should be arranged with all sterile trays wrapped and placed in position near the procedure table. All sterile trays should at all times remain above waist level and away from items that could contribute to their **contamination**, such as curtains and other nonsterile equipment. Sterile supplies should be nearby but out of the immediate area where the procedure will take place. The room should be well organized and free of unnecessary items. The temperature of the room should be adjusted to provide comfort to the patient as well as those persons involved in the procedure.

When the room has been prepared and the equipment has been assembled, the patient may be escorted into the procedure room. The patient should be instructed on disrobing, if appropriate, and supplied with a gown or drape to afford privacy.

Once the patient has disrobed, the medical assistant should knock before entering; once the patient is ready, enter the room. The patient may then be positioned as appropriate for the procedure and draped, taking care to leave exposed only those parts of the anatomy that need to be for the procedure.

Positioning and Draping

Some of the common positions used for surgical procedures are outlined below as a guide for the medical assistant. Physicians have distinct preferences for certain positions in various procedures. It is always prudent to ask the physician about preferences prior to preparing the patient. This avoids delays and embarrassment until you become familiar with the procedures.

DORSAL RECUMBENT

The patient is placed in the supine position on a flat table. This position affords easy access to the anterior surface of the body and is used for most general procedures. All areas of the anatomy should be covered except the head and the portion of the anatomy involved in the procedure. A pillow may be placed under the patient's head if this can be done without interfering with the procedure to be performed (Figure 9.1).

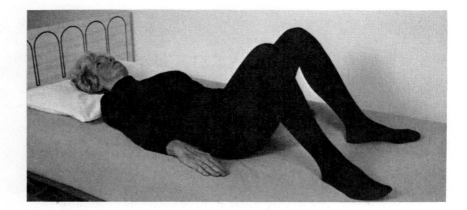

Figure 9.1 The dorsal recumbent position (Reproduced with permission from Hegner and Caldwell, *Nursing Assistant, A Nursing Process Approach*, 6th Ed., Delmar Publishers Inc., 1992)

LEFT LATERAL RECUMBENT

The patient is placed on a flat surface on the left side with the right knee drawn upward toward the chest. This position is used for gastroscopy, proctoscopy, and some gynecological procedures, particularly when the lithotomy position is impractical due to age or physical disability. All portions of the anatomy should be covered, with the exception of the head and the portions of anatomy on which the procedure is being performed (Figure 9.2).

LITHOTOMY

The patient is placed supine with the head slightly elevated. The feet are placed in stirrups with the legs spread apart. This is the most common position for gynecologic procedures and examinations. The upper thorax is draped with a sheet extending to the knees. Drapes are then placed over each leg, covering the inner thigh and leaving only the head and pelvic area exposed (Figure 9.3).

KNEE–CHEST

The patient kneels on the procedure table. A pillow is placed under the head, and the knees are drawn under the thorax. Weight is supported by the knees and elbows. A pillow may be placed under the abdomen for additional support. This position is primarily used for proctoscopy. If the patient is unable to tolerate this position

Figure 9.2 Left lateral recumbent position (Reproduced with permission from Hegner and Caldwell, *Nursing Assistant, A Nursing Process Approach*, 6th Ed., Delmar Publishers Inc., 1992)

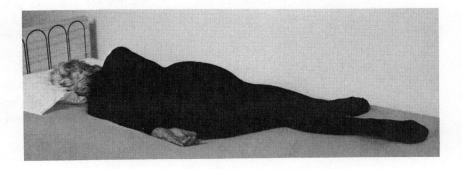

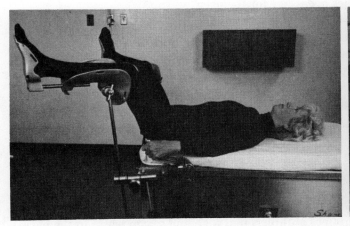
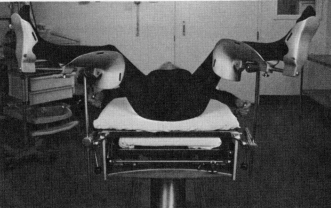

Figure 9.3 Lithotomy position (Reproduced with permission from Hegner and Caldwell, *Nursing Assistant, A Nursing Process Approach*, 6th Ed., Delmar Publishers Inc., 1992)

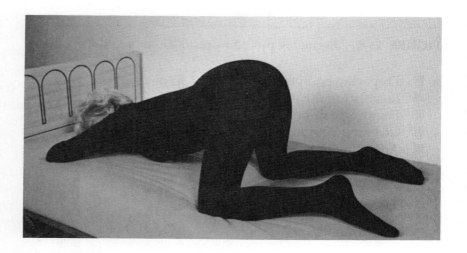

Figure 9.4 Knee-chest position (Reproduced with permission from Hegner and Caldwell, *Nursing Assistant, A Nursing Process Approach*, 6th Ed., Delmar Publishers Inc., 1992)

because of age or physical disability, the left lateral recumbent position may be used. Drape the patient from the shoulders to the buttocks. Use a second drape with towel clips or hemostats to cover the thighs and lower legs.

This position is difficult for almost any patient to tolerate for long periods, so do not position the patient in this manner until just prior to beginning the procedure. Some offices and clinics have tables that are bowed upward in the middle, allowing the same positioning with less discomfort for the patient (Figure 9.4).

If preparation of the patient is required, the medical assistant should explain the procedure during preparation. This is an ideal time to reassure the patient, allowing them time and opportunity to ask questions. Answer the patient's questions in a forth-right and honest manner without going into great detail. As the preparation is being completed, you can use this time to talk with the patient and set their mind at ease.

PROCEDURE FOR SURGICAL PREPARATION (PREP)

1. **Assemble the supplies necessary for the prep.**
   A. Surgical double-edge razors (at least two)
   B. Antimicrobial soap
   C. Basin of warm water
   D. Wash cloth and towel
   E. Betadine or other antimicrobial solution
   F. Pack of 4 × 4 gauze pads (12)
   G. Small basin
   H. Forceps
   I. Sterile towels
   J. Latex gloves
2. **Wash and dry your hands thoroughly.**
3. **Put on latex gloves.**
4. **Mix a generous portion of antimicrobial soap and warm water in the basin.**
   Use the wash cloth and thoroughly wash the area to be prepped, allowing a generous margin around the edge of the area. On completion, pat the area dry with a towel.

5. With the skin surface dry, **shave the body hair from the area** being careful not to cut or nick the patient's skin. Use a towel to remove stray hair from the area. In some facilities, a **depilatory** may be used in lieu of shaving.

6. **Open the pack of 4 × 4 gauze pads.** Place them in the remaining clean basin. Pour Betadine solution liberally over the pads, saturating them thoroughly. Take the sterile forceps and remove the top pad. Place the pad in the center of the prep area and with a circular motion wipe the area toward the outer edge of the prep area. Cover the area only once with the pad and discard in a trash can. Take the next pad and repeat the procedure. Continue until all pads have been used and the prep area has been liberally coated with the antimicrobial agent (Figure 9.5).

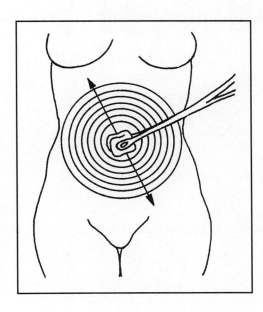

Figure 9.5 Application of antimicrobial agent to prep area, using circular motion from center of area toward perimeter (Reproduced with permission from Keir, Wise, and Krebs-Shannon, *Medical Assisting,* 2nd Ed., Delmar Publishers Inc., 1989)

7. **Cover the area with a sterile towel(s).**

8. **Clean up the area,** discard trash, place linen in the proper receptacle, clean other equipment and place in proper area.

9. **Remove and discard your latex gloves.**

Set Up and Maintain A Sterile Field

Once the patient has been positioned and draped, you may begin to set up the sterile field. Equipment and supplies will already have been placed in the room during the initial room preparation.

PROCEDURE FOR SETTING UP A STERILE FIELD

1. **Wash and dry your hands thoroughly.**

2. **Move sterile packs on tables closer to the procedure area,** taking care to allow the physician room to work while keeping trays and tables within reach.

3. **Unwrap sterile packs,** starting with the tail opposite from where you are standing, then the tail to the right, the tail to the left, and finally the tail nearest you. Avoid touching any item within the sterile field (Figure 9.6).

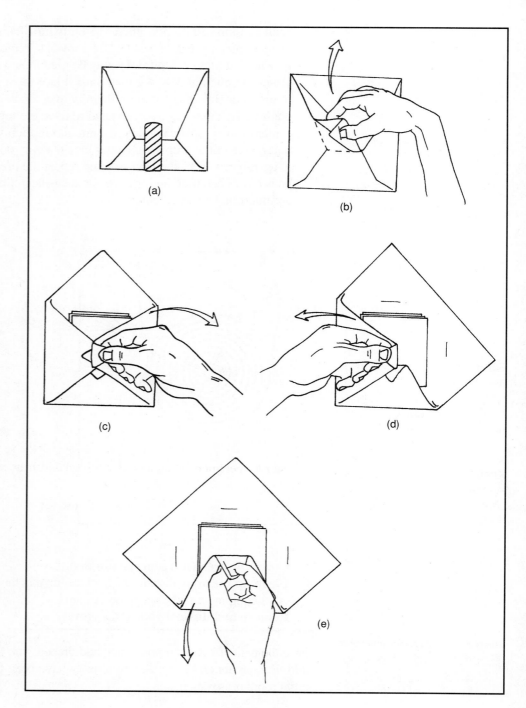

Figure 9.6 Proper procedure for unwrapping a sterile package (Reproduced with permission from Narrow and Buschle, *Fundamentals of Nursing Practice*, 2nd Ed., John Wiley & Sons, Inc., 1982)

4. If sterile liquids are needed during the procedure (saline irrigants, Betadine, etc.), **open the bottles, taking care to avoid contact with the neck of the bottle**. Once the bottle has been opened, hold the bottle waist high over a trash can on the floor near the sterile field and pour a small amount of liquid out of the bottle. This is known as "lipping" the bottle and is designed to remove contaminants from the edge of the bottle prior to pouring into the sterile field. Holding the

bottle over the receptacle in the sterile field, gently pour the liquid into the container without making contact with any item in the sterile field or splashing the liquid out of the container (Figure 9.7).

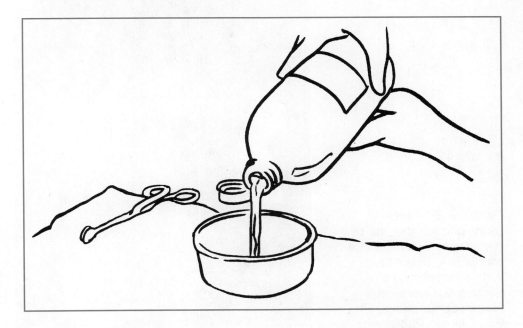

Figure 9.7 Proper technique for pouring sterile liquids (Reproduced with permission from Gomez and Hord, *Fundamentals of Clinical Nursing Skills*, John Wiley & Sons, Inc., 1988)

5. Open any items to be placed in the sterile field, taking care to avoid contact with the sterile contents. Hold the package four to six inches over the sterile field and allow the objects to drop on the field. These items may include sutures, syringes, sterile specimen containers, or additional instruments not included in the basic trays (Figure 9.8).

6. **If it is necessary to remove objects from the sterile field, long-handled sterile transfer forceps should be used.** Grasp the object firmly with the forceps and lift away from the field. Watch sleeves and other parts of clothing to avoid contamination of the field. When reaching into a sterile field, imagine that there is a wall about a foot high surrounding the field and that you have to reach over

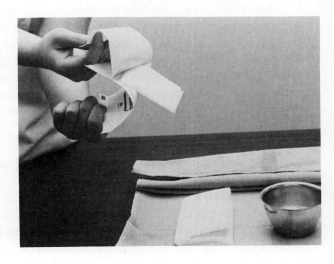

Figure 9.8 Proper technique for dropping sterile items into the sterile field (Reproduced with permission from Simmers, *Diversified Health Occupations*, 2nd Ed., Delmar Publishers Inc., 1988)

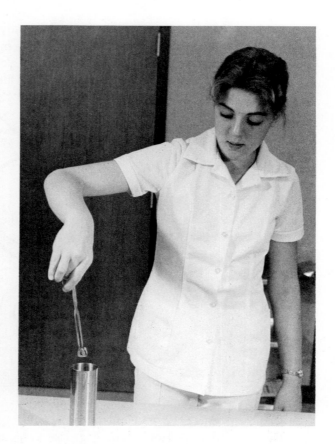

Figure 9.9 Proper technique for the use of transfer forceps within a sterile field (Reproduced with permission from Simmers, *Diversified Health Occupations*, 2nd Ed., Delmar Publishers Inc., 1988)

the wall to move objects in and out. This technique keeps your body away from the field (Figure 9.9).

7. **Avoid reaching across a sterile field once it has been opened** to avoid accidental contamination.

8. In surgical areas, **all items below waist level are to be considered contaminated.**

9. **Some facilities prefer that the field be covered with a sterile drape until the procedure begins. If this is the case, unwrap the drape using the last fold of the cover to hold the drape material.** Allow the drape to unfold without stirring air and gently cover the field, being careful to avoid contaminating the field. In most cases, this step will be unnecessary, as the procedure should begin soon after the field is established. This procedure should never be done if liquids have been poured into containers on the sterile field.

Scrubbing for Surgery

Thorough hand washing remains the best defense against the transmission of disease (refer to Chapter 3 for the description of proper hand washing technique). In surgical areas, the water flow at the sink is controlled by the knees or feet. Avoid touching items around the sink after you have scrubbed. The hands should be dried with a sterile towel at the end of the procedure. Remember, friction, not soap and water, is the most important aspect of proper hand washing.

In the surgical setting, there is no place for long fingernails or jewelry. These are receptacles for microorganisms and present a danger to the patient. Long fingernails must be cut short, and jewelry is not acceptable. One possible exception is a plain gold wedding band without stones (which could puncture or tear your gloves).

Your hands are clean, the room and patient are prepared. It is now time to gown and glove to begin the procedure.

Gowning and Gloving

PROCEDURE FOR GOWNING AND GLOVING

1. **Open two packs of sterile gloves** and place the envelopes containing the gloves on a table with the cuff end toward you. This should orient the gloves with the right glove on the right side and left glove on the left. One should be your size, and one the physician's size. Surgical gloves should fit tightly and conform to the contour of your hand without any loose material (Figure 9.10).

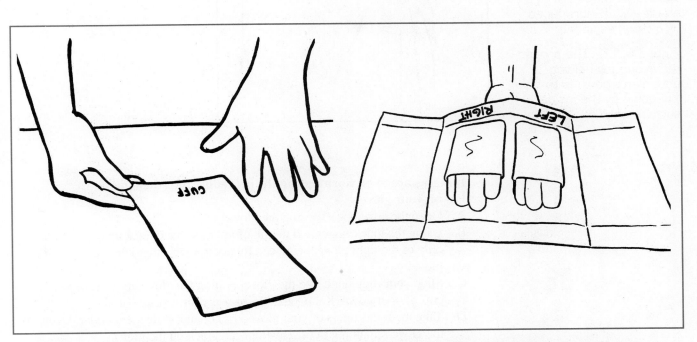

Figure 9.10 Package of sterile gloves laid open in preparation for wearing (Adapted with permission from Gomez and Hord, *Fundamentals of Clinical Nursing Skills*, John Wiley & Sons, Inc., 1988)

2. **Put on your gown.** Surgical gowns close in the back at the neck and waist. Put your arms in the sleeves and position the gown so it is comfortable and allows freedom of movement. The knitted cuffs of the sleeves must be close to your wrists. Tie the tails of the gown behind your neck. Tie the waist ties securely to prevent them from coming loose during the procedure.
3. **Hold the physician's gown from the front so the physician can just walk into the gown.** Tie the tails behind the neck and waist securely (Figure 9.11).

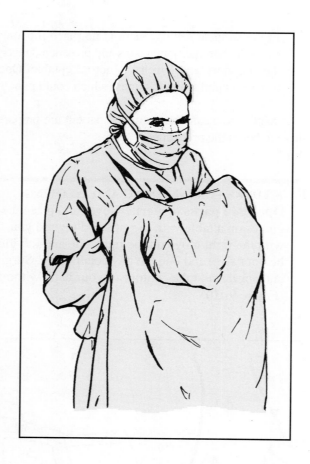

Figure 9.11 The proper technique for holding physician's gown is to hold the gown by the inside surface only

4. **If masks are to be worn during the procedure, put them on now.**
5. **Put on your gloves.**
   A. Open the envelope exposing the gloves.
   B. Using the index finger and thumb of your left hand, pick up the cuff portion only of the right glove, being careful not to touch any other portion of the glove.
   C. Slide your right hand into the glove, pulling the glove up over the knitted cuff of your gown. Keep the glove above your waist level.
   D. Take the four fingers of your gloved right hand, slide them under the cuff of the glove remaining in the envelope, and pick up the glove.
   E. Slide your left hand into the glove, keeping the glove above the level of your waist. Avoid contaminating the glove with skin surfaces while putting them on.
   F. By grasping the extreme end of the cuffs of the gloves, you may now turn the gloves up over the sleeve of your gown (Figure 9.12).
6. **Assist the physician in putting on gloves** (some physicians may prefer to wear two pairs of gloves).
   A. Pick up the physician's right glove by sliding the four fingers of your right hand under the cuff. Hold the glove above the level of your waist, with the fingers hanging downward, and present the glove to the physician so the right hand may be inserted into the glove. When the hand is in the glove, turn the cuff upward over the sleeve of the gown (Figure 9.13).

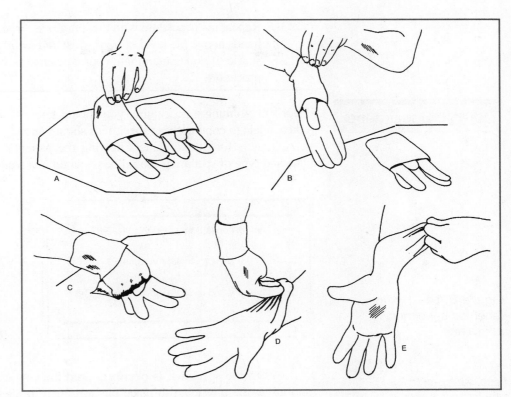

Figure 9.12 Proper sterile gloving technique (Reproduced with permission from Keir, Wise, and Krebs-Shannon, *Medical Assisting,* 2nd Ed., Delmar Publishers Inc., 1989)

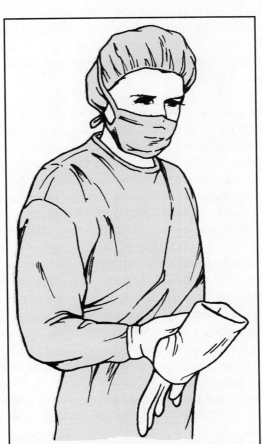

Figure 9.13 Assisting the physician in putting on sterile gloves

B. Repeat the procedure with the left glove. From this point on, keep your hands above the level of your waist and avoid touching any item that is not sterile. If you contaminate your gloves, remove them and repeat the gloving procedure.

Sterile Specimens

Prior to beginning a procedure, you should know which specimens will need to be taken. Vials to contain these specimens should already have been placed in the sterile field. Labels for the containers bearing the patient's name, physician's name, and date and type of specimen should be prepared in advance (Figure 9.14).

name: Jones, Mary C, date: 11-29-89

doctor: Dr. John Adams

specimen: Wound exudate, abdomen. For C & S

Figure 9.14 Sample label for specimen container

When the specimen is obtained, hold the container close to the area involved and allow the physician to place the specimen in the container. Add any necessary reagents or solutions while observing sterile technique. Cover the container with the cap and place the container in a plastic bag after applying the appropriate label.

If there is a procedure for routing the specimen to the laboratory, call the runner and send the specimen. If you need to work further in the sterile field, change your gloves.

Electrocautery and Cryosurgery

Electrocautery involves the use of a hot electrode to cut tissue or cauterize a bleeding vessel. In order to do this, there must be a flow of low-grade current through the patient's body, and a grounding plate must be attached to the patient's skin, usually well away from the area involving the procedure. An area of the skin, generally on the thigh, is shaved and conduction gel applied to the skin surface. The metal grounding plate is then placed directly over the gel and pressed firmly in place. Many grounding plates have an adhesive backing allowing them to stick to the skin. Many physicians prefer also to tape the plate in place. The better the grounding contact, the more efficiently the cautery device works. Any excess gel is wiped off.

Portable, battery-powered cautery instruments, approximately the size of a large penlight, are available. These are used primarily for nasal cauterization to stop **epistaxis** or for cauterizing small vessels during minor surgical procedures.

When cautery instruments are in use, a suction wand is often held near the site to vacuum the odors and smoke created by the cauterization. This prevents noxious odors from permeating the room.

Cryosurgery is in many ways similar to electrocautery, but instead of heat, extreme cold is used. Chilled cryoprobes are used in combination with cryospray containing liquid nitrogen, nitrous oxide, or freon to destroy areas of tissue or to cauterize a bleeding vessel. By fast freezing, tissues are destroyed or **hemostasis** is achieved.

Cryosurgery is used for intracranial applications, destruction of cutaneous structures (**warts**, **moles**, etc.), and some gynecologic procedures. A special cryoprobe, a cryoextractor, is used for the removal of cataract lenses in the eye.

Postoperative Care

Once the procedure is completed, inform the patient that the procedure is over and remove the excess drapes. Keep the patient warm and reassured. You may need to apply dressings to the surgical site. The physician usually will give instructions on the type of dressing to be applied at the completion of the procedure. If not, you should ask. Once you have completed a procedure several times with the same physician, you will become used to the techniques and be able to perform without difficulty.

Postoperative instructions generally are preprinted for each procedure. Take the time to go over the instructions step by step with the patient and, if possible, a family member or other caregiver. Once you are assured that they understand, give them a copy. Remember to ask if there are any questions. Assist the patient as necessary to get dressed. After the recovery period is complete, assist the patient to their vehicle.

Clean the procedure room thoroughly, discard linens in the proper receptacle, place hazardous wastes in the proper containers, place sharps in the proper containers, and restock the supplies used so that they will be available for the next procedure. Clean the instruments with a soft brush and antimicrobial agent and place them in the proper area to be resterilized. Get the room ready for the next patient. Return equipment to its proper place and take a few minutes to collect yourself before beginning the next procedure, time permitting of course.

1. Describe the four most common positions used in office surgery. Give an example of when each might be used.

2. List the steps in the surgical prep.

3. What is meant by "lipping a bottle"? Why is it done?

4. How are objects placed in a sterile field?

5. How are objects removed from a sterile field?

6. Below what level are items considered contaminated?

7. When opening a package of sterile gloves, why do you place the "cuff" ends of the envelopes toward you?

8. If masks are to be worn during the procedure, when should they be put on?

9. How do you avoid contaminating sterile gloves while putting them on?

10. What should you do if your gloves come in contact with a nonsterile item and become contaminated?

11. What information should appear on a sterile specimen label?

12. What is electrocautery used for?

13. Name two uses for cryosurgery.

14. How are noxious odors controlled during electrocautery?

15. Where are grounding plates placed?

CHAPTER 10

The Healing Process

OBJECTIVES

On completion of this chapter, you will be able to:
- Change operative site or other wound dressings.
- Identify the phases of wound healing.
- Identify various suturing methods.
- Describe the healing process.
- Identify the equipment needed to remove sutures.
- Identify at least four types of suture materials.
- Remove sutures.

Vocabulary— Glossary of Terms

Chromocized	Treated with a chromium compound.
Cicatrix	A scar.
Debridement	Removal of foreign material or contamination from a wound.
Debris	Trash; rubbish.
Discontinuity	A break or interruption in tissue.
Encysted	Encapsulated.
Fibrin	Insoluble protein formed from fibrinogen during clot formation.
Granulation	The formation in wounds of tissue composed of capillaries, fibroblasts, and inflammatory cells.
Hemostasis	Cessation or control of bleeding.
Laceration	A torn or ragged wound.
Necrotic	Pertaining to dead tissue.
Phagocyte	White cells capable of destroying bacteria and other debris by ingestion.
Septic	Infected; containing dead tissue and microorganisms.
Thrombocytes	Clotting cells.

Trauma	Injury.
Wound	Injury caused by physical means with discontinuity of tissue.

Wounds

A wound is an internal or external **discontinuity** in body tissues. It may occur intentionally, as in surgery, as self-inflicted **trauma**, or accidentally, as in a fall or vehicular accident. Wounds may also be **septic** (infected with pathogens) or aseptic (clean).

Open wounds demonstrate an opening in the skin that exposes underlying tissues; they may be produced by cutting, dull, or blunt instruments. Cutting instruments create an incised wound that normally has a clean edge. Open wounds may also be **lacerated** where the tissue has been torn by a dull or blunt instrument.

Penetrating or puncture wounds are caused by sharp, slender objects such as ice picks or knives and also include animal and snake bites. Wounds are also produced by falls and contact with extremely hot or cold objects and with caustic agents such as acids (Figure 10.1).

Wounds heal in three phases. Phase one, called lag phase, occurs when the blood vessels contract to produce **hemostasis** and **thrombocytes** form a network in the wound. Through a series of chemical reactions **fibrin** is released to establish clotting, which will result in scab formation. Approximately twelve hours later, **phagocytic** leukocytes will begin to clear away debris and bacteria. Within one to four days, the fibrin threads will begin to pull the edges of the wound together underneath the clot.

The second phase of the healing process is called proliferation; it is the new growth period, which lasts for approximately five to twenty days. During this phase, tissues repair themselves, new cells form, and complete contraction of the wound occurs providing no sepsis has occurred.

During the third phase, called remodeling, the cells produce a fibrous protein substance called *collagen* that strengthens wounded tissues and forms cicatricial tissue. The scar tissue (**cicatrix**) that is thus formed is not true skin and is devoid of normal blood supply and nerves. Clean, surgical wounds that have been sutured closed heal quickly and may heal with equivocal scarring. This type of healing is called healing by *first intention*. Tissues that have been severely damaged or kept open or that fail to close are said to heal *by granulation*, or from the bottom up. This **granulation** process is also referred to as healing by *second intention*.

Wound sepsis is the accumulation of **debris** from the breakdown of cellular components and pathogens. If the leukocytes are unable to clear this material away, suppuration or pus formation will occur. **Necrotic** and septic materials must be removed from wounds. This process is called **debridement** and may take place naturally, manually, or surgically.

Most wounds are kept covered during a portion of the healing process; however, there are strong arguments for open wound healing. Wounds that are left open stay dry, which inhibits bacterial growth and reduces infection. Preexisting infections remain localized. Open wounds are not irritated by contact with the dressing or bandage.

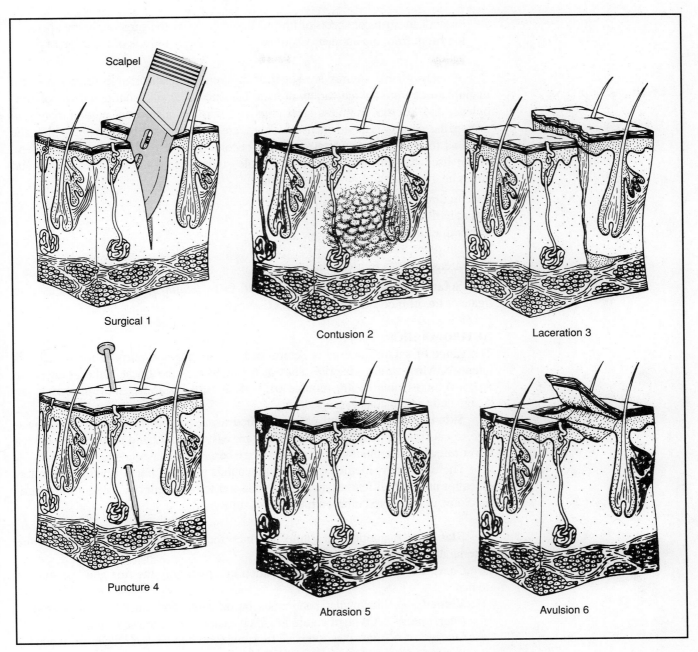

Scalpel

Surgical 1

Contusion 2

Laceration 3

Puncture 4

Abrasion 5

Avulsion 6

Figure 10.1 Types of wounds

Suture Materials

Surgical wounds normally are closed by suturing the various tissues together. Suture materials are classified as *absorbable* (absorbed or digested by the body cells during the healing process) or *nonabsorbable* (must be removed).

Absorbable suture is of two types:

1. Surgical gut or catgut, which is made from sheep or beef intestine. Chromic gut is **chromicized** or made tissue-resistant by means of a tanning process that retards its rate of absorption or digestion.

2. Fascia lata, strips or sheets of fibrous tissue taken by the surgeon, in the operating room from the aponeurosis of the lateral oblique muscle of the thigh of the patient.

Nonabsorbable sutures are superior in strength to absorbable sutures and are manufactured from a wide variety of materials, including silk, cotton, nylon, polypropylene, and Dacron. Stainless steel clips and wire are also used, predominantly in orthopedic surgery. Buried in tissues, they are not removed but remain within the body as foreign bodies, which generally become **encysted** and create no problem. When used as skin sutures, nonabsorbable sutures are removed after the wound edges heal roughly following this schedule:

Face in three to five days
Trunk in five to eight days
Extremities in five to ten days
Scalp in seven to ten days
Joint areas in ten to fourteen days

Suture materials may also be referred to as *ligatures*, since they are used to ligate or tie off blood vessels and other tissues.

SUTURE GAUGE

The gauge of suture material is determined by the area and purpose for which it is intended. Most suture materials start at 6-0, which is the finest. Other gauges are 5-0, 4-0, 000 (triple 0), 00 (double 0), 0, 1, 2, 3, 4, 5. Some suture materials are designated as fine, coarse, or medium.

Skin closure is frequently accomplished using Steri-Strips and has the advantage of causing no tissue reduction. They are easy to apply and remove and have a lower infection rate than wounds sutured together.

There are many methods of suturing wounds together. Each surgeon has preferences for use with different types of wounds and for different types of suture materials. Some of the more common methods of suturing are:

Blanket.   A continuous suture in which the needle is passed over the suture material at each stitch.
Continuous.   A type of running stitch in which only the first and last stitches are tied.
Halsted.   A subcuticular, continuous, buried suture concealed by the epidermis.
Interrupted.   A type of suture in which each stitch is tied separately.
Mattress.   A suture that is applied back and forth through both edges of a wound.
Purse String.   A continuous stitch passed in and out through the edges of a wound. The ends are then pulled together and tied.
Quilted.   A continuous mattress suture in which each stitch is tied as it is formed and the next stitch is passed in the opposite direction (Figure 10.2).

Dressing Changes and Surgical Site Care

The surgical site or wound site will need to be kept clean and as moisture free as possible to reduce infection. This is accomplished with bandages and dressings, which also act to control bleeding, hold wound edges together, absorb draining, hide disfigurement, and maintain constant pressure on a wound. Cleaning can be accomplished with any antibacterial agent, such as soap and water or hydrogen peroxide. Cleaning is frequently followed with application of a film of antibacterial or antibiotic ointment such as Polysporin.

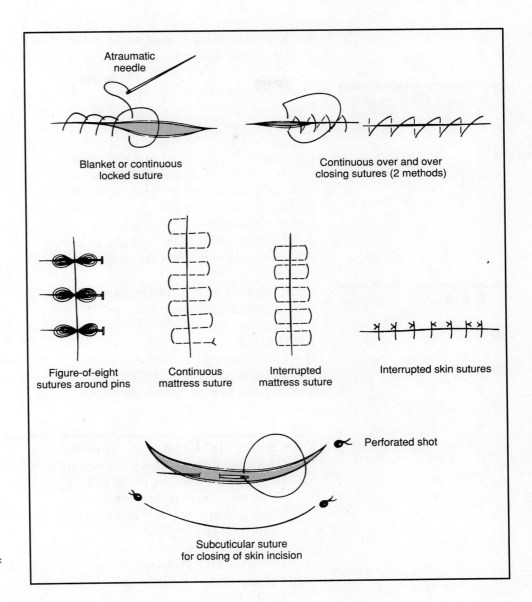

Figure 10.2 Methods of suturing

PROCEDURE FOR DRESSING CHANGE

1. **Wash and dry hands thoroughly.** Apply sterile gloves or nonsterile gloves.
2. **Protect the areas adjacent to the site from spills.**
3. **Clean the site with cotton-tipped applicators** soaked with skin antiseptic using a circular motion from the inside out, avoiding the wound edges.
4. If an ointment is to be used, **spread the ointment on with a sterile tongue depressor.**
5. **Make sure that the medication used and the dressing cover an area larger than the wound.**
6. **Secure the dressing with bandage or tape.**
7. **Remove equipment, supplies, and gloves.** Wash and dry hands thoroughly.

8. **Record dressing change on the patient chart**, including information about bleeding or discharge, appearance of the wound and the medication applied.

Patient Education

Patients should be instructed in caring for their wounds. Postoperative patients should be instructed in the care of the operative site and how to change dressings, should this be necessary between visits to the medical office. If there are restrictions on bathing or getting the injury or operative site wet, this must be included in the instructions. Orthopedic patients may need instructions on cast care.

It is always preferable to demonstrate a procedure and to provide patients with both verbal and written instructions. This will prevent errors due to faulty memory of the instructions. If the patient is not capable of following instructions, perhaps a family member or close friend can be instructed. With some patients, it may be preferable to provide them with the necessary supplies and equipment rather than relying on them to purchase the correct items.

Suture Removal

Suture removal is normally performed by the physician. In some instances, this function may be delegated to the medical assistant.

MATERIALS

One suture removal kit containing suture removal scissors and a thumb forceps
Skin antiseptic
Several gauze sponges, preferably 4 x 4

PROCEDURE FOR REMOVING SUTURES

1. **Check the patient's chart for the number of sutures that were inserted.**
2. **Explain the procedure to the patient.**
3. **Open the suture removal kit.**
4. **Wash and dry your hands thoroughly.**
5. **Glove with sterile gloves.**
6. **Clean the sutured area** using a skin antiseptic.
7. **Grasp the knot of the suture** with the dressing forceps without pulling.
8. **Cut the suture at skin level.**
9. **Gently lift the suture** toward the wound and out, using the thumb forceps.
10. **Check that the entire suture has been removed.**
11. **Continue until all sutures have been removed.**
12. **Clean the area once again** with the antiseptic.
13. **Apply a dressing** or Steri-Strips, as needed.
14. **Instruct the patient** to keep the area clean and dry.
15. **Dispose of equipment**, supplies, and gloves.
16. **Wash and dry hands thoroughly.**
17. **Record the number of sutures removed and the condition of the wound on the patient's medical record.** Record the appearance of the wound site and any dressing materials applied. The number of sutures removed should equal the number of sutures that were inserted.

1. Describe phase one of the healing process.

2. Proliferation is another term for which phase of the healing process?

3. During which phase of the healing process is the cicatrix formed?

4. What is the purpose of suturing surgical wounds?

5. Differentiate between absorbable and nonabsorbable sutures.

6. Name at least five types of nonabsorbable suture materials.

7. What is catgut made from?

8. What determines the gauge of suture material?

9. Define the term ligature.

10. Name at least three types of suture methods.

11. What information needs to be recorded on the patient's medical record following a dressing change?

12. What information needs to be recorded on the patient's medical record following suture removal?

13. List the equipment necessary to remove sutures.

14. Define hemostasis and laceration.

15. Why is some catgut tanned or chromocized?

16. Describe instances in which ligatures may be utilized.

17. What would you do if while removing sutures you can locate only eight, yet the chart indicates that ten were inserted.

18. How would you handle patient education for wound care if the patient does not understand or read English?

CHAPTER 11

Pharmacology

OBJECTIVES

On completion of this chapter, you will be able to:
- Classify drugs.
- Compute dosages.
- Interpret prescriptions.
- Differentiate systems of measurement.
- Identify and define the abbreviations used in prescription writing.

**Vocabulary—
Glossary of Terms**

Anesthesia	Insensitivity to pain.
Anorectic	Pertaining to lack or loss of appetite.
Antacid	A substance that neutralizes an acid.
Antibiotic	A substance that destroys or inhibits the growth of microorganisms.
Anticoagulant	A substance that inhibits or prevents coagulation.
Anticonvulsant	A substance that inhibits or prevents convulsions.
Antidepressant	A mood elevator.
Antidiarrheal	A substance that counteracts diarrhea.
Antidote	A substance that counteracts a poison.
Antiemetic	A substance that counteracts vomiting.
Antihistamine	A substance that counteracts histamine.
Antiseptic	A disinfectant; inhibits growth of microorganisms but does not necessarily destroy them.
Antitussive	A substance that relieves or prevents coughing.
Cathartic	A substance that causes evacuation of the bowels by increasing bulk or peristalsis.
Decongestant	A substance that reduces swelling and congestion.
Diuretic	A substance that increases urine production.

Elixir	A clear, sweet medicinal agent that contains a flavoring substance; frequently is hydroalcoholic.
Emetic	A substance used to induce vomiting.
Emulsion	A preparation in which small globules of one liquid are distributed throughout a second liquid.
Expectorant	A substance that promotes ejection of mucus and other fluids from the respiratory system.
Generic	Public or common name of a drug that is not protected by a trademark.
Hemostatic	A substance capable of controlling blood flow.
Hypnotic	A substance that induces sleep.
Laxative	A mild cathartic.
Relaxant	A substance that reduces tension.
Sedative	A substance that allays excitement.
Spirit	A volatile or distilled liquid.
Systemic	Affecting the body as a whole.
Tincture	A preparation of chemical substances in an alcohol or hydroalcoholic mixture.
Tranquilizer	A drug used to treat anxiety states, neuroses, and mental disorders.
Vasoconstrictor	A substance that constricts blood vessels.
Vasodilator	A substance that dilates blood vessels.

Drugs and Chemical Substances

Pharmacology is a broad term that covers all knowledge of drugs and their actions. A drug is any substance that causes chemical changes in the body. Drugs are used medically in diagnosis, cure, palliation, treatment, and prophylaxis. They include chemical substances, animal products, food substances, and plant parts or products. They may be obtained naturally or synthesized in the laboratory. In this chapter we emphasize the action of drugs within the body and their absorption and excretion.

Drugs are powerful chemical substances that can help or harm; the responsibility of the medical assistant in the administration of drugs is second only to that of the physician who prescribes them. It is the responsibility of the medical assistant to see that the right medication in the right amount is administered to the right patient at the right time by the right route.

The medical assistant is also responsible for knowing the action of the drug within the body, the correct dosage of the drug, the various methods of administration, symptoms of overdosage, and the abnormal reactions that can occur. The attitude of the medical assistant regarding this important facet of medical assisting can be critical in relationships with patients and in the employer–employee relationship.

Any individual who manufactures, dispenses, prescribes, or administers any substance identified as a *controlled substance* must register annually with the Drug Enforcement Administration (DEA) of the Department of Justice, which is responsible for enforcement of the Comprehensive Drug Abuse Prevention and Control Act of 1970, Title II, commonly known as the Controlled Substances Act. Initial application is made on DEA Form 224, which can be obtained from the DEA, Registration Section, P.O. Box 28083, Central Station, Washington, D.C. 20005. Complete listings of the drugs in each of the five schedules are available from the DEA office or can be found in the Code of Federal Regulations, Title 21. The basic schedules are as follows:

Schedule I

Includes drugs or other substances that have a high potential for abuse, as well as drugs that have no currently accepted medicinal use in the United States or for which there is a lack of accepted guidelines for safe use. Examples are heroin, marijuana, and LSD.

Schedule II

Includes drugs that have a high potential for abuse or abuse of which may lead to severe psychological or physical dependence or that may be used only with severe restrictions. Examples are morphine, codeine, Percodan, Ritalin, Nembutal and Quaalude.

When ordering Schedule I and II drugs, the physician must use a special order form (DEA Form 222) that is preprinted with the name and address of the physician. This form is issued in triplicate. One copy is to be kept in the physician's file, and the remaining copies are forwarded to the supplier who, after filling the order, keeps one copy and forwards the third copy to the nearest DEA office.

Prescription orders for Schedule II drugs must be handwritten and signed by the physician. Some state laws require that special prescription blanks with more than one copy be used. The physician's registration number must appear on the prescription blank. The order may not be given to a pharmacy over the telephone except in an emergency as defined by DEA. A prescription for Schedule II drugs may not be refilled.

All prescriptions for controlled substances must be dated and signed on the day issued and must bear the full name and address of the patient as well as the DEA registration number of the physician.

Medical assistants must know the laws of their state on controlled substances. State regulations frequently are more restrictive than federal regulations and may require a separate state registration. If controlled substances are to be handled in the medical office, the Code of Federal Regulations, Title 21, should be obtained from the nearest federal government bookstore and studied carefully. Controlled substances will also need to be kept under lock and key.

Schedule III

Includes drugs that have less potential for abuse than Schedule I and II drugs or for which abuse may lead to moderate or low physical dependence or high psychological dependence. Examples are various drug combinations that contain codeine, paregoric, amphetamine-like compounds, or butabarbital.

Schedule IV

Includes drugs with a low potential for abuse relative to the drugs in Schedule III or for which abuse may lead to limited physical or psychological dependence. Examples are Librium, Valium, and Darvon.

Schedule III and IV drugs require either a written or oral prescription by the prescribing physician. If authorized by the physician on the initial prescription, the patient may have the prescription refilled up to the number of authorized refills, not to exceed five times or beyond six months from the date that the prescription was issued.

Schedule V

Includes drugs whose potential for abuse is relatively low compared to those under Schedule IV or for which there may be very limited physical or psychological dependence. Examples include cough medications containing codeine and drugs such as Lomotil.

Classification of Drugs

Drugs are available in two basic forms, liquid and solid. Solid preparations include capsules, tablets, suppositories, ointments, and lozenges. Liquid preparations include syrup, **emulsion, elixir,** solution, **spirit, tincture,** liniment, lotion, and spray.

Generally drugs are classified by the action they have on the body. These classifications include but are not limited to analgesics, **anorectics, antacids, antibiotics, anticoagulants, anticonvulsants, antidepressants, antidiarrheals, antidotes, antiemetics, antihistamines, antiseptics, antitussives, cathartics, decongestants, diuretics, emetics, expectorants, hemostatics, hypnotics, laxatives,** muscle **relaxants, sedatives, tranquilizers, vasoconstrictors,** and **vasodilators.**

Drugs are sometimes classified by action, such as to treat infections, harden and contract tissues, increase blood supply to a body part, irritate tissues, destroy tissues, relieve pain, produce **anesthesia,** soothe, check bleeding, promote healing, coat and protect tissues, produce counterirritation, destroy or expel intestinal worms, supply a deficient secretion, or neutralize solutions in the digestive system.

Drugs are also classified by local action, which is the effect produced by a drug at the point of application on the skin or mucous membrane. Classification may also be by **systemic** action, which is the action of a drug on some tissue or organ remote from the site of application through absorption or the entrance of the drug into the bloodstream.

Drugs are manufactured and developed at a rapid pace. Being familiar with the drugs that you are required to administer is a full-time job. Below are listed some of the more common preparations, giving their action and proprietary and **generic** names.

Trade Name	Generic

Analgesics: Used for the relief of pain

Aspirin	Acetylsalicylic Acid (ASA)
Darvocet	Propoxyphene napsylate and acetaminophen
Demerol	Meperidine
Dilaudid	Hydromorphone
Duramorph	Morphine sulfate (MSO_4)
Percocet	Oxycodone and acetaminophen
Percodan	Oxycodone and ASA

Trade Name	Generic
Stadol	Butorphanol
Tylenol	Acetaminophen

Antacids: Used to relieve gastric distress

Maalox	Aluminum hydroxide and magnesium hydroxide
Mylanta	Aluminum hydroxide and magnesium hydroxide
Riopan	Magaldrate

Antibiotics: Used to fight infection

Ancef	Cefazolin
Flagyl	Metronidazole
Keflin	Cephalothin sodium
Kefzol	Cefazolin
Mefoxin	Cefoxitin
Omnipen, Polycillin	Ampicillin
Pen VK	Penicillin/potassium
Septra	Bacitracin
Zinacef	Cefuroxime

Anticoagulants: Used to slow or prevent blood clotting

Coumadin	Wafarin sodium
Liquaemin	Heparin

Anticonvulsants: Used to control seizure activity

Depekane	Valproic acid
Dilantin	Phenytoin
Luminal	Phenobarbital
Tegretol	Carbamazepine

Antidepressants: Mood elevators

Elavil	Amitriptyline
Valium	Diazepam
Xanax	Alprazolam

Antidiarrheals: Used to control diarrhea

Lomotil	Diphenoxylate and atropine

Antiemetics: Used to relieve nausea/vomiting

Benadryl	Diphenhydramine
Compazine	Prochlorperazine maleate
Tigan	Triethobenzamide
Vistaril	Hydroxyzine pamoate

Antihistamine: Used to decrease stomach acid production

Tagamet	Cimetidine
Zantac	Ranitidine

Antihypertensives: Used to lower blood pressure

Aldomet	Methyldopa
Apresoline	Hydralazine
Catapress	Clonidine

Trade Name	Generic
HCTZ	Hydrochlorthiazide
Lopressor	Metoprolol tartrate
Minipres	Prazosin

Antiinflammatory: Used to retard the immune response
(commonly referred to as Nonsteroidal antiinflammatory drugs)

Motrin	Ibuprofen
Naprosyn	Naproxen

Cardiotonics: Used to improve heart muscle contractility

Lanoxin	Digoxin

Diuretics: Used to remove excess fluid from the system

Aldactone	Spiralactone
Bumex	Bumetanide
Edacrin	Ethacrynic acid
HCTZ	Hydrochlorthiazide
Lasix	Furosemide

Hypnotics: Used for sleep

Dalmane	Flurazepam
Halcion	Triazolam
Restoril	Temazepam

Laxatives: Used to improve bowel function/relieve constipation

Colace	Docusate sodium
Milk of Magnesia (MOM)	Magnesium hydroxide magma

Muscle Relaxants: Used to relieve muscle spasm

Flexeril	Cyclobenzaprine
Robaxin	Methocarbamol
Soma	Carisprodol

Tranquilizers: Used to relieve anxiety

Haldol	Haloperidol
Thorazine	Chlorpromazine

Vasoconstrictors: Used to elevate blood pressure

Dopamine	Intropin
Epinephrine	Adrenalin
Levophed	Norepinephrine

Vasodilators: Used to dilate vessels / lower blood pressure

Nitrostat	Nitroglycerin

Drug References

All drugs in the United States are standardized, and there are three reference books that are recognized as the authoritative treatises. The first is the *United States Pharmacopeia* (U.S.P.), which not only includes a list of approved drugs, but also describes and defines them as to source, chemistry, properties, methods of assay, storage, dosage, compounding directions, and general use. The Pharmacopeia is customarily revised every five years in order to include new drugs and exclude those no longer in use. Two important standards for inclusion in the U.S.P. are that the drug must be useful clinically and available in pure form.

The most complete and up-to-date reference listing of drugs is the *Hospital Formulary*. This reference provides information about the characteristics of drugs and their clinical usage. It is updated more frequently than any other reference.

The *Physician's Desk Reference* (PDR) is the most commonly used reference book in the physician's office. It is published annually by the pharmaceutical manufacturers and updating supplements are provided, as needed, throughout the year. Commercial products are listed by their trade names, generic names, and therapeutic uses.

Mathematics Review

In order to correctly calculate a prescribed dosage, you must observe basic rules of mathematics. Following these rules will allow you to accurately perform dosage calculations with a minimum of difficulty.

1. Always convert all measurements to "like" values. It is not possible to calculate a dosage in which "grams" is supplied for a prescribed dose in which "milligrams" is required, without first converting both entities to milligrams.
2. An equals sign (=) implies that both sides of the equation (i.e., the sum of all terms to the left of the sign and the sum of all terms to the right of the sign) are equal. Therefore, in the process of solving for a value (x), any function performed on the left of the equation must also be performed on the right.

Example

$$100x = 1000$$

To solve for the value (x), both sides of the equation must be divided by 100.

$$\frac{100x}{100} = \frac{1000}{100}$$

The answer is $x = 10$.

Example:

$$0.1x = 10$$

To solve for the value (x), both sides of the equation must be multiplied by 10.

$$(10)\,0.1x = (10)\,10$$

The answer is $x = 100$

Systems of Measurement

Combinations of several systems of measurement are used in the delivery of medication. The most common are the apothecary system, the metric system, and the household system. Anyone who has at one time or another measured a cup of flour or a teaspoon of sugar is familiar to some degree with the household system. With the advent of the shift to the metric system some have been exposed to measures such as liters and kilograms, but few outside the medical community have had reason to become familiar with the apothecary system of measure.

Following is a table to help familiarize you with these systems and teach you how to convert measurements between the systems. Always check measurements when in doubt and refer to the appropriate portion of the table. Soon the measurements will come naturally.

Metric Equivalents		
1 kilogram (kg)	=	1000 grams
1 gram (Gm)	=	1000 milligrams
1 milligram (Mg)	=	1000 micrograms (Mcg)
1 liter (l)	=	1000 milliliters or cubic centimeters
1 milliliter (ml)	=	1 cubic centimeter (cc)

Apothecary	Metric	Household
	Weight	
$^1/_2$ grain (gr)	30 milligrams (mg)	
1 grain (gr)	60 milligrams (mg)	
10 grains	600 milligrams (mg)	
15 grains	1 gram (gm)	
1 dram	4 grams	
2.2 pounds (lb)	1 kilogram (kg)	2.2 pounds (lb)
	Volume	
1 minim	0.06 ml or cc	1 drop
15 minims	1 ml or cc	15 drops
1 fluid dram	4 ml or cc	1 teaspoon
1 fluid ounce	30 ml	1 ounce (oz)
1 pint	500 ml	2 cups
1 quart	1000 ml	4 cups

Dosage Calculations

Frequently in the medical community we find that drug manufacturers have made the job of dosage calculation somewhat easier for those administering medications in the field. Today many medications are supplied in the "unit dose" format. This is a system in which the manufacturer supplies medications in units that conform to recognized standard doses of the particular medication. In many cases this eliminates the need for calculation of the prescribed dose. However, because physicians do not always prescribe the same dosages that the manufacturer supplies, there is occasionally a need for computation. Dosages vary, depending on the patient's age, body size, and general physical condition.

When calculating a medication dosage, the first step is to read the label and determine the concentration of the drug on hand (e.g., Demerol 100 mg in 2 cc). The next step is to read the prescribed dosage (e.g., give Demerol 60 mg I.M.). Once you have determined the amount of drug on hand and the amount ordered, you may calculate the dose by means of a simple proportion, as follows:

STEP 1

$$\frac{100 \text{ mg}}{2 \text{ cc}} = \frac{60 \text{ mg}}{x \text{ cc}}$$

When setting up the proportion, remember to observe these rules.

1. Always place the dose on hand on the left.
2. Keep the quantity of drug above the line on both sides of the equation.
3. Keep the volume of the drug below the line on both sides of the equation.
4. The right side of the equation is the quantity of the drug desired.
5. x represents the number of cc's you want to give to the patient in order to deliver the desired dose.

By cross-multiplying the equation and reducing the equation to its simplest terms, you are able to arrive at the correct dose by solving for the value x.

STEP 2

$$100 \times (x) = 60 \times 2$$

STEP 3

$$100x = 120$$

STEP 4

$$\frac{100x}{100} = \frac{120}{100}$$

STEP 5

$$x = \frac{120}{100}$$

STEP 6

$$x = 1.2$$

The correct dosage to give would be 1.2 cc in order to deliver a dose of 60 mg.

It is unlikely that you will ever give a dose that would require the use of more than two vials, two ampules, or two pills. If you arrive at an answer that would require a dosage of this size, you should check your math or ask one of your coworkers to check your math for you. For instance, if in the above problem you arrived at a dosage that was 12 cc, this would require six ampules of medication in order to give your dose, which would come to a total of 600 mg. You should be suspicious of this type of dosage and recheck your math. You also should be aware that it would be very unlikely to give a dose of Demerol greater than 100 mg to anything smaller than a very large elephant. The maximum recommended dose for a human is generally 100 mg.

Prescriptions

Prescriptions are the method by which the physician communicates with the pharmacist regarding the amount, method, and frequency of a medication that he desires the patient to use. Prescriptions are written with symbols and abbreviations derived from a universal standard in pharmacology. In order to read prescriptions, you must become familiar with the language used and where information may be found.

ABBREVIATIONS
The following is a list of common abbreviations used in prescribing medication.

a.c.	after meals
A.D.	right ear
A.S.	left ear
A.U.	both ears
b.i.d.	twice per day
/c	with
gtt(s)	drop(s)
h	hour
h.s.	at bedtime

I.M.	intramuscular
I.V.	intravenously
npo	nothing by mouth
O.D.	right eye
O.S.	left eye
O.U.	both eyes
p.c.	after meals
p.o.	by mouth
p.r.n.	as required
q	every
qd	every day
qid	four times per day
qod	every other day
/s	without
s.l.	sublingual
s.q. or Subq	subcutaneously
stat	immediately
t.i.d.	three times per day
ung	ointment

READING PRESCRIPTIONS

A prescription is a legal document. It is an order from a physician to a pharmacist to dispense a medication to a particular patient, to be taken following specific directions. All prescriptions must have the following components to be a valid legal document:

1. The patient's name and address. Ages should be given for children.
2. The "superscription" or symbol Rx (from the latin word for recipe).
3. The "inscription," listing the medication and strength.
4. The "subscription," directing the pharmacist to dispense a certain quantity.
5. The "signa" or "sig," giving the patient instructions on taking the medication.
6. The physician's signature, address, and license number. If the prescription is for a controlled substance (Schedule I or II), the physician's DEA number must be included.
7. The number of refills authorized, if any, and any special instructions to be placed on the label by the pharmacist.

The information is placed on the proper form (Figure 11.1) and delivered to a pharmacist by the patient. The order is filled, and the patient receives the medication in a labeled container bearing the instructions for use.

Example: Dr. Robert Smith gives Mrs. Gladys Jones a prescription for an antibiotic. The following information is contained in the prescription:

Mrs. Gladys Jones
2322 Greentree Lane, Yourtown, USA.
Rx: Keflin, 500 mg Capsules
Sig: 1 cap p.o. q.i.d.
Disp: #40
Refill: 0   *Robert Smith, M.D.*
Generic Equivalent may be   *222 Doctor Lane, Yourtown, USA*
substituted.   *A123456789*

DEA NUMBER (MAY BE PRINTED) TELEPHONE NUMBER

PHYSICIAN'S NAME
ADDRESS ZIP

PATIENT'S NAME ______ DATE ______

ADDRESS ______

Rx

Sig:

Refill ______ Times

Please label ( )

______
PHYSICIAN'S SIGNATURE

Figure 11.1 Sample prescription blank (Adapted with permission from Keir, Wise, and Krebs-Shannon, *Medical Assisting,* 2nd Ed., Delmar Publishers Inc., 1989)

The information on the prescription tells the Pharmacist to give Mrs. Jones a bottle of forty 500-mg capsules of Keflin with instructions to take one capsule by mouth four times per day. There are no refills, and the pharmacist may fill the prescription using the generic equivalent of Keflin, which may be less expensive for the patient.

The pharmacist bottles the capsules, with a label on the container giving Mrs. Jones instructions in plain language, on how the medication is to be taken.

Authorizing Refills

Some states allow medical assistants to authorize prescription refills for patients, with the approval of the physician. If this is the case in the state of your employment, you are responsible for following the instructions of the physician exactly.

A medical assistant would never be called upon to authorize a refill for a medication with a potential for abuse. Medications that a patient takes regularly for a heart condition or hormones that a woman takes regularly after a hysterectomy are examples of medications that a medical assistant is generally authorized to approve refills.

The situation usually involves a patient who, for a variety of reasons, has not seen the physician for a period of time, usually at least several months. The patient has run out of a medication used regularly and has gone to the pharmacy to have the order refilled, only to discover that the prescription has expired. To delay refilling the patient's medication until an appointment can be scheduled and a new prescription issued could be detrimental to the patient's condition. A compromise is made. The physician directs the medical assistant to authorize the pharmacist to refill the medication for a short period, usually thirty days or less, and to instruct the pharmacist to inform the patient that an appointment must be made for a checkup prior to the expiration of the refill. Thus, the patient is not deprived of needed medication and the physician is able to evaluate the patient to determine if any changes are needed in the patient's continuing care.

Many offices have standard lists of those medications for which a medical assistant may authorize a refill and the period that the refill may cover. Such refills are generally done on a "one-time" basis.

1. What federal agency is responsible for the control of pharmaceutical substances in the United States?

2. Describe the criteria for a Schedule II drug and give an example.

3. For what purpose are triplicate prescription forms used?

4. What authorizes a physician to prescribe drugs?

5. What type of records are kept on drugs that a physician prescribes?

6. The physician orders 40 mg Demerol I.M. You have Demerol 50 mg in 2 cc. How Many cc's do you give?

7. The physician orders 2,500 units Heparin s.q. You have Heparin 5,000 units in 1 cc. How many cc's do you give?

8. The physician orders Capoten 6.25 mg p.o. You have 25-mg Capoten tablets that are double scored. What do you do?

9. The physician orders Ancef 600 mg I.M. You have Kefzol 1 gram in 10 cc (after reconstitution). What do you do?

10. What items must appear on a prescription?

11. What is a diuretic? An analgesic?

12. How many milligrams make a gram?

13. How many cc's make an ounce?

14. What is a dram?

15. What is a minim?

16. Why should grams be converted to milligrams when calculating a dosage in milligrams?

17. The physician orders Demerol 75 mg I.M. You have Demerol 50 mg in 1 cc. How many cc's do you give?

18. The physician orders ASA gr *x* p.o. You have 325-mg aspirin tablets. How many tablets do you give?

19. The physician orders Nifedipine 100 mg p.o. You have 10 mg. Nifedipine capsules on hand. What do you do?

CHAPTER 12

Administration of Medications

OBJECTIVES	On completion of this chapter, you will be able to:
	• Demonstrate the proper technique in administering parenteral medications.
	• List the absolute rules concerning medication administration.
	• Identify the various routes of medication administration.
	• List the five "rights" of medication administration.

**Vocabulary—
Glossary of Terms**

Buccal	Medication placed in the cheek for absorption.
Contraindications	Conditions limiting the use of a particular drug.
Inuction	Application of topical medication to the skin surface.
Sublingual	Medication given under the tongue in order to dissolve.

Absolute Rules for Administration of Medications

Throughout the history of medicine in the United States, the patient has put a great deal of trust in the physician and other members of the medical community. The feeling that a physician's purpose is to cure your ills and make you feel better has allowed many patients to follow blindly the doctor's recommendations. Modern times have seen the advent of consumer awareness, and the term *caveat emptor* (let the buyer beware) has found its way into the delivery of medical care as well as the commercial market place. More patients are aware of the types of medications and their actions than ever before. More patients question the rationale for treatment than ever before.

The fact that patient awareness has increased, however, does not relieve the medical assistant of responsibility when treating the patient, especially concerning the administration of medications. It is the medical assistant's responsibility to know what medication is being given, what effect it will have on the patient, and how the patient is to receive the medication.

You will be called upon to administer some medications the patient could buy without a prescription at the corner pharmacy. Others may be potent prescription drugs, which if given incorrectly could cause death or serious harm to the patient. Even if the medical assistant follows the instruction of the physician to the letter, if the dosage is incorrect or out of the ordinary, any harm that comes to the patient is at least the moral responsibility, if not the legal responsibility, of the person who *physically administered* the medication. It is not only your responsibility, but your right, to question an order that appears to be abnormal. If the explanation received does not satisfy your doubt, it is also your right to refuse to administer the medication. By being sure of your actions, you not only protect the patient, you also protect yourself. Observing the following rules will help ensure proper administration of medications.

1. Know the drug category and action of a medication before you administer it. If you are unsure, look it up in a reliable reference. Don't count on your coworkers to educate you.

2. Know the recommended dosage of any drug that you administer before you give it. If there is a discrepancy, verify the dosage with the physician and document your actions in the patient's medical record.

3. Fulfill the five "rights" before giving a patient a medication:
   a. Right Patient
   b. Right Medication
   c. Right Dose
   d. Right Time
   e. Right Route

4. When preparing to give a medication, check the label *three times:*
   a. When you first pick up the bottle.
   b. When you draw or pour the medication.
   c. When you return the bottle to its place.

5. Be aware of your patient's allergies. If a patient tells you of an allergy to a drug that you are preparing to give, check with the physician before administering the drug.

6. Be familiar with the **contraindications** of drugs that you administer. Question orders when contraindications are present.

7. Listen to your patient. If the patient does not recognize a medication that you are preparing to give, yet it is a medication that the patient takes regularly, recheck your medication.

By following these rules, you will eliminate or minimize medication errors. If you consider the consequences of your actions, you will be a safe practitioner, which is, or should be, the goal of the medical community as a whole.

Routes of Administration

Routes of administration fall into four broad categories; topical, oral, rectal, and parenteral. Within each of these categories are subcategories. The medical assistant must be as familiar with the recommended route of administration as with all other facets of medications.

Topical administration applies to medications that are applied to the skin surface. They include but are not limited to creams, salves, lotions, ointments, tinctures, soaps, and shampoos. These medications are often ordered by the terms "local application" or "**inuction**," as well as "topical." Vinyl gloves should be used when administering medications in this manner to prevent absorption of the medication through the hands.

Oral administration applies to medications taken via the mouth. This includes medications given by **sublingual** or **buccal** routes as well as medications that are swallowed. Sublingual medication is placed under the tongue; buccal medication is held in the cheek. In both cases the medications are allowed to dissolve, being absorbed rapidly by the mucous membrane of the mouth. In both cases medication enters the system very rapidly as a result of the high capillary bed concentration in oral mucosa.

Oral medications include tablets, pills, capsules, spansules, suspensions, elixirs, and syrups. Tablets are either scored or unscored. If a tablet is scored, the manufacturer guarantees an equal disbursement of medication throughout the entire tablet. In these cases a tablet may be split to give a partial dose (e.g., one half or one quarter). If the tablet is not scored, then the medication is not guaranteed to be evenly disbursed, and so a portion of the tablet may not be given as a substitute for a smaller dose (Figure 12.1).

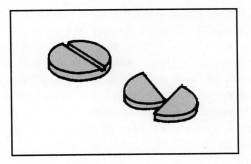

Figure 12.1 Scored tablets (Adapted with permission from Keir, Wise, and Krebs-Shannon, *Medical Assisting*, 2nd Ed., Delmar Publishers Inc., 1989)

Pills often are "enteric coated" to protect the lining of the stomach by releasing the medication in the lower intestine. These pills are intended to be swallowed whole and are never to be chewed by the patient.

Most of us are familiar with capsules, but there is a subtle difference between a capsule and spansule. Outwardly, they look very similar. The form of medication inside the gelatin capsule is what makes the difference between the two. Capsules are filled with medication in a powdered or liquid form. If a patient has difficulty swallowing a capsule, the ingredients can be removed and dissolved in a liquid. The spansule, however, is filled with hundreds of tiny multicolored time-release pills, designed to spread the dose of medication over a specified period or span of time. Hence the name *span*sule. To dissolve these pills in liquid would defeat the mechanism of time release, thereby exposing the patient to the risk of overdose. Caution should be used in administering capsules and spansules.

Suspensions have medication partially dissolved in a solvent. Before measuring a dose of a suspension, shake the mixture thoroughly to distribute the medication uniformly throughout the carrier.

Elixirs are medications dissolved in a liquid containing a sugar and alcohol base. These medications are rarely, if ever, given to children because of their alcohol content. Syrups are medications dissolved in a mixture of sugar and water to enhance the flavor and so make the medication more palatable.

The rectal route is used for unconscious patients, patients who would otherwise tolerate the medication poorly if administered orally, or in those instances when the medication if taken orally would be inactivated by digestive enzymes. Suppositories have medication suspended in a firm, molded base, often cocoa butter, and are rapidly absorbed into the system through the rectal mucous membrane. Suppositories should always be lubricated before insertion and delivered well into the rectal vault. Gloves should always be worn when giving suppositories. Medications may also be administered vaginally when appropriate.

The fourth route of administration is the parenteral route, which covers anything given by injection. There are various types of parenteral administration: intravenous, intramuscular, subcutaneous, and intradermal.

Intravenous administration of medication falls into the realm of responsibility of the physician and the registered nurse. It is not within the scope of practice of the medical assistant. There are no circumstances under which the medical assistant can legally give intravenous medication. There are no exceptions.

Intramuscular medication can be given by a medical assistant under the supervision of a licensed physician. Intramuscular injections (I.M.) are given deep into the body of a large muscle at sites chosen for their lack of blood vessels and nerve fibers. Some of the common sites for I.M. injection include the middle deltoid muscle, the upper-outer gluteus medius, the ventral gluteus medius, and the vastus lateralis (Figure 12.2). Never inject more than 3 cc of fluid in a single I.M. injection, never more than 2 cc at the deltoid site, and smaller amounts in infants and children. Within the area of each of these muscles is an injection site chosen to reduce the danger of hitting a nerve or artery. The anatomical landmarks for intramuscular injection outlined in Figure 12.2 are the guidelines you must use in choosing your injection site. The vastus lateralis and ventral gluteus are the preferred sites for I.M. injections to infants and children.

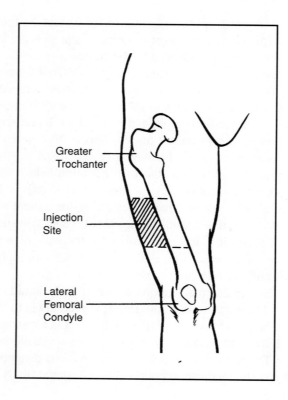

Figure 12.2 Common I.M. injection sites: (A) Vastus lateralis (Reproduced with permission from Gomez and Hord, *Fundamentals of Clinical Nursing Skills*, John Wiley & Sons, Inc., 1988).

Greater Trochanter

Injection Site

Lateral Femoral Condyle

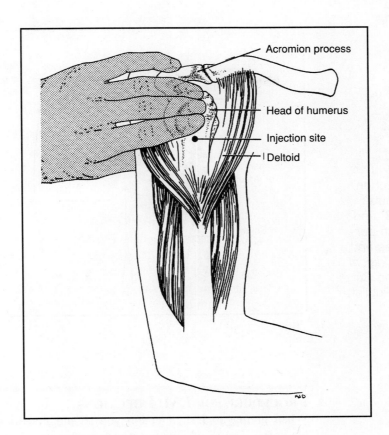

Figure 12.2 continued
Common I.M. injection
sites: (B) Middle deltoid.

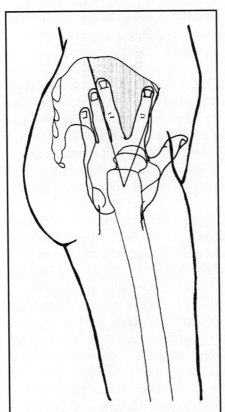

Figure 12.2 continued
Common I.M. injection
sites: (C) Ventral gluteus
medius (Reproduced with
permission from Narrow
and Buschle, *Fundamen-
tals of Nursing Practice*,
2nd Ed., John Wiley &
Sons, Inc., 1982).

Figure 12.2 continued
Common I.M. injection
sites: (D) Upper outer
gluteus medius (B) and
(D) (Reprinted with per-
mission from Reiss and
Evans, *Pharmacological
Aspects of Nursing Care,*
3rd Ed., Delmar Publish-
ers Inc., 1990)

PROCEDURE FOR I.M. INJECTIONS

When giving an I.M. injection you should first locate the site by the anatomical landmarks. Areas of scar tissue, edematous areas, and traumatized areas should be avoided. Medication is poorly absorbed in such areas. Choose a needle with as small a gauge as possible and long enough to reach well into the muscle (22 gauge × 1½" is the most common for adults; larger gauge is used when injecting thicker medications). Prep the site using an alcohol wipe in a spiral pattern, starting at the injection site and working outward. After verbally preparing the patient, introduce the needle with one brisk motion into the area to its full length at a 90-degree angle to the skin surface. Before injecting the medication, you *must* aspirate for blood. If blood returns in the syringe, the tip of the needle is in a blood vessel. When this happens you must withdraw the needle slightly and aspirate again. Once there is no blood return with aspiration it is safe to inject the medication slowly. Once the injection is complete, withdraw the needle rapidly and massage the injection site briskly with the alcohol swab.

A special technique, designed for use when injecting unusually caustic medications and medications that stain tissue, is the *Z-track* technique. The same principles apply with this technique as with intramuscular injections, the one difference being that just before the needle is introduced to the musculature, traction is applied to the skin adjacent to the injection site. Introduce the needle and after aspirating for blood, inject the medication. Before removing the needle, release the traction on the skin surface and withdraw the needle rapidly. The theory behind this technique is simply that the traction displaces underlying layers of tissue when the needle is introduced. When traction is released and the needle is removed, the tissue layers resume their normal position, preventing the escape of the medication to the upper tissues by way of the needle track. Some clinicians prefer to use the Z-track technique routinely for all I.M. injections (Figure 12.3).

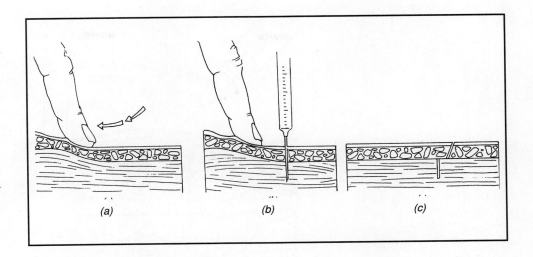

Figure 12.3   Correct method for Z-track injection: (A) Skin pulled to one side and held there. (B) Needle in place. (C) Z-track sealed when the skin is released. (Reproduced with permission from Narrow and Buschle, *Fundamentals of Nursing Practice*, 2nd Ed., John Wiley & Sons, Inc., 1982)

(a)   (b)   (c)

PROCEDURE FOR SUBCUTANEOUS INJECTIONS

Subcutaneous injections (subq or s.q.) introduce medications to the fatty layer of tissue beneath the skin surface. Usually injections are 1 cc or less. For these injections a smaller gauge needle is used (25 to 27 gauge × ⅝"). Injections are given with the needle at a 45-degree angle to the skin surface in areas where fatty tissue is in good supply (e.g., lateral thighs, buttocks, abdomen, outer surface of upper arm, and upper two thirds of the back) (Figure 12.4). There is very little vasculature imbedded in subcutaneous tissue, so it is not necessary to aspirate for blood prior to injection. Cleanse the area with an alcohol wipe in the same manner as preceding an I.M. injection. After locating the site, proceed with the injection. It is recommended to rotate sites when patients receive frequent injections to prevent scarring of tissue. Subcutaneous heparin is always given in the abdomen.

It is a good practice to have another practitioner check dosages of heparin and insulin before subcutaneous injection to verify that the dosage is correct. These medications, if given incorrectly, can cause the patient serious harm. The quantities involved are very small, and the chance for error is great.

PROCEDURE FOR INTRADERMAL INJECTIONS

Intradermal injections are used primarily for allergy testing and tuberculin testing. A fine needle similar in size to that used for subcutaneous injection is used. The skin is prepped with an alcohol wipe and the needle inserted just below the skin surface. A very small amount of fluid is injected until a small blister appears on the skin surface. The needle is then withdrawn (Figure 12.5).

In addition to the routes discussed already, medications may be introduced to body cavities or wounds by other methods. *Instillation* introduces medication to a cavity or wound and allows it to be absorbed. *Irrigation* is the act of flushing a body cavity or wound with a solution containing medication and allowing the fluid to escape into a container.

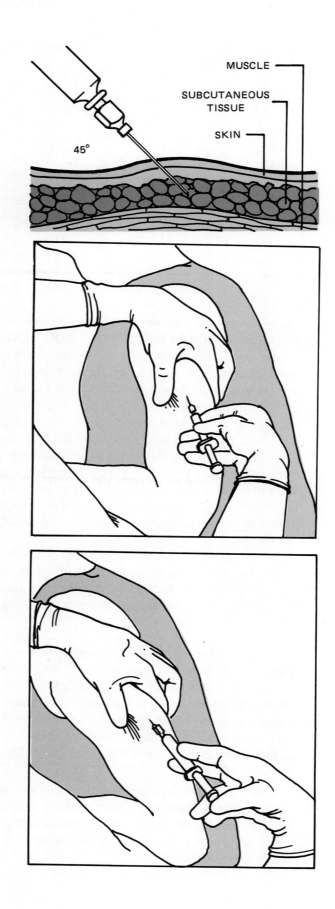

Figure 12.4 Correct technique for subcutaneous injection (Reproduced with permission from Keir, Wise, and Krebs-Shannon, *Medical Assisting*, 2nd Ed., Delmar Publishers Inc., 1989)

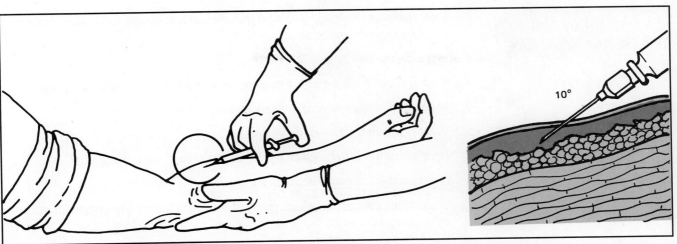

Figure 12.5 Correct technique for intradermal injection (Reproduced with permission from Keir, Wise, and Krebs-Shannon, *Medical Assisting,* 2nd Ed., Delmar Publishers Inc., 1989)

Documentation

When administering medications, documentation is extremely important. If a medication is given for the relief of pain or other discomfort document this action, but also document the effect that the medication has on the patient. If the medication relieved the pain, chart this fact.

Routes of medication are important as well. Document the location of an injection and any special technique used, e.g., 25 mg Demerol, I.M., LUOG by Z-track injection.

Remember that all services you perform are relevant to the patient's condition and at some time may fall under the scrutiny of a court of law; you will be well advised to chart in detail those services that you render. Remember, "If it wasn't charted, it wasn't done." Errors and omissions may be corrected only at the time of occurrence.

1. How many times should you read the label on a medication container before administering the medication?

2. What are the five "rights"?

3. Who is most liable for injury to a patient as a result of a medication error?

4. Name two sources of drug reference information.

5. What is meant by the "Z-track" method?

6. If a medication is to be given by the buccal route, where is it given?

7. Describe the difference between a capsule and a spansule.

8. Under what circumstances are medical assistants allowed to give medication by intravenous route?

9. What should be documented after a medication is given for the relief of pain?

10. Who may give intravenous medications?

11. At what angle to the skin surface is the needle held for a subcutaneous injection?

12. Under what circumstances may a tablet be broken in order to give a partial dose of medication?

13. What should always be used when a suppository is given?

14. What is the most common site for I.M. injection in adults?

15. Where are most I.M. injections given to infants and small children?

16. Name two drugs that should have their doses verified by another person prior to administration.

17. Name three areas to avoid when giving an I.M. injection.

CHAPTER 13

Specimen Collection

OBJECTIVES

On completion of this chapter, you will be able to:

- Demonstrate proper technique in obtaining a specimen by venipuncture.
- Obtain a laboratory specimen by capillary puncture.
- Identify the purpose of venipuncture.
- Identify the equipment and supplies necessary to perform venipuncture.
- Identify the vessels most commonly used for venipuncture sites.
- Identify the purpose of capillary puncture.
- Identify the equipment needed to perform a capillary puncture.

Vocabulary— Glossary of Terms

Anemia	A **hematocrit** below normal level.
Artery	A vessel carrying blood from the heart to tissues; pulses are felt when palpating arteries.
Autolet	A holder for **lancets**.
Hematocrit	The percentage of red blood cells as compared to the total blood volume. Normal value for males is 45 to 52% and for females 37 to 48%.
Hematoma	Bleeding into soft tissue, formation of a bruise.
Hemoglobin	A protein found in erythrocytes, responsible for the transport of oxygen in the blood. Normally the value of the patient's hemoglobin is approximately one-third the value of their hematocrit. Normal value for males is 13 to 18 grams/100 ml, and for females 12 to 16 grams/100 ml.
Hemolyze	To destroy erythrocytes, releasing hemoglobin.
Intima	The innermost portion of the wall of a vessel.
Lancet	A sharp, sterile instrument used for capillary puncture.
Neonate	A newborn infant.
Phenylalinine	An amino acid.

PKU	Phenylketonuria. A recessive hereditary disease, caused by the body's inability to metabolize **phenylalinine** to tyrosine. If untreated, can result in severe mental retardation. Treatment involves a diet low in phenylalinine. Treatment must be started prior to the age of three years. Infants are routinely tested at birth in most states.
Polycythemia	A hematocrit above normal level.
Tourniquet	Any item that when wrapped around a body part slows the flow of blood and causes pooling in the veins. Tourniquets are usually made of an elastic material.
Tortuous	Twisting and turning, following an irregular path.
Vein	A vessel that carries blood from tissues to the heart; no pulse is felt when palpating a vein.

Venipuncture	**V**enipuncture is defined as the surgical puncture of a **vein**. As one of the most common diagnostics in the practice of medicine, it offers the physician a variety of information with which to diagnose and treat the patient's complaints.

The status of the patient's blood can be determined by the complete blood count (CBC). This will indicate the presence of infection as indicated by elevated white cell count, the presence of **anemia** by a low red cell count, the presence of blood dyscrasias by low platelet count, the ability of the blood to carry oxygen by the level of **hemoglobin**, and a variety of abnormalities including some types of leukemia by the population of various types of white blood cells present.

Blood samples can identify systemic infection, prerenal failure, low levels of electrolytes and other chemicals, and tell us how well some medications are functioning in relation to our individual systems. We can also type and cross-match blood for purposes of transfusion. Often diseases are diagnosed solely on the results of tests done on the blood.

Medical assistants are allowed to perform venipuncture only for the purpose of obtaining laboratory specimens. They are not allowed to start intravenous lines or give medications or solutions intravenously. Medical assistants are not allowed to make **arterial** punctures for any reason, not even to obtain laboratory specimens.

EQUIPMENT AND SUPPLIES

Blood may be drawn using a needle and syringe or by the vacutainer system. In both cases, the other necessary equipment is identical.

Before drawing blood, the medical assistant should assemble:

1. Vacuum tubes for collection with the appropriate additives for the test desired (see Chapter 14, "Laboratory Examinations").
2. A **tourniquet** (a piece of penrose drain stock is often used).
3. Alcohol pledgets (benzalkonium chloride must be used if drawing blood to test for alcohol in excess of legal limit).
4. Bandaids
5. Sterile needle device used in the draw.
    a. vacutainer holder and double needle (Figure 13.1)
    b. syringe and sterile luerlock needle (Figure 13.2)

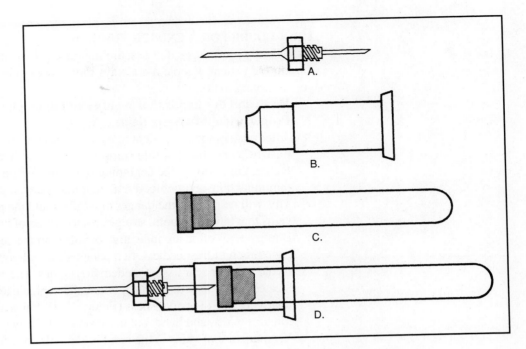

Figure 13.1 Components of the Vacutainer system: (A) Needle. (B) Holder. (C) Vacuum tube. (D) Assembled unit. (Reproduced with permission from Walters, Estridge, and Reynolds, *Basic Medical Laboratory Techniques*, 2nd Ed., Delmar Publishers Inc., 1990)

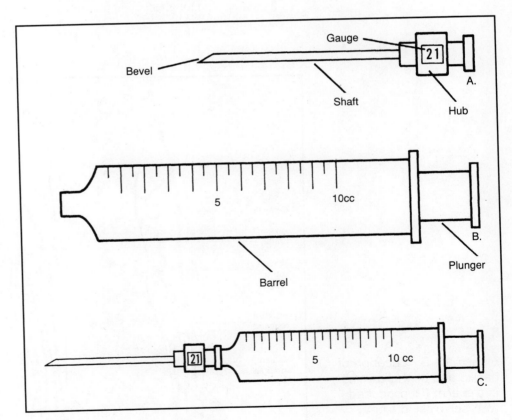

Figure 13.2 Components of needle and syringe system: (A) Hypodermic needle. (B) Syringe and needle assembled. (Reproduced with permission from Walters, Estridge, and Reynolds, *Basic Medical Laboratory Techniques*, 2nd Ed., Delmar Publishers Inc., 1990)

6.   It is also wise to have ammonia ampules or smelling salts nearby for the occasional patient who becomes light-headed or faints at the sight of their own blood.

7.   Prepare labels for the tubes prior to the procedure.

PROCEDURE FOR VENIPUNCTURE

As with any procedure, after assembling the equipment necessary, explain the procedure to the patient. People are always more cooperative when they understand what you are trying to do.

1. **Wash and dry hands thoroughly and put on gloves.**
2. **Properly identify the patient.**
3. After positioning the patient in a chair, with the arm supported, **observe the patient's arm for possible venipuncture sites.** If the patient complains of feeling faint prior to the beginning of the procedure or relates a history of fainting while having blood drawn, it may be wise to have the patient lie down. This will help avoid the danger of a fall should the patient faint. Observe for veins that have a smooth, straight contour, free of bumps and **tortuousness.** Bumpy areas often are indicative of valves in the vessel that can be damaged by penetration of the needle. Often patients can tell you where the "best" sites are. Avoid areas of scar tissue or edematous areas. The most common sites are located in the antecubital area, where the cephalic and basilic veins are large and relatively free of tortuousness (Figure 13.3). Veins also may be used in the forearm, wrist, and hand, but these sites are always secondary choices. Venipuncture of veins in the hand is generally painful for the patient due to increased skin toughness and proximity of nerves and tendons to the venous structures.

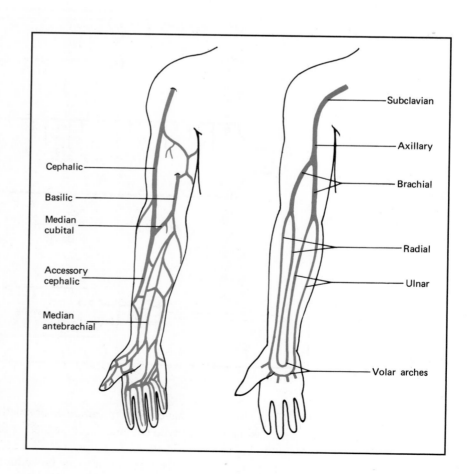

Figure 13.3 Location of basilic and cephalic veins in the arm (Reproduced with permission from Burke, *Human Anatomy and Physiology in Health and Disease*, 3rd Ed., Delmar Publishers Inc., 1992)

4. Once you have identified a potential site, or if you have difficulty locating a potential site, **apply a tourniquet** approximately six inches above the anticipated site for venipuncture (Figure 13.4). Tie the tourniquet tight enough to allow filling of the veins but never tight enough to occlude the distal arterial pulses. Initially, you will probably have to palpate pulses, but with experience you will develop a "feel" for the tension needed with the tourniquet. Obese people and dark-skinned people offer the greatest challenge in locating a vein. Often you may not locate the vein visually, but by palpating with the pads of your first three fingers you can generally locate a soft, "springy" area, the telltale location of a vein. If the tourniquet has been on for a while during your search for a vessel, release the tourniquet for a few seconds and reapply before performing the procedure. If the vein has been difficult to locate, make a mental note of some landmark in the general area to allow you to find it quickly during the procedure. When all else fails, look at your own veins and compare their location to the patient's arm for a starting point. Try to be discreet when using this technique, since it's not known for building your patient's confidence.

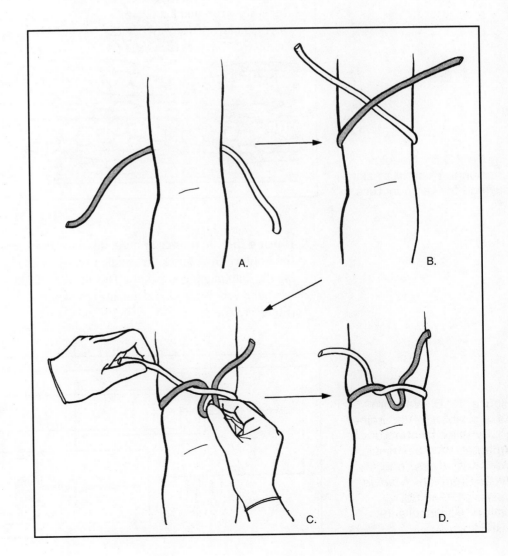

Figure 13.4 Application of a tourniquet (Reproduced with permission from Walters, Estridge, and Reynolds, *Basic Medical Laboratory Techniques, 2nd Ed.,* Delmar Publishers Inc., 1990)

5. **Cleanse the site with alcohol** (benzalkonium chloride if drawing to determine a legal blood alcohol level), using a circular pattern starting at the anticipated site of puncture and moving outward.

6. **Locate the vein beneath the skin surface and hold the barrel of the syringe or the vacutainer holder so that the needle is oriented at a 30-degree angle to the skin surface** with the beveled edge of the needle pointed upward (Figure 13.5). Do not remove your gloves thinking you cannot feel veins with gloves on. Latex gloves are very thin, and human beings are very adaptable. You will learn to palpate veins with gloves on if you work at it. The danger of disease from contact with a patient's blood is much too great a risk to work without gloves.

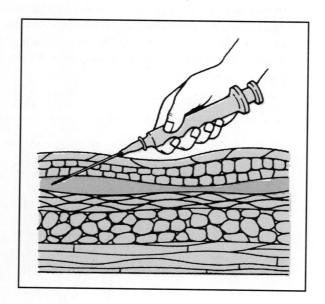

Figure 13.5 Needle position in relation to skin surface for venipuncture

7. **If using the vacutainer system, advance the vacuum tube to the guideline of the holder.** This causes the needle to fully imbed in the stopper without puncturing the diaphragm completely. This prevents leakage of blood into the holder when the vein is punctured and also prevents leakage of vacuum from the tube (Figure 13.6).

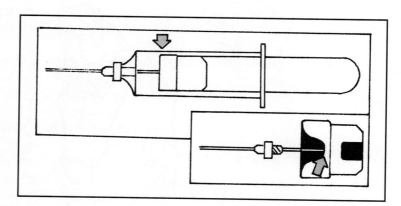

Figure 13.6 Vacuum tube position in Vacutainer holder prior to puncture (Adapted with permission from Keir, Wise, and Krebs-Shannon, *Medical Assisting,* 2nd Ed., Delmar Publishers Inc., 1989)

8. **If using a syringe and needle, depress the plunger of the syringe completely**, so that no air is in the barrel of the syringe.
9. **Enter the skin with a smooth firm movement**. The needle may be positioned directly over the vein or slightly to one side of the vein, depending on your personal preference. As soon as the needle is imbedded in tissue, advance the vacutainer tube with the thumb to puncture the diaphragm of the stopper (Figure 13.7).

Figure 13.7 Vacuum tube advancement to puncture diaphragm of tube after tissue penetration (Adapted with permission from Keir, Wise, and Krebs-Shannon, *Medical Assisting,* 2nd Ed., Delmar Publishers Inc., 1989)

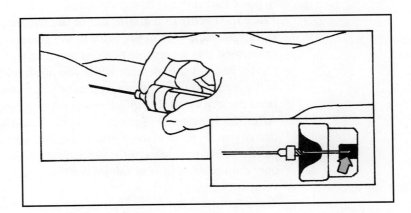

10. **Advance the needle smoothly and gently toward the vein**. As **intima** is penetrated, there will be slight resistance. Often a small "pop" is felt. Move the barrel of the syringe or the vacutainer holder closer to the skin surface and advance the needle slightly so that it is well seated in the vein. Particularly with patients who are obese, veins tend to "roll" or move away from the needle. In these cases, it is sometimes helpful to apply gentle traction with the fingers to the skin proximal to the puncture site in order to hold the vessel in place. If you are unable to locate a vein, you may make another attempt after applying a fresh sterile needle. The general rule for attempting to perform a venipuncture is: "If you cannot locate a vein in two attempts, let someone else try." Some patients are difficult to draw, and some days are better than others. Avoid traumatizing the patient because of your inability to hit a vein.
11. **With the vacutainer system blood will begin to flow into the tube at this point.** (If unable to locate the vein, you may conserve the vacuum in the tube by withdrawing the tube from the needle prior to withdrawing the needle from tissue.) Tubes may be changed as necessary while holding the needle and vacutainer holder firmly in place.
12. **If a syringe and needle are being used, apply gentle traction** to the plunger of the syringe, allowing the syringe to fill at a slow, steady rate. Too much traction can **hemolyze** the specimen, making the blood unusable for some tests. The syringe and needle method is frequently used when drawing blood from a small vein since vacutainer pressures can cause damage to small veins and so are seldom used in this instance.
13. **If the patient faints during the procedure, withdraw the needle immediately**, apply a pressure dressing to the site, and assist the patient to a lying position. If unable to arouse the patient, break an ammonia ampule and wave it

gently under the patient's nose. Before continuing, the patient should be examined by a physician.

14. **If the patient complains of dizziness or feels faint after the procedure it is usually helpful to have the patient place the head between the knees, increasing the flow of blood to the head.**

15. **When the specimen(s) have been obtained, release the tourniquet immediately.** Place a cotton ball or rolled gauze pad over the puncture site and apply gentle pressure while withdrawing the needle. Tourniquets should never be left in place longer than one minute.

16. **Place the needle in a holder out of the way to prevent a "needle stick" injury and apply firm pressure to the puncture site while elevating the extremity.** It is acceptable to enlist the assistance of the patient, allowing the patient to apply the pressure while you finish with the specimens. If the site is in the antecubital area, place a piece of gauze over the site and have the patient bend the arm upward at the elbow to apply pressure to the site.

17. **After thirty seconds of pressure, apply a bandaid to the site** with the cotton ball or gauze still in place, forming a small pressure dressing, and instruct the patient to leave the bandaid in place for an hour or two. Following this procedure eliminates or at least minimizes the development of a **hematoma** at the venipuncture site.

18. **Transfer blood from the syringe to vacuum tubes. Label all vacuum tubes** with the patient's name, physician's name, date, test desired, and your initials and route specimens to the lab for processing.

19. **Discard all sharps in the proper container, discard soiled items in the appropriate contaminated waste container, remove gloves, and wash and dry hands thoroughly.**

Capillary Puncture

Capillary puncture is used when only a very small amount of blood is needed to perform a laboratory test. The capillary beds are composed of a network of minute vessels that link arterioles to venules (Figure 13.8). The capillary bed is the area in which the exchange of oxygen from arterioles to tissue takes place and the exchange of waste products from tissue to venules takes place. This area is an excellent source for measuring the body's balance of nutrients and waste products.

One of the tests performed from capillary puncture measures the ability of the **neonate** to metabolize **phenylalinine**, an amino acid. The test, for **PKU** (phenylketonuria), is required by law in most states in the United States and most provinces in Canada. This disease, if not discovered and treated, can result in mental retardation.

The **hematocrit**, representing percentage of red blood cells as compared to the total blood volume, may also be tested by capillary puncture. A low hematocrit is found in anemia, and a sharply elevated hematocrit is indicative of **polycythemia**, often associated with advanced Chronic Obstructive Pulmonary Disease.

Hemoglobin, a protein found in erythrocites, is responsible for the transport of oxygen in the blood stream. With the aid of a hemoglobinometer, the level of hemoglobin can be determined from capillary puncture.

Depending on the equipment available, other components of the complete blood count (CBC) can be determined. These include white cell counts, platelet counts, total granulocyte count, total mono/lymph count, percentage granulocytes, and percentage mono/lymph.

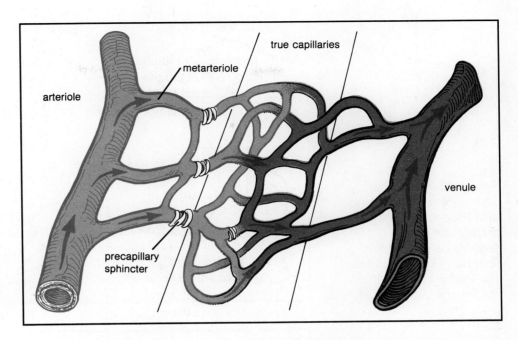

Figure 13.8 Capillary bed (Reproduced with permission from Fong, Ferris, and Skelley, *Body Structures and Functions,* 7th Ed., Delmar Publishers Inc., 1989)

The level of blood glucose also can be determined by capillary puncture, using either reagent strips or glucometers. Until very recently, diabetic patients were forced to rely on urine testing for home monitoring of blood sugar levels. But by the time sugar is detected in the urine, blood sugar levels can be dangerously high; and urine testing is not as accurate as blood testing for glucose. With new technology, glucometers are available to the general public for a reasonable price. These machines boast an accuracy rating of plus or minus two percent on a drawn blood sugar. This allows the diabetic to monitor sugar levels at home with more accuracy, making control of the disease an easier task, particularly in the case of the brittle diabetic.

EQUIPMENT AND SUPPLIES

The equipment and supplies needed for capillary puncture are compact and easily carried in a small hand tray. Prior to beginning the procedure, the medical assistant should assemble:

1. Alcohol pledgets
2. Sterile **lancets**
3. **Autolet** device (optional; Figure 13.9)
4. Gauze pads
5. Latex gloves
6. Supplies for the particular test that you are to perform (supplies vary with the test performed and are covered under the area of individual tests).

Capillary blood may be obtained from the earlobe or the fingertips of the two middle fingers in an adult or from the heel of the foot or great toe in infants. The index finger is avoided because of the large concentration of neuroreceptors found at the tip; the thumb is generally too calloused; and the little finger affords a very small area of capillary beds and likely will not yield a large enough sample to perform the test desired. When using the middle two fingers of the hand, avoid the area of the pad at the fingertip. This area contains a large concentration of sensitive neuroreceptors and will cause lingering pain for the patient. Use the sides of the fingertip between the nail and pad. The earlobe is much less sensitive than the fingertip (Figure 13.10).

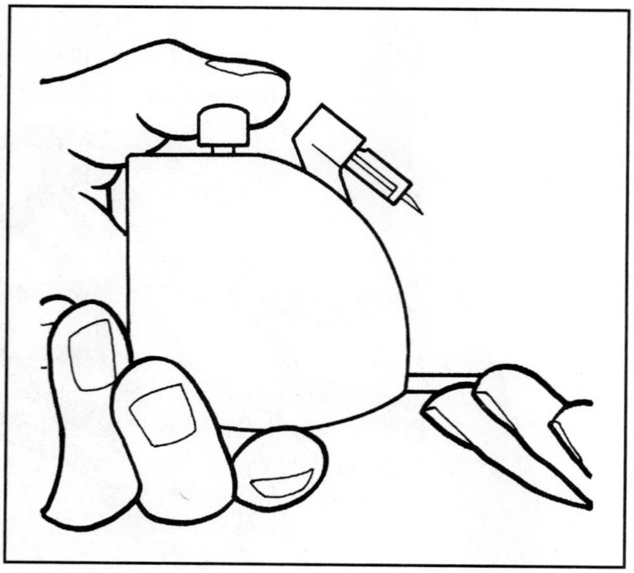

Figure 13.9 Autolet device for capillary puncture (Reproduced with permission from Keir, Wise, and Krebs-Shannon, *Medical Assisting,* 2nd Ed., Delmar Publishers Inc., 1989)

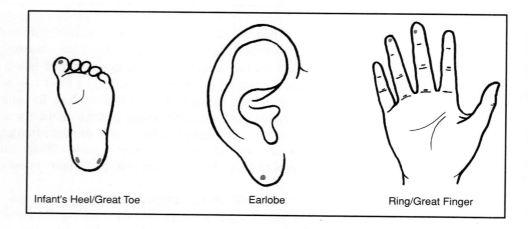

Figure 13.10 Sites for capillary puncture (Adapted with permission from Keir, Wise, and Krebs-Shannon, *Medical Assisting,* 2nd Ed., Delmar Publishers Inc., 1989)

Infant's Heel/Great Toe   Earlobe   Ring/Great Finger

PROCEDURE FOR CAPILLARY PUNCTURE

The procedure for obtaining a capillary specimen is the same for all tests, but the handling of the specimen varies with each test. To obtain a capillary specimen, the medical assistant should follow these steps.

1. **Wash and dry hands thoroughly and put on gloves.**
2. **Properly identify the patient, and explain the procedure.**
3. **Examine the patient and select a site.** Avoid areas with scarring or edema. Ask the patient if the patient has a preferred site.
4. **If the patient is an adult, show them to a seat; if the patient is an infant, have one of the parents hold the child.**
5. **Cleanse the site with alcohol and allow to air dry.** If instructing the patient to perform this procedure at home, teach them to clean the area thoroughly with soap and water. When used repeatedly, alcohol causes the skin to become thick and hard.
6. **If an Autolet is to be used, place a sterile lancet in the device and remove the protective cover from the sharp edge.** Avoid contamination of the sharp

edge. If the tip is contaminated, discard the lancet and use another. Lancets for use in Autolet devices come in various lengths and are color coded. Choose the correct length for the situation. The short lancet will not be effective for a mechanic with calloused hands, and the longer lancets will be more than is necessary for an infant or elderly woman. Cock the device. Hold the area adjacent to the site firmly with the thumb and forefinger of one hand; use the other hand to press the Autolet against the desired site and trigger the device, allowing the lancet to pierce the skin.

7. **If the lancet is to be used alone, remove the protective cover from the sharp edge.** Avoid contamination of the sharp edge. If the tip is contaminated, discard the lancet and use another. Hold the area adjacent to the site firmly with the thumb and forefinger of one hand; hold the lancet between the thumb and forefinger of the other hand with the sharp tip pointed downward. Puncture the site with a steady downward motion and withdraw the lancet. Be firm, not brutal.

8. **Holding the finger down will increase the flow.** Discard the first drop of blood by wiping with a small gauze pad. This keeps serous fluid from contaminating the sample. Gentle pressure adjacent to the site with the finger will increase the blood flow. Too much pressure will dilute the specimen with serous fluid and cause contamination. Remember to keep a firm hold on the area until the specimen is collected. This is particularly important with infants; they don't know much, but they generally know that they don't like this procedure.

9. **When the sample has been collected, clean the area once again with an alcohol pledget** and have the patient or parent hold a small gauze pad over the site while you continue with the specimen. Be sure to check that the bleeding has stopped.

10. **Discard all used materials in the proper receptacle.** Remember that lancets are sharp, so they go in the sharps container.

11. **Remove and discard gloves; wash and dry your hands.**

PKU

In addition to the equipment needed for the PKU procedure, you will need the PKU blood test form supplied by the local department of public health. There is an area on the card in which a drop of blood is to be placed in each of three circles. The goal is to saturate these three areas completely with the sample. Please remember to use a sufficient amount of blood to accomplish this. This test is generally performed in the hospital nursery shortly after birth, but there may be occasions when the test will be performed in the physician's office.

Procedure for PKU Test
1. **Obtain the form for the test from the parent of the child.**
2. **Make the capillary puncture as directed,** using the heel or great toe of the infant, while the parent holds the child.
3. **After discarding the first drop, allow one drop to fall on the card in each of the three circles.** This requires having a firm grip on the child. With practice, either it will become easier or your ability to hit a moving target will improve.

4. **Forward** the PKU form to the public health agency by mail; analyze the test, report the results to the physician, and place them in the child's medical record (Figure 13.11).

Blood Glucose

Blood glucose may be measured after fasting (the patient has not eaten or drunk for a period of eight to twelve hours prior to the test), as post prandial (two hours after a meal), or randomly (at any time). Normal values vary based on the type of test performed.

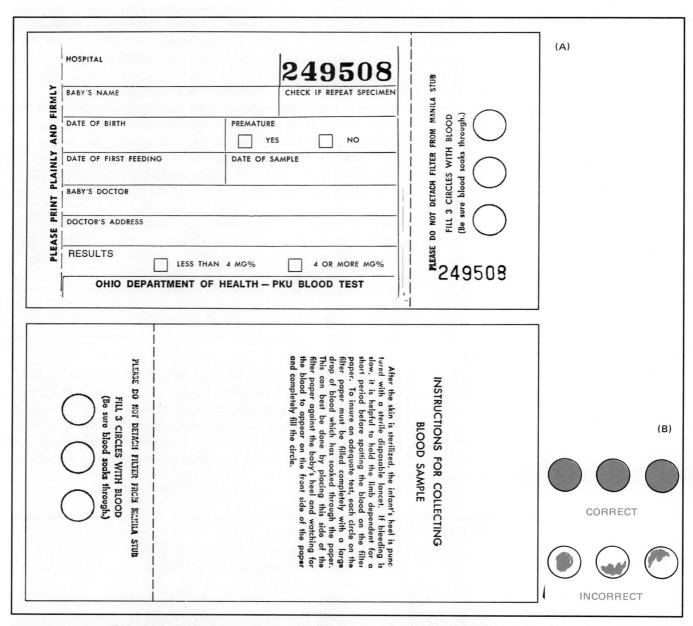

Figure 13.11 PKU blood test form: (A) Instructions and questions. (B) Circles. (Reproduced with permission from Keir, Wise, and Krebs-Shannon, *Medical Assisting,* 2nd Ed., Delmar Publishers Inc., 1989)

In addition to the equipment for collecting the capillary specimen, you will need a bottle of reagent strips or a glucometer system.

PROCEDURE FOR BLOOD GLUCOSE TEST

1. **Make the capillary puncture as directed**.
2. **Discard the first drop of blood.**
3. **If using reagent strips, read the directions carefully on the container before beginning the test**. Most strips require that a hanging drop of blood be placed on the test pad of the strip. After waiting a specified amount of time, wipe the specimen off the pad with a cotton ball or tissue and take a reading after waiting a short period. The test pad changes color and is compared to a scale on the side of the container. Record the results in the patient's chart.
4. **If using a glucometer system, become familiar with the instructions before attempting to perform the test**. Most systems have a reagent strip that must be placed in the machine with the sample in place. The reagent strips have a number code on the side of the container that must agree with the number code in the machine in order for the test to be accurate. You may need to calibrate the machine before performing the test. Most glucometers require that a hanging drop of blood be placed on the test area. Some require that the blood be wiped from the reagent strip prior to placing in the machine; others do not. The machine generally gives a digital readout of the patient's blood glucose level. Record this value in the patient's chart. Most of the glucometers on the market are able to read a level within a certain range; values above or below this range must be obtained by a venous draw. Be familiar with the equipment that you use and follow the manufacturer's instructions (Figure 13.12).

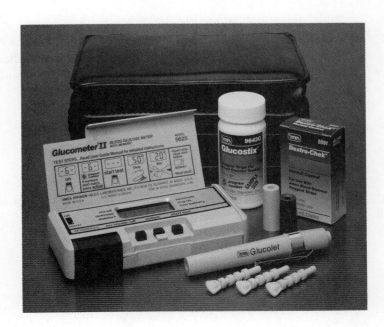

Figure 13.12
Glucometer (Courtesy Miles Laboratory)

GLUCOSE TOLERANCE TEST (GTT)

The glucose tolerance test measures the patient's ability to metabolize sugar. Usually the patient is placed on a high carbohydrate diet for seventy-two hours prior to the test. The night before the test, the patient is required to fast—nothing by mouth, not even water. It is generally the responsibility of the medical assistant to explain the diet and the pretest fast to the patient. Be explicit! Cover the instructions one by one and question the patient to be sure the patient understands what to do.

On the morning of the test, the patient arrives and a fasting blood sample and urine sample are collected. The blood glucose specimen is often collected by the capillary method. The patient is given a solution containing 100 grams of glucose and must drink all of the solution.

One half-hour later, another urine sample and blood glucose are measured. At the one hour point and every hour thereafter, the urine and blood are tested for glucose. At the end of six hours, the test is complete. The method of testing glucose varies from one office to another, but the most popular method is by capillary testing because of the number of samples needed and the accuracy of glucometers (Figure 13.13).

DATE	PATIENT		ADDRESS	

☐ GLUCOSE TOLERANCE TEST _____ HOURS

TIME	BLOOD SUGAR	URINE SUGAR	ACETONE	PATIENT'S CONDITION (SYMPTOMS)
FASTING	mg/100ml			
½ HR	mg/100ml			
1 HR	mg/100ml			
2 HR	mg/100ml			
3 HR	mg/100ml			
4 HR	mg/100ml			
5 HR	mg/100ml			
6 HR	mg/100ml			
PHYSICIAN		PHONE	TECHNOLOGIST	

Figure 13.13 Glucose tolerance test form (Reproduced with permission from Keir, Wise, and Krebs-Shannon, *Medical Assisting*, 2nd Ed., Delmar Publishers Inc., 1989)

BLOOD COUNTS

Capillary puncture may be used to measure various components of the blood count. For these tests microhematocrit tubes or blood capillary tubes and pipettes are needed in addition to the other equipment outlined for a capillary puncture. The procedure is outlined in Chapter 14, "Laboratory Examinations."

**REVIEW/
SELF-EXAMINATION**

1. For what purpose may a medical assistant perform venipuncture?

2. Under what circumstances may a medical assistant perform an arterial puncture?

3. Name two methods used for collecting specimens by venipuncture.

4. What difference in technique is used when drawing a sample to test for legal blood alcohol level?

5. What is the longest length of time that a tourniquet should be left in place?

6. What should you do when you cannot see the vein?

7. How long should pressure be applied to the venipuncture site?

8. At what angle to the skin surface should the needle be oriented when preparing to make a venipuncture?

9. What action should you take if you must make a second venipuncture?

10. How many attempts can you make to locate a vein before you ask someone for assistance?

11. When should a tourniquet be removed?

12. What prevents blood from leaking into the vacutainer holder?

13. Where is the most common site to make a venipuncture?

14. What areas should be avoided when choosing a venipuncture site?

15. What action should you take if a patient faints during the procedure?

16. What action should you take if the patient complains of dizziness after the procedure?

17. What is the purpose of capillary puncture?

18. What sites are used for this procedure?

19. Name three tests performed by capillary puncture.

20. What difference in the procedure should be taught to patients for home use? Why?

21. What component of blood is responsible for oxygen transport?

22. When are PKU tests performed? Why?

23. What agency is responsible for the PKU test?

24. What is the normal range for hematocrit in males? Females?

25. What is a glucose tolerance test?

26. Why is the first droplet of blood discarded when performing capillary puncture?

27. What is a lancet?

28. What areas should be avoided when performing capillary puncture?

CHAPTER 14

Laboratory Examinations

OBJECTIVES

On completion of this chapter, you will be able to:
- Perform three routine laboratory tests.
- Demonstrate specimen collection techniques.
- Demonstrate correct handling of specimens.
- Explain the rules for laboratory safety.
- Identify common laboratory tests.
- Explain the need for proper collection and handling of specimens.

**Vocabulary—
Glossary of Terms**

Acid	Sour; pH 1–7, acid causative.
Agglutinin	Antibody that agglutinates an antigen.
Agglutinogen	A substance that stimulates the production of agglutinin.
Bacteriology	Study of bacteria.
Base	Nonacid part of a salt; pH 7–14, alkaline.
Basophil	Cell with attraction for basic dye.
Biohazard	Biological threat.
Caustic	Burning.
Corrosive	Destructive to tissues.
Culture	Propagation of microorganisms or living tissue on special media.
Dyscrasia	Abnormal or pathological blood condition.
Eosinophil	Granulocyte with affinity for eosin dye.
Erythrocyte	Red blood cell; biconcave disk that acts as oxygen transport.
Excreta	Waste material.
Hematocrit	Volume percentage of erythrocytes in whole blood.
Hemoglobin	Oxygen-carrying pigment of erythrocytes.

Leukocyte	White blood cell.
Lymphocyte	Mononuclear leukocyte.
Monocyte	Mononuclear, phagocytic leukocyte.
Neutrophil	Polymorphonuclear leukocyte.
Pipette	Glass or plastic tube used in measuring or transferring liquid in small quantities.
Platelet	Thrombocyte.
Reagent	A substance used to produce a chemical reaction.
Serum	Clear liquid portion of blood.
Thrombocyte	Clotting cell.
Volatile	Capable of evaporating rapidly; unstable.

T he Clinical Laboratory Improvements Act of 1988 (CLIA) has had an impact on more than 300,000 medical laboratories, including those in physician offices, under federal standards and regulations written by the Department of Health and Human Services, released in 1990. These regulations are aimed at assuring the quality and accuracy of medical tests. Under the new regulations, every laboratory, regardless of its location, must be federally certified as meeting quality standards. Laboratory tests are divided into three categories. High-risk tests such as Pap smears and simpler tests such as cholesterol screening. Low-risk tests such as dipstick urinalysis are exempt from regulation. This means that most laboratory tests will have to be performed in certified laboratories by certified laboratory technicians and will no longer be performed by nonlicensed or noncertified personnel in the medical office or screening sites. Laboratories failing to comply with federal requirements for quality control and personnel qualifications could have their certification revoked or suspended. Each state will specify and adopt standards to comply with the federal requirements.

The regulations mean that much of the testing previously performed by the medical assistant in the medical office will now have to be performed by licensed or certified laboratory technicians. The medical assistant will still be responsible for the collection and handling of specimens to be processed by the laboratory. Physician office laboratories (POLs) probably will be required to maintain a licensed or certified laboratory technician on staff to assure that the quality of the in-house laboratory testing meets the federal requirements.

Testing that will continue to be performed by the medical assistant is covered in this chapter. In addition, some testing that has been performed by the medical assistant in physician office laboratories, is also included, with the understanding that once the states implement the Clinical Laboratory Improvements Act (CLIA) some of these tests may no longer be performed by the medical assistant. The medical assistant is responsible for knowing state law and which laboratory tests a medical assistant may perform.

Laboratory examinations are performed on body **excreta**, fluids, **serums**, scrapings from internal or external lesions, or biopsy materials. This material is always considered a possible source of contamination, and its handling requires extreme care to prevent contamination of the individual performing the examinations. Most accidents that occur in a laboratory do not just happen but are the result of carelessness. Use of the Universal Precautions System is of paramount importance in the collection and handling of laboratory specimens.

Laboratory Safety Rules

Personnel working in the laboratory should be reminded continually of safety precautions. The exercise of caution and good technique combined with common sense will overcome many of the potential hazards of the laboratory. Adherence to the following rules will prevent many laboratory accidents:

1. *Wear disposable gloves at all times when collecting and handling laboratory specimens.* This is to protect you as well as the patient from the transmission of AIDS and other diseases. If there is a high risk from possible spill or other accident, wear a disposable gown, mask, and eye protectors.

2. *All containers should be labeled properly.* The term **biohazard** denotes infectious material or agents that present a risk or potential risk to human health. Biological infections frequently are transmitted by accidental oral aspiration of material via a **pipette**, by accidental inoculation with contaminated needles or instruments, by sprays from syringes, or by accidents with a centrifuge. Cuts and scratches from contaminated glassware are also sources of infection. Chemicals that are used to perform tests also should be labeled properly.

3. *Chemicals and reagents used to perform laboratory examinations should be stored properly.* Many of these agents are inflammable solvents, such as ether and acetone, and have a potential for fire and explosion. Others are **caustic, corrosive**, poisonous, or **volatile**, such as strong **acids** and **bases**.

4. *Handle all chemicals and reagents with care.* Many of these chemicals and reagents have toxic fumes and a potential to burn and cause blindness.

5. *Keep working fire extinguishers available* for any type of chemical or other fire and be sure that everyone is instructed in their correct use.

6. *Be sure that the work area is kept clean and free from clutter.* A strong bleach solution can be used to clean the area of spills. All glassware should be cleaned with soap and water following use. Discard any glassware that is damaged or broken. Stainless steel containers should be cleaned with a strong detergent solution, such as 3% phenolic detergent, then rinsed and dried thoroughly.

7. *Pipet all solutions using mechanical suction.* Never use mouth suction.

8. *Never store or use inflammable substances near an open flame, heater, or water heater.*

9. *Wipe up spills immediately.* Spills on the floor can result in serious falls.

10. *Pour liquids carefully to prevent spills.*

11. *Wear gloves when cleaning glassware* in case there is broken or damaged glassware.

12. *Wash hands frequently, especially after handling patient specimens.* Always wash hands before leaving the laboratory.

13. *Know the basic first-aid procedures for laboratory accidents,* such as cuts and burns.

Collection of Specimens

In collecting blood for morphologic studies in hematology, capillary or peripheral blood can be obtained from the fingertip, earlobe, heel, or big toe. This kind of sampling is called *microsampling* and is preferred for the newborn infant or small child who has a small blood supply, so removal by venipuncture would deplete too much blood. These methods may also be employed with adults when collection of a small quantity of blood is preferable. Collection from most adults and older children is by venipuncture using a Vacutainer and the appropriate tube(s).

Disposable blood-diluting units such as Unopette, which consist of a prefilled reservoir containing a premeasured diluting fluid, capillary pipette, and pipette shield are available. Unopettes are available for counting **erythrocytes, leukocytes,** and **plateletes.** Package inserts contain detailed instructions that when correctly followed result in accurate dilution.

The Vacutainer system is the most commonly used venous blood collection method. It consists of evacuate tubes of various sizes with color-coded tops indicative of the tubes' contents, sterile disposable double-ended needles of different lengths and gauges, and reusable plastic adapters that hold the needle and guide the tubes. They are available in both pediatric and adult sizes. Vacutainer stopper colors are indicative of the following contents:

Color	Contents
Red	None
Royal blue	Chemically clean
Black/red mottled	Serum-separator gel
Black/yellow mottled	Clot activator, separator gel
Light blue	Citrate
Lavender	EDTA (anticoagulant)
Black	Balanced oxalate
Green	Heparin
Gray	Fluoride

All tubes with contents must be mixed thoroughly by gentle inversion following blood collection. Always check the specimen requirements provided by the laboratory that will be performing your tests.

PROCEDURE FOR SPECIMEN COLLECTION
1. **Have the necessary equipment available.**
2. **Explain the procedure to the patient or to the parent(s) or guardian of the child.**
3. **Wash and dry hands thoroughly. Put on gloves.**
4. **If using a Vacutainer, be sure to use the appropriate tube(s).**
5. **Record the information on the patient's chart** as to the date and time the specimens were collected and for which test. Sign your name or initial your entry (Figure 14.1).

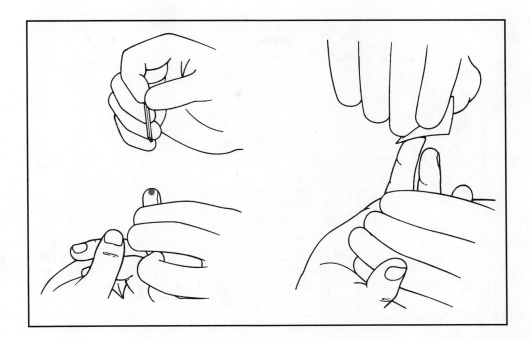

Figure 14.1 Collecting a blood specimen: (left) puncturing the finger; (right) using sterile gauze to stop the bleeding

HANDLING OF SPECIMENS

Once specimens are properly collected, they may be labeled with the patient's name, date of collection, and any other information necessary, then sent to a clinical laboratory for testing. Blood counts performed in a clinical laboratory are among the tests that are now computer automated.

Each specimen container should be labeled with the patient's name, age, date and time of collection, and specific test requested. When submitting specimens to a laboratory, accompany them with a requisition containing the following information:

1. Physician—name, address, telephone number, account number (if any).
2. Patient—full name, address, telephone number, insurance information, date of birth, and sex.
3. Date and time of collection.
4. Specific test required.
5. Tentative diagnosis.
6. Any medications currently being taken by the patient.
7. Indicate if STAT results are required.

If the laboratory the medical office uses is located in the same city or general area, it will probably have a daily specimen pickup service. Have all specimens properly labeled and requisition slips ready for the laboratory at the appointed time.

Specimens to be mailed must be packaged carefully to prevent damage to contents and contamination of handlers. Lids should be taped shut. Tubes and vials and other containers should be wrapped in absorbent material. All specimens should be placed in a second container for transport. The requisition slip normally is placed inside the outermost wrapping (Figure 14.2).

Slide Agglutination Tests

The adult human has about 5–6 liters or 10–12 pints of blood, consisting of formed elements or blood cells that make up about 45% of blood volume and a liquid portion called *plasma* that makes up about 55% of blood volume. Red blood cell membranes contain a myriad of different proteins and carbohydrates that are capable

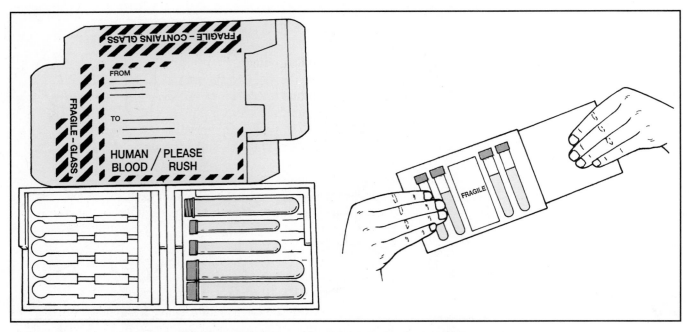

Figure 14.2 Specimens prepared for the laboratory

of provoking antibody formation. For this reason it is necessary to know the blood type of a pregnant woman and of an individual prior to transfusion.

Karl Landsteiner, an Austrian-born American pathologist, discovered in 1900 the ABO system of typing blood. Under this system there are four main blood types, A, B, AB, and O, and several minor types. The letters refer to the kind of **agglutinogen** present in the red blood cells. The major antigens are called A and B; the major antibodies are anti-A and anti-B. The genes that determine the presence or absence of A or B activity reside on chromosome number 9. Type A blood has A agglutinogen, B has B agglutinogen. AB has both A and B agglutinogen, and O has no agglutinogen. All humans have in their serum **agglutinins**, which react with all types of agglutinogen not present in their own cells. Thus, A blood has anti-B agglutinin, B blood has anti-A agglutinin, AB has no agglutinin, and O has both anti-A and anti-B agglutinin. When agglutinins, in sufficient concentration, come in contact with the corresponding agglutinogen, *agglutination* (clumping) of the red cells occurs, followed by rapid destruction of these cells, which often results in death.

In recent years, additional blood types have been found, and probably even more will be discovered. Their importance is still under dispute, but they are sometimes used with other groups in determining paternity.

The Rh or *rhesus factor* was first discovered on the red cells of the rhesus monkey and is found in conjunction with any one of the main blood types. Presence of the Rh factor is designated as Rh+, its absence as Rh−. The serum of an Rh− person does not contain significant amounts of anti-Rh agglutinins unless there has been previous exposure to Rh+ blood. This previous exposure may have been a transfusion or injection of Rh+ blood or pregnancy with an Rh+ fetus. With exposure to Rh+ blood, the Rh− person gradually builds up a high titer of anti-Rh agglutinins. In some cases, anti-Rh agglutinin readily crosses the placental barrier, which results in erythroblastosis fetalis (destruction of the infant's red cells) in Rh+ babies born to Rh− mothers.

PROCEDURE FOR ABO, RH SPECIMEN COLLECTION

1. **Have the necessary equipment available.**
2. **Explain the procedure to the patient.**
3. **Wash and dry your hands thoroughly. Put on gloves.**
4. **If using vacuum tube method of collection,** utilize a red-stoppered tube, which does not contain an anticoagulant.
5. **If using venipuncture with the syringe method, transfer the specimen to a collection tube that does not contain an anticoagulant.**
6. **Remove and dispose of gloves.**
7. **Wash and dry hands thoroughly.**
8. **Prepare specimens for processing by the laboratory.**
9. **Record the specimen collection method on the patient's chart and sign or initial your entry.**

PROCEDURE FOR ABO AND RH TYPING

1. **Remove the antiserum from the refrigerator,** where it should be stored. Check the antiserum package expiration date. Discard if out of date. Read the directions carefully. Allow the antiserum to reach room temperature.
2. **Wash and dry hands thoroughly. Put on gloves.**
3. **Assemble necessary equipment and supplies.** The equipment will include two clean, lint-free slides, a colored wax pencil, wooden applicator sticks, an optional rocker board, and the antiserum.
4. **Follow the antiserum package directions explicitly.** Prepare the slides by using the colored wax pencil to label the slides with the patient's name. Using the wax pencil, make two large circles on one of the slides and one large circle on the other. Make sure the outline of the circles is thick enough to prevent the blood from breaking out of the circle. Label the circles A, B, and Rh as indicated.
5. **Place one drop of anti-A serum in the circle marked A, one drop of anti-B serum in the circle marked B, one drop of anti-Rh serum in the circle marked Rh.** Using freshly drawn blood, place one drop of the patient's blood next to the drop of antiserum in each circle. Using a separate wooden applicator for each circle, quickly mix each drop of blood within the circle boundaries.
6. **Gently rock the slides by hand or on the rocker board for one minute.**
7. **Observe for agglutination as directed.** Record the information on the patient's chart, including date and time the test was performed, the antiserum used, and your name or initials.

    Group A blood—positive reaction with anti-A antiserum.
    Group B blood—positive reaction with anti-B antiserum.
    Group O blood—negative reaction with both anti-A and anti-B antiserum.
    Rh factor as positive (+) or negative (−).
8. **Clean supplies and equipment as needed.**
9. **Store supplies and equipment in appropriate place.**
10. **Remove and dispose of gloves. Wash and dry hands thoroughly.**
    (Figure 14.3).

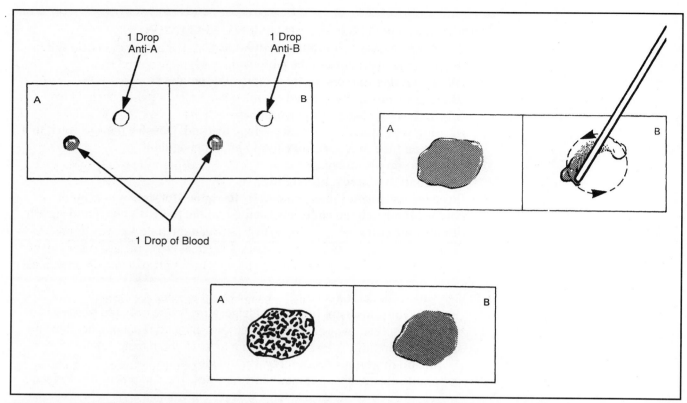

Figure 14.3 Slide test method for blood typing (Reproduced with permission from Walters, Estridge, and Reynolds, *Basic Medical Laboratory Techniques,* 2nd Ed., Delmar Publishers Inc., 1990)

Another commonly performed agglutination test is the serum test for infectious mononucleosis. There are a variety of kits prepared by various manufacturers for performing this test using serum or plasma rather than whole blood. The mono test will probably continue to be performed in the medical office by the medical assistant (Figure 14.4).

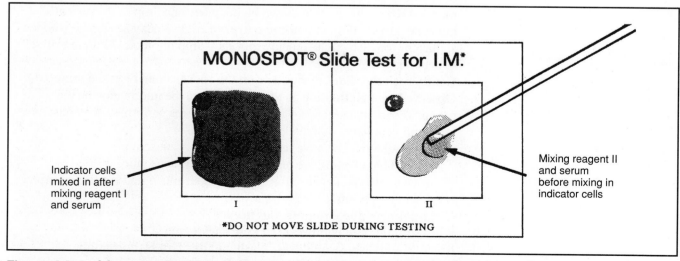

Figure 14.4 Monospot R slide test for infectious mononucleosis (Reproduced with permission from Walters, Estridge, and Reynolds, *Basic Medical Laboratory Techniques,* 2nd Ed., Delmar Publishers Inc., 1990)

PROCEDURE FOR MONO TEST: GENERAL DIRECTIONS

1. **Remove the test kit from the refrigerator.** Check the expiration date and discard if out of date. Allow the contents to reach room temperature.
2. **Once the contents have reached room temperature, wash and dry hands thoroughly and apply gloves.**
3. **Read directions thoroughly and follow explicitly.**
4. **Fill the disposable capillary tube to the calibration mark** as directed with serum or plasma from a centrifuged blood specimen.
5. **Using the bulb provided in the kit, deposit the specimen in the middle circle of the glass slide** also provided in the kit.
6. **Place one drop of negative control in the right circle and one drop of positive control in the left circle.**
7. **Mix the test reagent by rolling gently between the palms of the hands.**
8. **Holding the reagent bottle dropper in a vertical position, add one drop of reagent to each area of the slide,** being careful not to touch the dropper to the slide.
9. **Mix each area thoroughly using separate utensils as provided.**
10. **Rock the slide gently for two minutes** by hand or using a rocker.
11. **Interpret the test results.** Agglutination is positive. No agglutination is negative.
12. **Record the results on the patient's chart** and sign your name or initial the entry.
13. **Dispose of kit and contents.**
14. **Clean work area.**
15. **Remove gloves. Wash and dry hands thoroughly.**

Blood Counts

Blood counts are helpful in diagnosing many diseases and in determining the overall health of the patient. The red cell or erythrocyte count in the normal adult is 4,000,000 to 6,000,000 per cubic mm. These are the cells that contain **hemoglobin**, which is the essential carrier of oxygen in the blood. Increase in the number of erythrocytes may indicate polycythemia vera, while a decrease may be indicative of hemorrhage or one of the anemias.

Platelets or **thrombocytes** are much smaller than red cells and are necessary for the clotting of blood. Normal range in the adult is 200,000 to 500,000 per cubic mm. Reduction in platelet count is seen in conditions such as purpura and aplastic anemia. Increase in platelets is seen in fractures and certain kinds of anemias.

White blood cells or leukocytes are important in the immune reaction of the body. Increase in count is seen in infections, allergies, and certain blood disorders, while a decrease in seen in blood **dyscrasias** and drug and chemical toxicity. Normal range in the adult is 4,000 to 11,000 per cubic mm.

There are several kinds of white blood cells, which can be identified microscopically, and it is helpful to know which types of cells are increased or decreased in the presence of a particular disease or group of diseases. The granulocytes, **eosinophils, neutrophils**, and **basophils** appear to increase in bacterial infections, parasitic infestations, allergic conditions, and some blood dyscrasias, while the agranulocytes, the **lymphocytes**, and **monocytes** may be increased in such conditions as measles and Hodgkin's disease.

Blood counts may be ordered in a variety of ways: an RBC or red blood cell count, WBC or white blood cell count, platelet count, CBC or complete blood cell count, or a total of RBCs, WBCs, and platelets. The CBC with differential is a complete blood cell count with a differential count of the white blood cells (Figures 14.5 and 14.6).

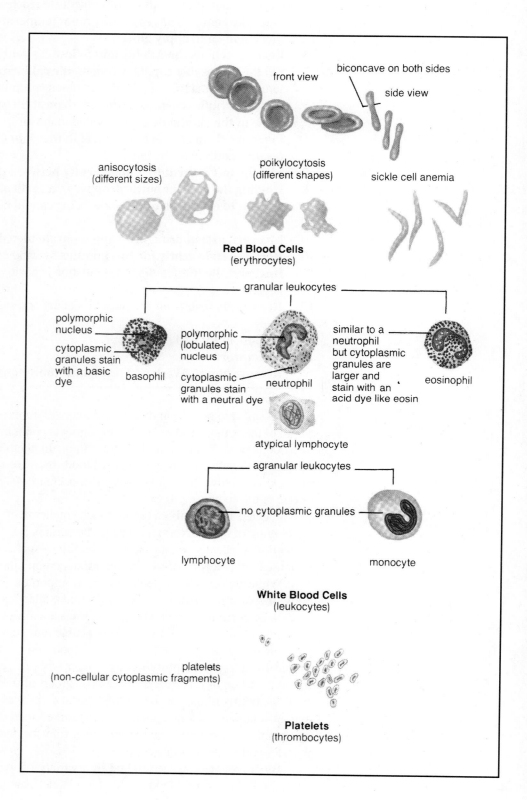

Figure 14.5 Maturation of blood cells (Reproduced with permission from Burke, *Human Anatomy and Physiology in Health and Disease*, 3rd Ed., Delmar Publishers Inc., 1992)

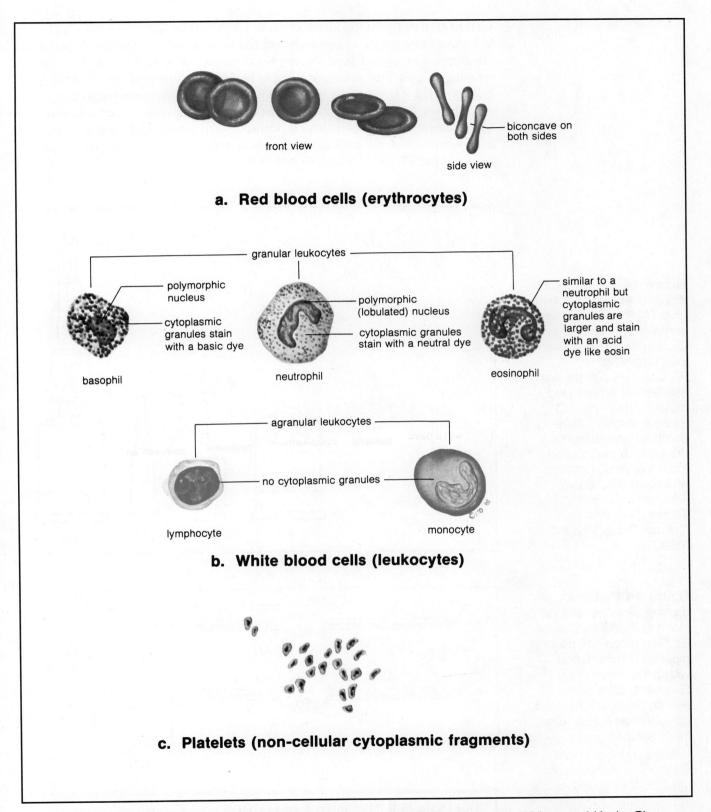

a. **Red blood cells (erythrocytes)**

biconcave on both sides

front view

side view

granular leukocytes

polymorphic nucleus

cytoplasmic granules stain with a basic dye

polymorphic (lobulated) nucleus

cytoplasmic granules stain with a neutral dye

similar to a neutrophil but cytoplasmic granules are larger and stain with an acid dye like eosin

basophil

neutrophil

eosinophil

agranular leukocytes

no cytoplasmic granules

lymphocyte

monocyte

b. **White blood cells (leukocytes)**

c. **Platelets (non-cellular cytoplasmic fragments)**

Figure 14.6   Blood cells and platelets (Reproduced with permission from Keir, Wise, and Krebs-Shannon, *Medical Assisting,* 2nd Ed., Delmar Publishers Inc., 1989)

COLLECTION OF SPECIMENS

In collecting blood for morphologic studies in hematology, capillary or peripheral blood can be obtained from the fingertip, earlobe, heel, or big toe. This kind of sampling is called microsampling and is preferred for the newborn infant or small child who has a small blood supply, so removal by venipuncture would deplete too much blood. These methods may also be employed with adults when collection of a small quantity of blood is preferable. Collection from most adults and older children is by venipuncture using a Vacutainer with lavender-stoppered tubes that contain the anticoagulant EDTA (Figures 14.7 and 14.8).

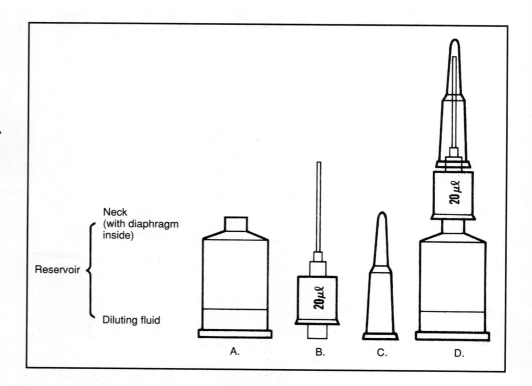

Figure 14.7 Parts of a disposable blood diluting unit: (A) Prefilled reservior containing premeasured diluting fluid and sealed with diaphragm. (B) Capillary pipette with overflow chamber and capacity marking. (C) Pipette shield. (D) Assembled unit. (Reproduced with permission from Walters, Estridge, and Reynolds, *Basic Medical Laboratory Techniques*, 2nd Ed., Delmar Publishers Inc., 1990)

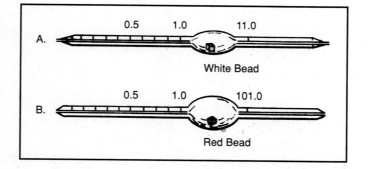

Figure 14.8 Blood diluting pipettes. (A) White blood cell diluting pipette. (B) Red blood cell diluting pipette. (Reproduced with permission from Simmers, *Diversified Health Occupations*, 2nd Ed., Delmar Publishers Inc., 1988)

PROCEDURE FOR SPECIMEN COLLECTION

1. **Have the necessary equipment available.**
2. **Explain the procedure** to the patient or to the parent(s) or guardian of the child.
3. **Wash and dry hands thoroughly. Put on gloves.**

4. **If using a Vacutainer, be sure to use the lavender-stoppered tubes that contain the anticoagulant EDTA.**
5. **Record the information on the patient's chart.** Sign or initial the entry.

HANDLING OF SPECIMENS

Once properly collected, specimens should be labeled with the patient's name, date of collection, and any other necessary information, then sent to a clinical laboratory for testing. Blood counts performed in a clinical laboratory are automated.

DIFFERENTIAL CELL COUNT

In order to study the morphology of blood cells, one must prepare blood smears by spreading a drop of blood on a clean glass slide. The best slides are prepared from capillary blood, but EDTA anticoagulant blood can be used provided the blood smear is prepared within two hours of collection (Figure 14.9).

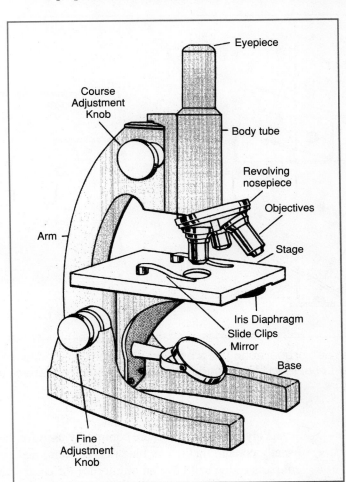

Figure 14.9 Monocular microscope (Reproduced with permission from Simmers, *Diversified Health Occupations,* 2nd Ed., Delmar Publishers Inc., 1988)

PROCEDURE FOR BLOOD SMEAR PREPARATION

1. **Wash and dry hands thoroughly. Put on gloves.**
2. **Place a drop of blood approximately one half-inch from the right end of a glass slide with a frosted end.**
3. **Using another glass slide, spread the drop of blood with a quick, smooth, sliding motion. Obtain at least three and preferably five slide smears. A**

good smear will cover up to three quarters of the slide and show a gradual transition from thick to thin with feathered edges. It will have a smooth appearance with no ridges, holes, streaks, or clumps. On microscopic examination, the cells should be evenly distributed.

4. **Allow the smear to air dry.**
5. **When the smear is dry, label the frosted end with the patient's name.**
6. **Fix the slides in methanol. This is done by dipping or dropping the fixative over the slide.** Many of the stains presently available contain the fixative in the stain, thus eliminating the need for this step in slide preparation.
7. **Remove gloves and wash and dry hands thoroughly.**
8. **Record information on the patient's chart. Sign name or initial entry** (Figure 14.10).

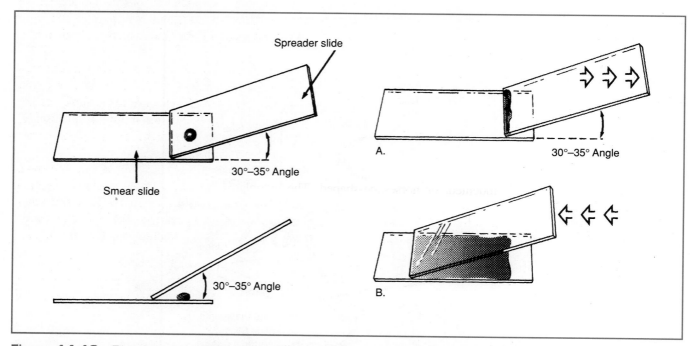

Figure 14.10 Blood smear preparation (Reproduced with permission from Walters, Estridge, and Reynolds, *Basic Medical Laboratory Techniques,* 2nd Ed., Delmar Publishers Inc., 1990)

Polychromatic stains are commonly used for the examination of blood cells and usually contain methylene blue (a blue stain) and eosin (a red-orange stain). Different parts of the cell have an affinity for different stains, which enables easier visualization and differentiation. The most commonly used differential blood stain is Wright stain.

Erythrocytes (red blood cells) are normally the most numerous cellular elements. They are anucleated, biconcave discs that should appear pinkish-tan as a result of the staining of the hemoglobin in the cell.

Thrombocytes (platelets) are the smallest of the cellular elements. Their shape is round to oval; they are anucleated, and they stain blue.

Leukocytes (white blood cells) are the largest of the cellular elements. There are five types of leukocytes, and each has its own characteristic appearance. Granulocytes contain granules in their cytoplasm and may possess segmented nuclei. *Neutrophils, eosinophils,* and *basophils* are granulocytes. Agranulocytes have few, if any, granules in their cytoplasm and nonsegmented nuclei. *Lymphocytes* and *monocytes* are agranulocytes.

Neutrophils, also known as polymorphonuclear neutrophils, segmented neutrophils, polys, and segs, are the most numerous of the leukocytes in adults. An immature form is called band or stab. The nucleus stains a dark purple; the cytoplasm is pale pink and contains fine pink or lilac granules. They are phagocytic in action and increase in many types of bacterial infections.

The nucleus of the eosinophil is divided into two or three lobes that stain purple. The cytoplasm of eosinophils stains pink and contains large round or oval red-orange granules. They are phagocytic in action and increase in allergic conditions such as asthma and hay fever and in certain parasitic infections such as amebiasis.

The basophil has a nucleus that is segmented and stains light purple. The large dark blue-black granules in the cytoplasm contain histamine, which is a part of the allergic response.

Lymphocytes are the second most numerous leukocyte in adults; in children they are the most numerous. The nucleus of the lymphocyte is usually oval or round and stains purple. The cytoplasm stains blue. Lymphocytes are responsible for the recognition of antigens and the production of antibodies for immunity to disease. They are commonly called lymphs and increase in viral infections and some bacterial infections such as tuberculosis, as well as in leukemias.

The largest white blood cell is the monocyte, whose nucleus may be oval, indented, or horseshoe-shaped. The cytoplasm stains gray-blue and may contain vacuoles. Monocytes are also called macrophages; they ingest bacteria and other debris. They increase in certain viral infections such as hepatitis, rickettsial infections such as Rocky Mountain spotted fever, and bacterial infections such as brucellosis (Figure 14.11).

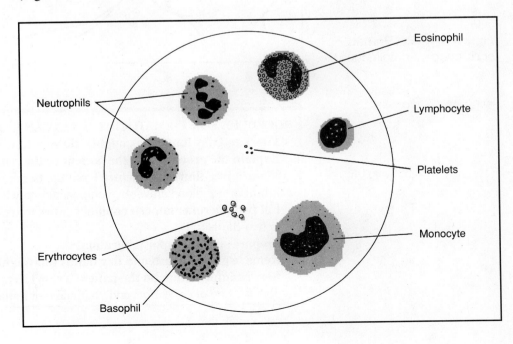

Figure 14.11 Microscopic view of a blood smear

HEMATOCRIT

The **hematocrit** (Hct) is frequently a more useful and reliable test than the erythrocyte count because there is less chance for error. The hematocrit is usually performed in association with the hemoglobin test, but in some instances, the hematocrit is performed with more regularity. This test normally is used to evaluate and classify various types of blood dyscrasias. Since the procedure requires only a small amount of blood, it is an ideal test for checking the progress of patients undergoing treatment for blood dyscrasia.

The hematocrit is a measurement of the percentage of packed erythrocytes in a volume of blood. While the normal values vary with the age and sex of the patient, the normal range is considered to be from 36% in women to 52% in men (Figure 14.12).

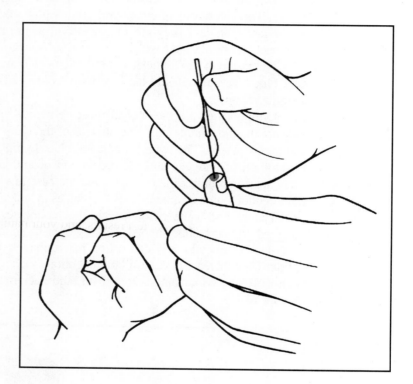

Figure 14.12 Hematocrit specimen collection

PROCEDURE FOR HEMATOCRIT SPECIMEN COLLECTION

1. **Wash and dry hands thoroughly. Be sure to wear disposable gloves.**
2. **Explain the procedure to the patient or the patient's parent(s) or guardian.**
3. **Make a free-flowing puncture from the finger of an adult or the heel of an infant** or use blood drawn by venipuncture to which EDTA has been added.
4. **Fill two microhematocrit capillary tubes to within 2 cm of the end** (one-half to two-thirds full).
5. **Prepare specimens for laboratory.**
6. **Remove gloves. Wash and dry hands thoroughly.**
7. **Record information on the patient's chart** as to the date and time of collection, method of collection, and your name or initials.

HEMOGLOBIN

Normal hemoglobin (Hgb) values vary throughout one's life but are generally considered to be within normal range if they are between 12 and 18 gm per 100 cc of blood.

Hemoglobin is the essential oxygen carrier of the blood and is also responsible for the red coloration of the blood. Decrease in hemoglobin values is frequently associated with iron-deficiency anemia. The most accurate method of measuring hemoglobin involves the use of a photometer and of a pipette and **reagent**.

Another method of determining hemoglobin value is the specific gravity technique. It requires no special instrument but gives only an estimate of hemoglobin concentration.

PROCEDURE FOR HEMOGLOBIN—SPECIFIC GRAVITY TECHNIQUE

1. **Wash and dry hands thoroughly and wear disposable gloves.**
2. **Put a drop of blood into a prepared copper sulfate solution of a particular density or specific gravity.**
3. **If the drop falls to the bottom of the container within sixty seconds, the specific gravity of the blood is greater than the specific gravity of the copper sulfate.** A normal amount of hemoglobin in the blood should cause the blood to fall rapidly. Blood with a low hemoglobin does not fall rapidly.
4. **Dispose of gloves. Wash and dry hands thoroughly.**
5. **Record information on the patient's chart** as to date and time of collection, method of collection, test results, and your name or initials.

ERYTHROCYTE SEDIMENTATION RATE

The erythrocyte sedimentation rate (ESR) measures the rate at which the erythrocytes separate from plasma and fall to the bottom of a special tube. While this test is not specific for any disease, increase in ESR is found in inflammatory conditions such as rheumatoid arthritis, rheumatic fever, some types of cancer, and hepatitis. Normal values are 15 to 20 mm/hour.

The Wintrobe method is commonly used; its equipment consists of a tube that is graduated from 0 to 100 mm and a special rack that holds the tube in a vertical position (Figure 14.13).

PROCEDURE FOR ESR USING WINTROBE METHOD

1. **Wash and dry hands thoroughly. Wear disposable gloves.**
2. **Using venous blood with the anticoagulant EDTA added, fill the Wintrobe tube to the zero mark with blood.**
3. **Place the tube upright in the rack for one hour.**
4. **At the end of the hour, measure the total distance the erythrocytes have fallen.** This is the length of the plasma column above the cells.
5. **Dispose of gloves. Wash and dry hands thoroughly.**
6. **Record type of test and findings on patient's chart,** as well as the date and time of the test and your name or initials (Figure 14.14).

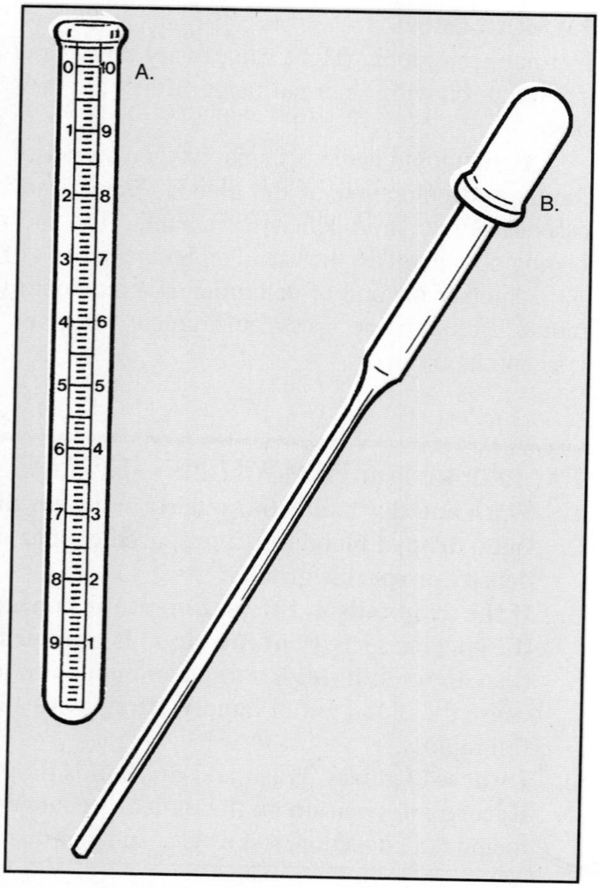

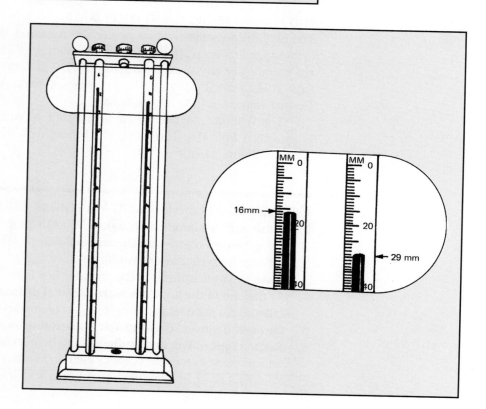

Figure 14.13 Materials used in the Wintrobe method: (A) Wintrobe sedimentation tube. (B) Long-stemmed pipette used for filling Wintrobe tube. (Reproduced with permission from Walters, Estridge, and Reynolds, *Basic Medical Laboratory Techniques,* 2nd Ed., Delmar Publishers Inc., 1990)

Figure 14.14 Reading a Wintrobe tube: the tube on the left reads 16 mm/hr, the one on the right 29 mm/hr (Reproduced with permission from Keir, Wise, and Krebs-Shannon, *Medical Assisting,* 2nd Ed., Delmar Publishers Inc., 1989)

Blood Chemistry

As mentioned earlier, it may be convenient for the medical office to do some fairly simple laboratory tests that can provide quick information to the physician to aid in diagnosis and treatment. Some of the blood chemistry tests also can be performed quickly using reagent strips available for this purpose. An example is the reagent strip used for testing blood glucose. However, the more complete chemistry tests, including serum total protein, protein electrophoresis, BUN, creatinine, uric acid, lipoproteins, bilirubin, etc., are performed in a medical laboratory.

If you are using reagent strip testing, use Universal Precautions, follow the package directions explicitly, and record the information on the patient's chart as to the date and time the test was performed, the type of test performed, test results, and your name or initials (Figure 14.15).

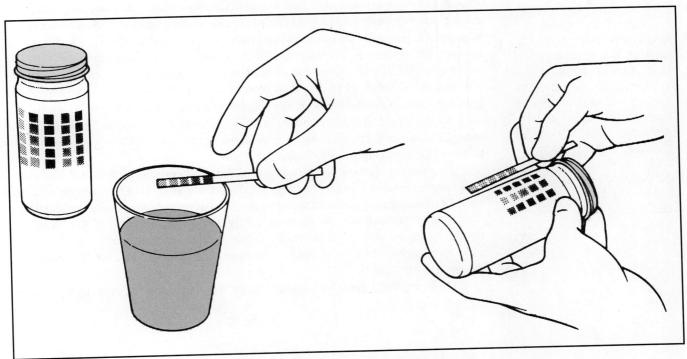

Figure 14.15   Reagent strip testing

PROCEDURE FOR SPECIMEN COLLECTION

1. **Have the necessary equipment available.**
2. **Wash and dry hands thoroughly. Put on gloves.**
3. **Explain the procedure to the patient.**
4. **Collect the necessary number of specimens using the appropriate technique and specimen containers.**
5. **Perform the test, following manufacturer's package directions.**
6. **Record the information on the patient's chart** as to the type of test performed, date and time of collection, test results, and your name or initials.
7. **Remove gloves. Wash and dry hands thoroughly.**

Bacteriology

In vitro **bacteriological** or microbiological testing is performed by means of smears and **cultures**. Specimens are obtained and grown on culture media in the laboratory in order to identify correctly the causative organism and to insure correct treatment of the patient. Material for testing may be obtained by swabbing the infected area, obtaining samples of body fluids, tissues, blood, or other materials. Remember that normal flora are capable of causing disease if present in abnormal proportions or in locations that are not normal.

Specimens collected for bacteriological examination should be handled carefully. Most are not particularly affected by slight changes in temperature, but they are susceptible to drying out. After collection, refrigerate specimens until culturing to prevent overgrowth of organisms.

CULTURES

Blood. The venipuncture site must be meticulously cleaned in order to avoid introducing skin organisms that would complicate the culture results. The blood specimen is usually anticoagulated using sodium polyethanol sulfonate (SPS), which will not damage the organisms, but may inhibit the growth of Neisseria organisms; if these are suspect, be sure to inform the laboratory so they can take appropriate counteractive measures. Draw 10 to 20 ml of blood from an adult and 1 to 5 ml from small children. Blood cultures are normally incubated for at least seven days.

Spinal Fluid. Aseptic lumbar puncture is the method used to obtain the specimen. Leakage or contamination of specimens is prevented by using screw-top containers; 1 or 2 ml is normally obtained.

Respiratory System. Sputum is one of the most commonly cultured specimens. It is usually obtained in the morning by deep coughing. Avoid collection of saliva and nasal discharge. Postural drainage may be of assistance in specimen collection.

Throat cultures are obtained by gently swabbing the back of the throat and tonsilar surfaces with a sterile swab. Throat cultures normally are placed immediately in a sterile tube containing a transport medium to preserve the organisms (Figure 14.16).

Other material may be obtained from the respiratory system by endoscopic aspiration or biopsy.

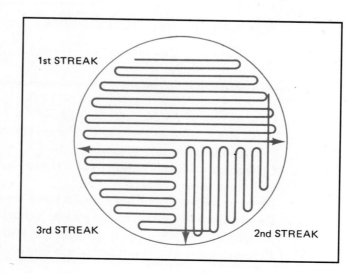

Figure 14.16 Pattern for smearing a culture plate (Reproduced with permission from Simmers, *Diversified Health Occupations*, 2nd Ed., Delmar Publishers Inc., 1988)

Urine. Midstream "clean-catch" specimens voided into a sterile container are the usual method of specimen collection. In some instances, sterile specimens are collected by catheterization.

Feces. Fecal specimens are usually collected in a large, clean container and then transferred to the container to be sent to the laboratory for examination. Feces specimens may also be obtained by swabs of the rectal area.

ANTIBIOTIC SENSITIVITY

One of the primary functions of microbiological or bacteriological examination is to assist the physician in the isolation of causative organisms and their susceptibility to antimicrobial agents or antibiotics.

In vitro testing for antibiotic sensitivity provides an estimate of the effectiveness of particular agents against specific organisms. This is usually accomplished by means of paper filters that have been impregnated with antimicrobial agents in known concentrations. Agar culture plates are inoculated with the bacteria being tested. The impregnated paper filter is then carefully placed on the culture plate, and the plate is incubated overnight. The following morning there will be a zone of growth inhibition around the disk that contains the agent to which the organism is susceptible.

SMEARS AND SLIDES

A number of testing procedures use direct smears on slides, such as the Papanicolaou (Pap) test and Gram testing. These tests are performed on a variety of body fluids, which may include throat and tracheal secretions, cervical secretions, etc. These materials are usually collected on a swab or spatula. Correct preparation of the slides is extremely important (Figure 14.17).

PROCEDURE FOR DIRECT SMEAR SLIDE PREPARATION

1. **Assemble the necessary equipment and supplies.**
2. **Wash and dry hands thoroughly. Put on gloves.**
3. **Label the slides with a diamond-tip pen** to prevent the label from being destroyed in the staining process.

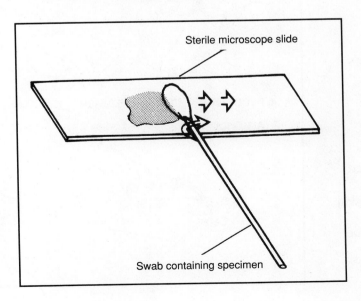

Sterile microscope slide

Swab containing specimen

Figure 14.17 Transferring a specimen to a slide (Reproduced with permission from Keir, Wise, and Krebs-Shannon, *Medical Assisting,* 2nd Ed., Delmar Publishers Inc., 1989)

4. **Roll the swab on the slide, making certain that all areas of the swab come in contact with the slide.** This should produce a thin, fairly even smear, which is necessary for evaluation. If a spatula is used, be sure to spread thinly.
5. **Allow the smear to air dry.**
6. **If required by the laboratory, spray with a fixative.** This normally would be used with a Pap smear. Other smears are fixed by "flaming," passing over the flame of a Bunsen burner.
7. **Record information on patient's chart** as to type of specimen collected, date and time of collection, and your name or initials.
8. **Process the specimen according to laboratory directions.**
9. **Remove and dispose of gloves. Wash and dry hands thoroughly.**

GRAM STAIN

The Gram stain is a procedure that frequently provides the physician with sufficient preculture information to initiate therapy. The stain is performed on a thin smear of material obtained by rolling a swab on a slide, making sure that all areas of the swab touch the slide. The slide should then be allowed to air dry (Figure 14.18).

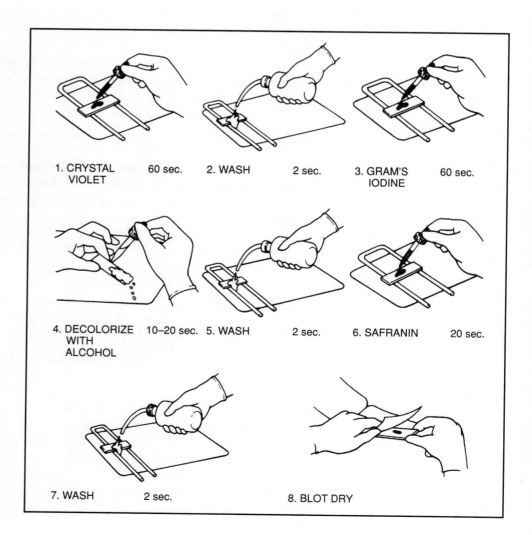

1. CRYSTAL VIOLET — 60 sec.
2. WASH — 2 sec.
3. GRAM'S IODINE — 60 sec.
4. DECOLORIZE WITH ALCOHOL — 10–20 sec.
5. WASH — 2 sec.
6. SAFRANIN — 20 sec.
7. WASH — 2 sec.
8. BLOT DRY

Figure 14.18 Gram-staining procedure (Adapted with permission from Keir, Wise, and Krebs-Shannon, *Medical Assisting,* 2nd Ed., Delmar Publishers Inc., 1989)

PROCEDURE FOR GRAM STAIN

1. **Wash and dry hands thoroughly. Wear disposable gloves.**
2. **Place the slide face up on a staining rack.**
3. **Flood the slide with crystal violet.** Time for thirty seconds.
4. **Flood the stain off with distilled water from the wash bottle.** Tip the slide to remove the water.
5. **Flood the slide with Gram's iodine (mordant).** Time for thirty seconds.
6. **Flood the iodine off with distilled water from the wash bottle.** Tip the slide to remove the water.
7. **Hold the slide nearly vertical and decolorize** by running the decolorizer (alcohol) down the slide until the smear stops, giving off purple stain in all but the thickest portions.
8. **Rinse the slide with distilled water** and return to the staining rack.
9. **Flood the slide with Safranin.** Time for thirty seconds.
10. **Rinse the slide well with distilled water.**
11. **Blot the slide dry with sheets of absorbent paper.** Label slide with patient's name.
12. **Clean the work area.**
13. **Dispose of gloves. Wash and dry hands thoroughly.**

HEMOCCULT TEST

The Hemoccult® test is a test for occult blood in the stool and is used to detect bleeding in the gastrointestinal system. The patient is provided with an addressed envelope containing slides, applicator sticks, and written instructions for obtaining the specimen. After collection, the specimen can be mailed or returned to the medical office (Figure 14.19).

PROCEDURE FOR HEMOCCULT TEST

1. **Wash and dry hands thoroughly. Wear disposable gloves.**
2. **Open the test window on the back of the slide and add two drops of developer to each test area.** Development of a blue color indicates positive results.
3. **Add developer to the on-slide performance monitor at the bottom of the slide window.** Check for correct reactions in the positive and negative control circles.
4. **Dispose of gloves. Wash and dry hands thoroughly.**
5. **Record results in the patient's chart** with your name or initials.

Urine Tests

The function of the urinary system is to eliminate from the body waste products of metabolism, such as urea and creatinine. Foreign substances such as chemicals are frequently detectable in urine (Figure 14.20). While microscopic examination of urine yields a tremendous amount of information, commercial chemical tests, such as multiple reagent strip testing, can yield immediate results, including information on the presence of glucose, ketones, bilirubin, leukocytes, phenylketones, protein, urobilinogen, occult blood, and others. Strips are also available for pH and specific gravity testing. Reagent strips can be purchased either individually or as combination tests. Reagent strip testing provides the physician with valuable information on the status of the patient's liver and kidney function, acid–base balance, and carbohydrate

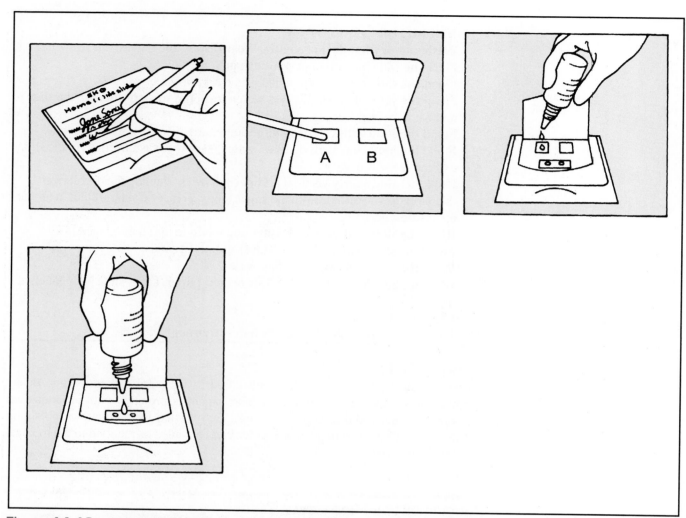

Figure 14.19   Steps for Hemoccult® test. (A) Identify the patient. (B) Collect small stool sample on one end of applicator and smear inside box A. (C) To develop test apply Hemoccult® developer and read results within 60 seconds. (D) To develop performance monitors, apply Hemoccult® and read result within 30 seconds.

metabolism. Each strip is designed to be used once and then discarded. Directions for the use of the strips are located on the package, along with a color-comparison chart for interpreting test results. When using commercial products, employ Universal Precautions and follow the manufacturer's directions explicitly. Record information on the patient's chart as to the date and time the test was performed, the type of test or tests performed, the test results, and your name or initials.

SPECIMEN COLLECTION

Urine specimens may be collected in a clean, dry container at any time of the day, but the preferred specimen for most examinations is the first voiding of the morning, since this specimen will be the most concentrated. Specimens should be refrigerated until tested. In most cases, specimens over eight hours old should be considered void for most tests. In some cases, preservative tablets can be used. Be sure to check with the laboratory that will be doing your testing.

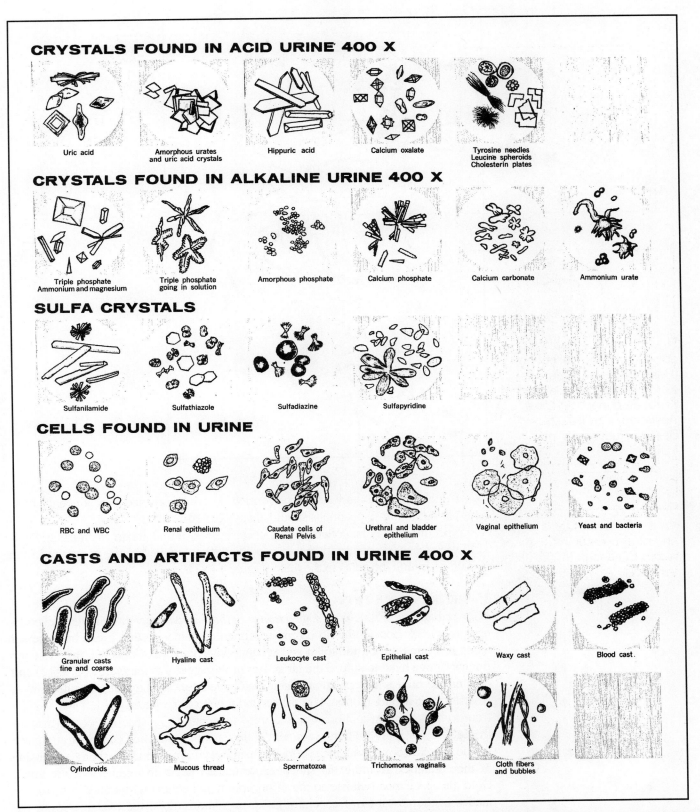

Figure 14.20 Crystals, cells, and casts found in urine sediment (Reproduced with permission from Keir, Wise, and Krebs-Shannon, *Medical Assisting,* 2nd Ed., Delmar Publishers Inc., 1989)

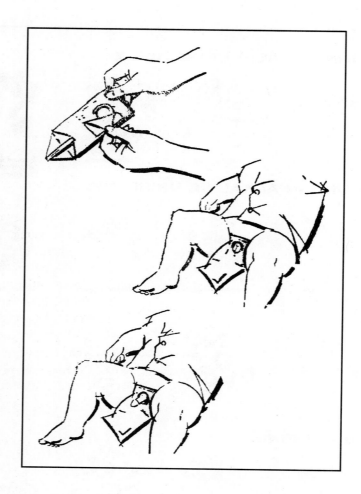

Figure 14.21 Pediatric urine specimen collection (Reproduced with permission from Keir, Wise, and Krebs-Shannon, *Medical Assisting,* 2nd Ed., Delmar Publishers Inc., 1989)

Certain quantitative tests are performed on urine collected over a twenty-four-hour period. Volume specimens should always be refrigerated.

Specimens may be collected by catheterization or midstream clean-catch. Pediatric specimens are collected in a sterile pouch that is taped to the perineum in the female or around the penis in the male (Figure 14.21).

PATIENT INSTRUCTIONS

Midstream Urine Specimen Collection—Female. Open the three towelette packages provided. Loosen the lid on the specimen container so that it can be removed using one hand. Sit on the toilet and separate your knees as far as possible. Use the fingers of one hand to spread the labia, lips of the vagina, as far apart as possible and continue to hold in this position. Using one towelette, cleanse the right side using a front-to-back wiping motion. Use the second towelette to cleanse the left side using a front-to-back wiping motion. Use the third towelette to cleanse the center using a front-to-back wiping motion. Remove the lid from the specimen container and place the lid top side down on a clean surface, being careful not to touch the rim or inside of the container. Holding the specimen container, begin to urinate into the toilet. Hold the specimen container in the urine stream and collect a specimen (one to two inches in the container is generally adequate), and remove the container from the stream. Finish urinating into the toilet. Replace the lid securely on the container. Wipe the exterior of the container with paper towels. Wash hands thoroughly with soap and water and dry with paper towel. Use towel to handle specimen container and place specimen in location provided or give to medical or laboratory assistant.

Midstream Urine Specimen Collection—Male. Open the towelette packages that have been provided and loosen the cap on the specimen container so that it can be removed using one hand. Retract the foreskin (if uncircumcised) and use one towelette to cleanse the glans. Use the second towelette to cleanse the urethral opening. Take the lid off the container and place top side down on a clean surface, being careful not to touch the rim or inside of the container. Begin urinating into the toilet, then hold the specimen container in the urine stream and collect a portion of the urine (one to two inches in the container is usually adequate). Finish urinating into the toilet. Replace the lid securely on the specimen container and wipe the outside of the container with paper towels. Wash hands thoroughly with soap and water and dry with paper towel. Use towel to handle specimen container and place container in location provided or give to medical or laboratory assistant.

Infant Urine Specimen Collection. Using antiseptic towelettes, cleanse the perineum and genital area carefully. Using a sterile urine pouch, tape the pouch in place over the penis or on the labia. Hold the infant so that the urine will flow into the pouch without touching the skin. Remove the pouch as soon as the specimen has been collected and transfer the specimen to a sterile container. Urine production can be stimulated in infants by placing their feet in cold water if necessary.

If the specimens are collected at home, be sure to note the date and time on the container and refrigerate the specimen until transported to the medical office or laboratory.

PREGNANCY TESTING

Pregnancy tests are designed to detect human chorionic gonadotropin (HCG), normally found in the urine of pregnant women. The urine sample tested should be the first urination of the morning. The hormone HCG appears in urine about one week after the missed onset of menstruation. The level of HCG rises for the first two months and then begins to decline about the third month of gestation and disappears altogether a few days following delivery. Using Universal Precautions, follow manufacturer's directions explicitly for the test product you use and record the information on the patient's chart—the date and time of the test, the test product used, and your name and initials.

REVIEW/
SELF-EXAMINATION

1. List eight rules for laboratory safety.

2. Identify five common laboratory tests.

3. What is a Vacutainer, and what is it used for?

4. What does a lavender-stoppered Vacutainer contain?

5. Which stopper Vacutainer has no contents?

6. Which stopper Vacutainer contains Heparin?

7. List the information needed on a specimen container label.

8. How are specimens to be prepared when they are to be mailed?

9. What are the major blood antibodies?

10. What are the major blood antigens?

11. What is meant by Rh factor?

12. Name a common reagent strip test performed on blood.

13. What is the normal adult range for
    a. RBCs?
    b. WBCs?

14. What three white blood cells contain granules in their cytoplasm?

15. List the three sites for obtaining capillary blood.

16. Unopettes are used to collect specimens for what type of testing?

17. Describe the simple test procedure used for estimating the amount of hemoglobin in the blood.

18. List at least eight reagent strip tests available for urine testing.

19. Why would the physician order a differential blood count?

20. Name the agranulocytic white blood cells.

21. Name the test used to evaluate and classify blood dyscrasias.

22. What is the normal hemoglobin range?

23. What is normal ESR value?

24. Name two conditions in which ESR might be elevated.

25. Name four chemical reagent tests that might be performed in the medical office.

26. Why should bacteriological specimens be refrigerated until culturing?

27. What is the purpose of the Gram stain?

28. On what is the Hemoccult test performed?

29. What are the two methods of urine specimen collection?

30. What is meant by clean-catch specimen?

31. Why would a physician be interested in the hemoglobin count of a patient?

32. What diagnostic information is provided by the ESR?

CHAPTER 15

Other Diagnostic Tests

OBJECTIVES

On completion of this chapter, you will be able to:
- Distinguish between artifact and dysrhythmia on the EKG.
- Demonstrate the correct technique in performing an EKG and mounting the tracing for the patient's medical record.
- Identify the anatomy and physiology of the heart and explain the conduction of electrical stimuli through the myocardium.
- Discuss the various forms of radiological studies.
- Demonstrate the technique of arterial blood gas interpretation.
- Explain the components of the pulmonary function study.

Vocabulary—Glossary of Terms

Anaphylaxis	An untoward reaction of the body to a foreign substance; usually begins with generalized redness and edema followed by respiratory difficulty and may even lead to death if not treated quickly.
Antiarrhythmic	A drug that restores normal heart rhythm by blocking conduction of an abnormal impulse through the myocardium.
Atria	The uppermost chambers of the heart.
Block	A delay in conduction of the electrical impulse through the normal pathways in the myocardium; may be caused by internal factors (disease) or external factors (medications).
Defibrillation	The application of electrical energy to the myocardium to interrupt abnormal electrical activity; countershock.
Diastole	The period when the heart is at rest and the ventricles are filling.
Dysrhythmia	Any cardiac rhythm other than sinus rhythm; abnormal rhythm.
Fibrillation	Chaotic electrical activity through the myocardium causing rapid, irregular muscle activity and serving little purpose.
Hypoxemia	A condition in which oxygen concentration in the circulating blood is below acceptable levels.

Idioventricular	Originating from within the ventricle.
Infarction	Death of tissue due to loss of blood supply.
Ischemia	A lower than acceptable level of oxygenation in tissue.
Myocardium	The smooth striated muscle that forms the heart.
Pulmonary	Having to do with the lungs and the exchange of gases.
Radiopaque	Having the ability to be detected by X ray.
Repolarization	In the heart muscle, a change of electrolyte concentration altering the polarity of the myocardium, making it ready to conduct another electrical stimulus through the pathway.
Sinus Node	The intrinsic pacemaker of the heart, located in the right atrium.
Systole	The contraction of the myocardium, when the highest pressures are exerted on the vasculature.
Ventricles	The lower chambers of the heart.

Electrocardiograms

In order to understand the function and purpose of the electrocardiogram (EKG), you must know something of the anatomy and physiology of the heart (Figure 15.1).

ANATOMY AND PHYSIOLOGY OF THE HEART

The heart is composed of smooth muscle tissue, very different from skeletal muscle tissue. It is located in the thoracic cavity to the left of the median. Approximately the size of the fist, the heart is divided into four chambers and is encased in a durable, protective pericardial sac.

Blood enters the heart at the right **atrium** from the venous system by means of the superior and inferior vena cava. The right atrium is the home of the **sinus node** or intrinsic pacemaker. Traveling through the tricuspid valve, the blood passes into the right **ventricle**, where it is delivered to the **pulmonary** arteries by way of the pulmonic valve. Passing through the lungs, it receives oxygen and is returned to the left atrium by the pulmonary veins. From the left atrium, it travels through the mitral valve and enters the left ventricle, the workhorse of the heart, where the greatest thickness of the **myocardium** is found. In **systole**, the blood is forced through the aortic valve into the aorta and to the distant reaches of the circulatory system. The entire journey occurs once every thirty minutes (Figure 15.2).

The electrical stimulation responsible for the reaction of the myocardium is measured by the EKG. Starting in the sinus node (SA node), the impulse travels to the area between the atria and ventricles where the atrioventricular junction (AV node) is located. From there through the Bundle of His, the impulse is relayed to the left and right bundle branches and into the Purkinje fibers embedded deep in the subendocardial layer of the ventricles. The electrical impulse is then delivered to the cells of the ventricles simultaneously. The entire cycle is completed in 0.8 second at a heart rate of seventy-five beats per minute (Figure 15.3).

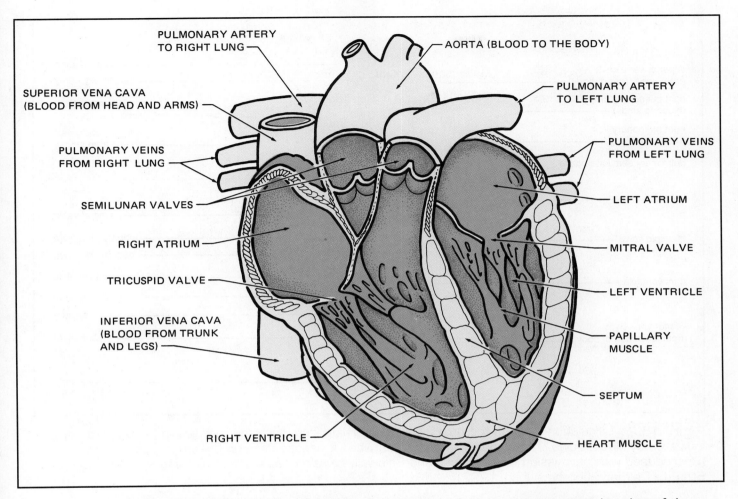

PULMONARY ARTERY TO RIGHT LUNG

AORTA (BLOOD TO THE BODY)

SUPERIOR VENA CAVA (BLOOD FROM HEAD AND ARMS)

PULMONARY ARTERY TO LEFT LUNG

PULMONARY VEINS FROM RIGHT LUNG

PULMONARY VEINS FROM LEFT LUNG

SEMILUNAR VALVES

LEFT ATRIUM

RIGHT ATRIUM

MITRAL VALVE

TRICUSPID VALVE

LEFT VENTRICLE

INFERIOR VENA CAVA (BLOOD FROM TRUNK AND LEGS)

PAPILLARY MUSCLE

SEPTUM

RIGHT VENTRICLE

HEART MUSCLE

Figure 15.1   The anatomy of the heart. Note the thickness of the left ventricle compared to that of the right. (Reproduced with permission from Burke, *Human Anatomy and Physiology in Health and Disease*, 3rd Ed., Delmar Publishers Inc., 1992)

INTERPRETING THE WAVEFORM

Using a series of ten electrodes placed at strategic locations on the body, this electrical activity is viewed from twelve different vantage points. This permits diagnosing a variety of conditions that affect the heart muscle and its ability to function in a normal manner.

The resulting waveforms are labeled with a series of letters denoting various portions of the cardiac cycle. "P" is the label given to the contraction of the atria and corresponds to **diastole** (when the ventricles are filling). The letters "Q," "R," and "S" are assigned to the mechanism of systole and are the result of the contraction of the ventricles. While the ventricles rest between heartbeats, the complex sodium and potassium pumps are in action at the cellular level, and the myocardium is in a stage of **repolarization**. This action is labeled the "T" wave and is widely considered to be the most vulnerable time of the cardiac cycle in which disaster may strike (Figure 15.4).

One of the most common variances from the norm in the EKG waveform is not caused by disease process, but by interference. Electrical interference, tremors, and

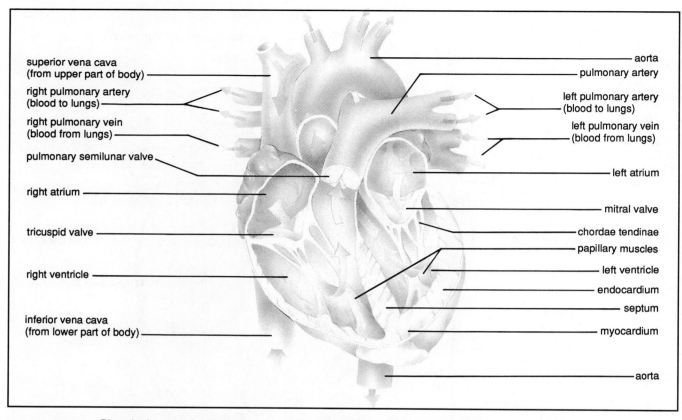

superior vena cava
(from upper part of body)

right pulmonary artery
(blood to lungs)

right pulmonary vein
(blood from lungs)

pulmonary semilunar valve

right atrium

tricuspid valve

right ventricle

inferior vena cava
(from lower part of body)

aorta

pulmonary artery

left pulmonary artery
(blood to lungs)

left pulmonary vein
(blood from lungs)

left atrium

mitral valve

chordae tendinae

papillary muscles

left ventricle

endocardium

septum

myocardium

aorta

Figure 15.2 Circulation through the heart. Blood returning from systemic circulation (deoxygenated) is indicated by blue arrows. The blood receives oxygen when it passes through the lungs (red arrows). (Reproduced with permission from Hegner and Caldwell, *Nursing Assistant, A Nursing Process Approach*, 6th Ed., Delmar Publishers Inc., 1992)

poor electrode contact cause a distortion of the waveform. This condition is called *Artifact*. Usually, artifact can be resolved by checking electrode placement, improving the degree of skin preparation at the electrode site, and reapplying the electrodes (Figure 15.5).

The body's supply of basic electrolytes also affects the EKG because the heart's ability to function properly is extremely dependent on the exchange of sodium (Na^+) and potassium (K^+) through the myocardium. Calcium (Ca^+) and magnesium (Mg^+) are important minerals in the depolarization and repolarization of all muscles in the body, especially the myocardium. Even small imbalances in these minerals can be responsible for serious cardiac problems.

Normal sinus rhythm indicates a healthy heart and is a rate of 60 to 100 beats per minute in the adult (Figure 15.6). This rhythm originates in the sinus node and follows the pathways noted previously. If the heartbeat originates in the sinus node but the heart rate that is generated is less than sixty beats per minute, then the condition is called sinus bradycardia. Sinus tachycardia is a heart rate greater than 100 beats per minute but still originating in the sinus node.

Should the sinus node fail as a result of a pathological condition, the heart has a back-up system at the atrioventricular (AV) junction. When this occurs, the AV

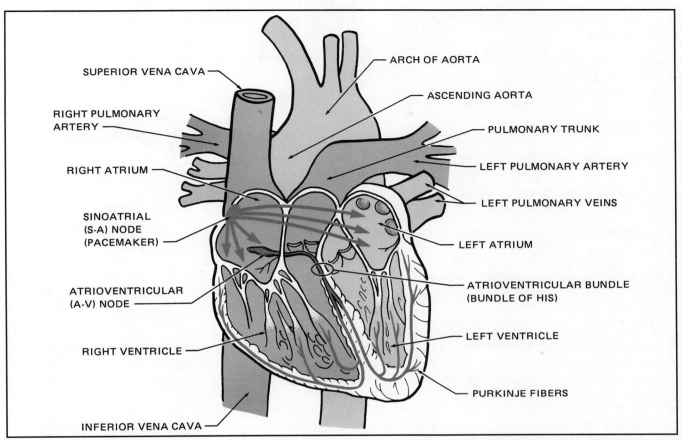

Figure 15.3 Electrical impulse pathway originating in the sinus node and traveling through the myocardium (Reproduced with permission from Keir, Wise, and Krebs-Shannon, *Medical Assisting,* 2nd Ed., Delmar Publishers Inc., 1989)

junction can develop a heart rate of forty to sixty beats per minute, enough to sustain life at rest. This condition is evidenced by abnormalities in the P–R interval on the EKG. These abnormalities vary, but simply stated they indicate that if the sinus node is generating an impulse, it is unable to stimulate the ventricles. In view of the point of origin, the rhythm is termed *junctional rhythm* (formerly referred to as nodal rhythm) (Figure 15.7).

In the event of failure of both the sinus and AV nodes, in some cases a focus in the ventricle will act as a pacemaker and usually can generate a rate of twenty to forty beats per minute but generally is not able to sustain life. This condition is known as **idioventricular** rhythm (Figure 15.8).

In addition to the problems that can occur with the various intrinsic pacemakers, there are also pathological conditions that affect the atria. An irritable focus or foci can cause the atria to beat independently of the sinus node and at remarkably rapid rates. Should this occur, the concern is not for the atria, which tolerate rates as great as 400 beats per minute, but for the ventricles, which have little tolerance for a rate greater than 150 beats per minute. Considering the design of the heart, it appears that the plan is for the ventricle to beat once for every atrial beat. In the case of rapid atrial rates, if the ventricles were to maintain the 1:1 ratio, the myocardium would

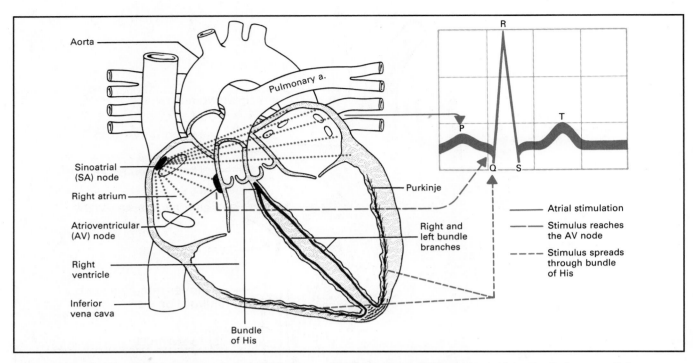

Figure 15.4 The components of the EKG wave—P, Q, R, S, and T—give an electrical picture of the cardiac cycle (Reproduced with permission from Burke, *Human Anatomy and Physiology in Health and Disease,* 3rd Ed., Delmar Publishers Inc., 1992)

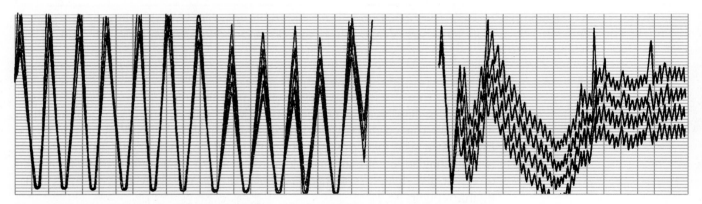

Figure 15.5 A representation of a typical EKG pattern caused by movement, poor lead placement, or electrical interference

Figure 15.6 A representation of a normal sinus rhythm. Note the consistency of the relationship between the waves in the cycle. All components of the waveform are present and identical.

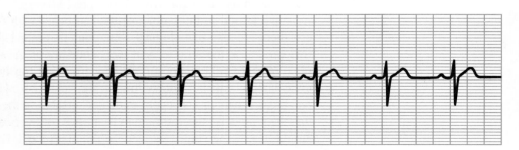

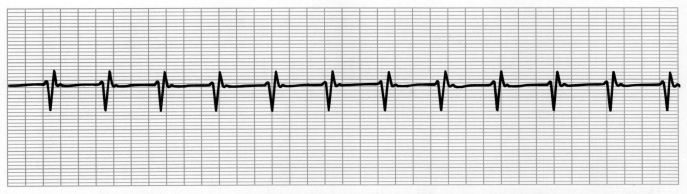

Figure 15.7   A representation of a junctional rhythm. Note the relationship of the P wave to the QRS complex.

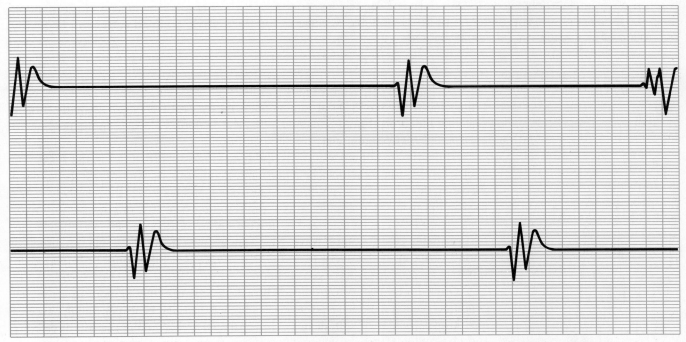

Figure 15.8   A representation of an idioventricular rhythm. Note the widened QRS complex and the absence of the P wave. The rhythm is much slower when originating in the ventricle.

soon fall into oxygen debt and death would result. Fortunately, this is a rare occurrence. The ventricles usually will beat at a slower rate, establishing a safer 2:1, 3:1, or 4:1 atrial–ventricular ratio.

At atrial rates of 150 to 250 per minute, a condition of atrial tachycardia exists. From 250 to 350 beats per minute, the condition is termed atrial flutter. At rates greater than 350 beats per minute, the condition is called atrial **fibrillation** (Figure 15.9).

All of the atrial **dysrhythmias** are characterized by the presence of multiple P waves in each cardiac cycle, with the possible exception of atrial fibrillation, in which the P waves occur so rapidly that they are rarely, if ever, discernible. In all cases, the concern again is not for the atria, but for the ventricles. Poor ventricular

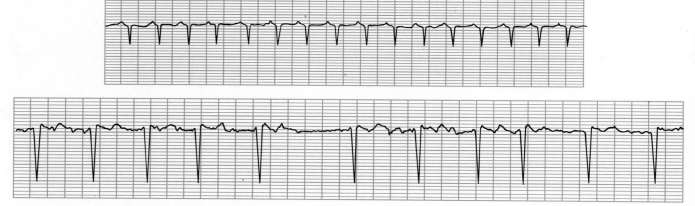

Figure 15.9 A representation of an atrial dysrhythmia. Note the increased rate of the atria (P waves) in the top strip (atrial tachycardia). Also note the classic sawtooth pattern of the flutter waves in the second strip (atrial flutter) and the absence of an identifiable P wave in the third strip, coupled with the irregularly occurring QRS complexes (atrial fibrillation).

filling due to the rapid atrial rate is often the cause of a rather dramatic drop in systemic blood pressure. Frequently, atrial dysrhythmias are seen in the presence of chronic obstructive pulmonary disease (COPD).

The atria are not alone in their ability to cause abnormalities in the EKG. The ventricles also can sometimes be a most unwelcome culprit. An irritable focus/foci in the ventricle can cause a "pacemaker-like" effect and take over the heartbeat. When this occurs in isolated circumstances, the resulting beat is a *premature ventricular contraction* (PVC), characterized by a wide, bizarre QRS complex and the absence of a verifiable contributing P wave. Many people experience these without difficulty, during sleep, in the recovery period after a myocardial **infarction**, or in periods of less than acceptable levels of oxygenation.

Often PVCs occur in groups. When in groups of three or more in a row, the condition (ventricular tachycardia at rates higher than 150 beats per minute, accelerated idioventricular rhythm at rates slower than 150 per minute) is life threatening and constitutes a medical emergency. If the mechanism deteriorates and becomes chaotic, the condition is ventricular fibrillation and is also a medical emergency. In both cases of medical emergency, the administration of **antiarrhythmic** drugs and/or electrical countershock (**defibrillation**) may be indicated to interrupt the cycle long enough for the sinus node to resume control of the heart rate (Figure 15.10).

Wayward pacemakers contribute to a large portion of the abnormalities in the EKG, as evidenced by problems originating from the atria and the ventricles. But there are other abnormalities originating from other areas of the heart.

Conduction difficulties comprise an array of problems in the EKG tracing. Difficulties in the pathway of electrical activity also appear on the EKG tracing. Abnormal transmission of the impulse from the sinus node to the ventricles causing a time lapse of greater than 0.2 second is termed a first-degree atrioventricular **block**. Abnormal transmission of the impulse from the sinus node to the ventricles in which not all P waves inspire a QRS complex is termed a second-degree atrioventricular block. When there is no relationship between the P wave and the QRS complex,

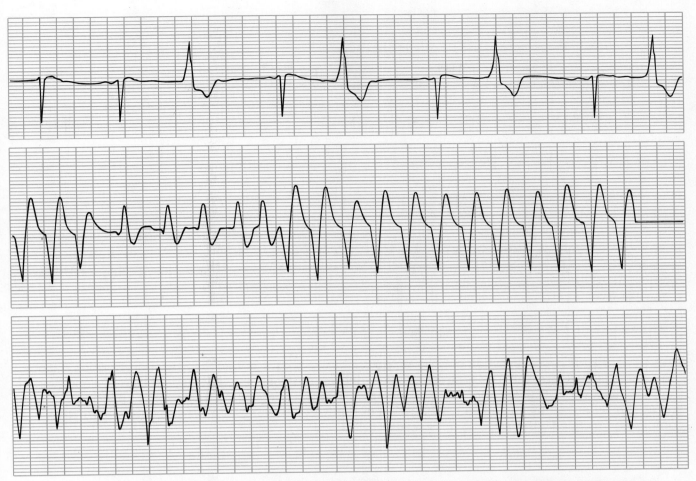

Figure 15.10 A representation of ventricular dysthythmias. In the top strip, the wide complexes are premature ventricular contractions. In the middle strip, the sawtooth ventricular pattern is ventricular tachycardia. The bottom strip is ventricular fibrillation; note the chaotic pattern.

there is a third-degree atrioventricular block. Second-degree block can be serious, and third-degree block is often, if not always, life threatening (Figure 15.11).

Difficulties with the transmission of electrical impulse involving the right or left bundle branches manifest in the widening of the QRS complex to a time frame of greater than 0.12 second. Based on the configuration of the wave form in the chest lead V_1 (see section on lead placement), it is easily established whether the difficulty lies in the left or right bundle branch (Figure 15.12).

The diagnosis of various forms of heart disease is among the most well-known functions of the EKG as a diagnostic tool. The recognition of myocardial **ischemia** by the elevation of the ST segment of the waveform, the evidence of acute myocardial infarction by the appearance of a significant Q wave (exceeding 1 mm in width or greater than one-third the height of the R wave), and the obvious signs of hypertrophic cardiomyopathy as a result of cor pulmonale (evidenced by the ventricular strain pattern) are examples of the value of the EKG in making accurate diagnoses. Lab work serves to support findings obtained in these noninvasive tests, which can be performed quickly and painlessly.

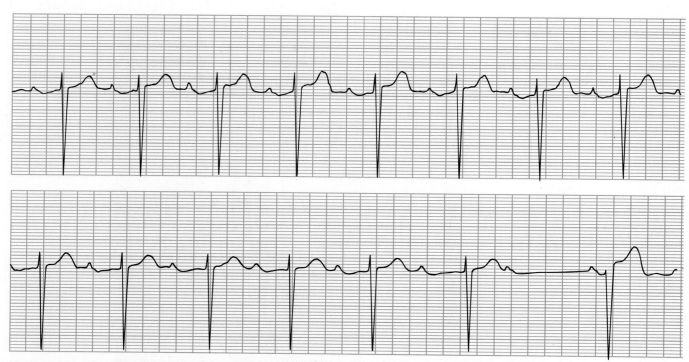

Figure 15.11 A representation of atrioventricular blocks that are identified by abnormalities associated with the P–R interval. The first strip is first-degree AV block and is identified by a prolongation of the P–R interval to >0.2 second. The second strip is second-degree AV block, Type I (Weinkeback) and is characterized by a gradual prolongation of the P–R interval over several beats until a QRS complex is "dropped"; the cycle then repeats itself.

Figure 15.12 A representation of left and right bundle branch blocks. Bundle branch blocks are identified by the width of the QRS complex being > 0.12 second. The strips must be interpreted in the V_1 or MCL_1 leads to distinguish between the left and right bundle. Note the configuration of the wave in the upper strip; the deep "V" pattern is indicative of the left bundle branch. The lower strip shows the RSR[1] or "rabbit ear" pattern indicative of a right bundle branch block.

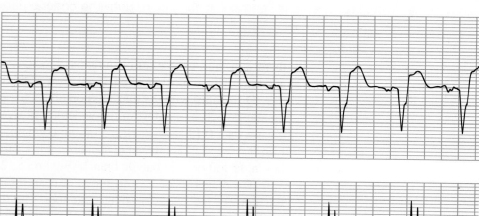

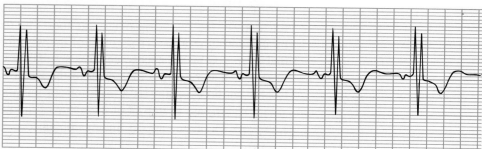

One of the more common misunderstandings related to the EKG tracing involves a patient who just has a perfectly normal EKG one day, and the next day falls victim to a myocardial infarction. The first tracing was normal because on the first day the patient's heart was normal; but next day genuine problems arose. There is seldom any relationship between one day's EKG and the next's.

Discussion of the EKG would be incomplete without mention of the pacemaker. Pacemakers usually are implanted in the fatty tissues of the chest or abdomen. Wires are imbedded in the myocardium and through small electrical charges are able to stimulate the heartbeat.

Today pacemakers come in a variety of styles. The ventricular demand pacemaker is used when the sinus node is failing. The pacemaker is programmed at a set rate (e.g., sixty beats per minute). Whenever the heart rate falls below the set rate, the pacemaker stimulates the ventricles to beat. Dual-chambered pacemakers are able to stimulate both the atria and the ventricles, if necessary. One of the newest pacemakers, the Activitrax, is able to sense the activity of the body and stimulate the ventricles at a rate appropriate to the activity level. If the person is involved in vigorous activity, the rate is increased, while the rate is slower while the person is sleeping.

Pacemakers show a distinctive waveform on the EKG. The electrical impulse from the pacemaker generates a straight, tall spike, while the QRS appears wide and bizarre, owing to cell-to-cell conduction through the myocardium (Figure 15.13).

Performing the EKG

The most important thing in obtaining a readable EKG tracing is proper preparation of the patient prior to placing leads.

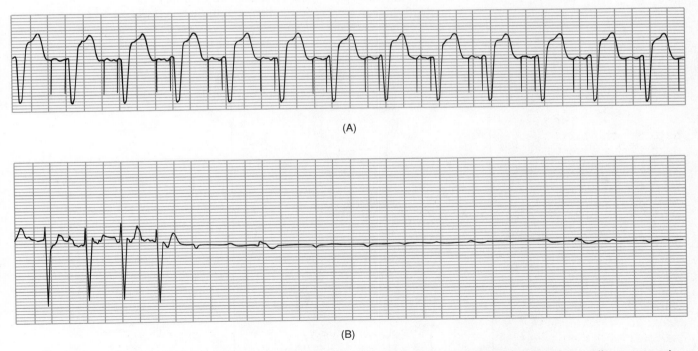

(A)

(B)

Figure 15.13 (A) A representation of a pacemaker. Note the sharp, straight pacemaker spikes caused by the electrical discharge of the pacemaker generator, followed by the wide QRS complex. This is typical of an AV sequential or dual-chambered pacemaker. (B) A representation of an asystole. Note the absence of the QRS; only P waves are shown.

PROCEDURE FOR PATIENT PREPARATION

1. **Explain the procedure to the patient.**
2. **Cleanse the areas for lead placement** with an alcohol-based solution to remove natural oils on the skin surface. Shave areas with excess hair to allow firm contact between the electrode and the skin surface.
3. When placing the electrodes, **identify the correct site and then place the electrode over the area desired**, smoothing the adhesive outward from the center to obtain firm contact between the conduction gel and the skin surface.

Regardless of the age of the machine, some facets of acquiring an EKG tracing remain constant. Lead placement never varies.

PROCEDURE FOR LEAD PLACEMENT

1. **Secure the arm leads** to the upper arm avoiding bony prominence (white on right and black on left).
2. **Place the leg leads** on the lower extremity proximal to the ankle on a fleshy area of the lower leg (green on right, red on left).
3. **Place the V-leads (chest)** as follows:

   V_1 at the fourth intercostal space at the right sternal border
   V_2 at the fourth intercostal space at the left sternal border
   V_3 at the fifth intercostal space at the midclavicular line
   V_4 at the sixth intercostal space using the nipple as a reference in most cases
   V_5 at the sixth intercostal space on the anterior axillary line
   V_6 at the fifth intercostal space at the midaxillary line (Figure 15.14).

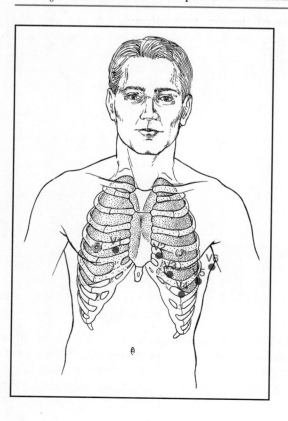

Figure 15.14 EKG chest lead placement

The only variation in this pattern occurs when the physician diagnosing the tracing suspects a right ventricular infarct. On the physician's order the V-leads are reversed to a mirror-image configuration (e.g., the V_1R lead starts at the fourth left intercostal space and the leads proceed around to the right flank using the same landmarks). Some physicians prefer to use the "right chest EKG" to confirm a posterior wall myocardial infarction. Many physicians also prefer that if serial EKG is to be done the chest wall be marked with a waterproof ink to ensure consistency in lead placement.

The tracing should be observed for signs of artifact. If this occurs, check lead placement and verify that the leads are in firm contact with the skin surface and that a conduction medium (gel) has been applied. Request that the patient lie still without talking or touching metal objects or family members.

Observe the size of the tracing. Press the calibration button. The tracing in lead II should be at least half the size of the reference mark made by calibration. If this is not the case, increase the sensitivity of the machine or check for correct lead placement.

There are a variety of machines currently in use for gathering EKG data. Each machine has its own unique characteristics. For our purposes, we limit the discussion to two basic varieties.

The first, the continuous strip machine, requires a roll of single-tracing EKG paper. With this machine, the operator is required to manually place each chest lead, using conduction gel to enhance the quality of the waveform. The person conducting the test is required to mark each lead using a universal code at the top of each strip. The lead selector must be adjusted for each lead.

More modern computerized units allow all leads to be placed at the same time. The machine uses a paper that prints all leads simultaneously and requires no mounting. One touch of a button and the EKG is fed out of the machine. Some of the newest machines incorporating state-of-the-art technology, use no conduction gel, but instead have adhesive foil pads that adhere to the patient and attach to the lead (Figure 15.15).

For a single-strip EKG, the following universal code has been adopted. Pressing the "marker" button on the machine makes marks along the upper margin of the tracing, corresponding to the following legend.

Lead I .	V_1 —— .
Lead II ..	V_2 —— ..
Lead III ...	V_3 —— ...
aVR __	V_4 —— ....
aVL __ __	V_5 —— .....
aVF __ __ __	V_6 —— ......

Mounting the EKG

The format for mounting the EKG is also standardized. A careful selection of strips that have a stable baseline and give an accurate picture of the cardiac status is of key importance. Once the strips have been selected, they are mounted on a standard form in the following pattern in lengths of approximately three-second duration:

LEAD I	LEAD aVL	V_1	V_4
LEAD II	LEAD aVR	V_2	V_5
LEAD III	LEAD aVF	V_3	V_6

LEAD II STRIP THE LENGTH OF THE MOUNTING CARD

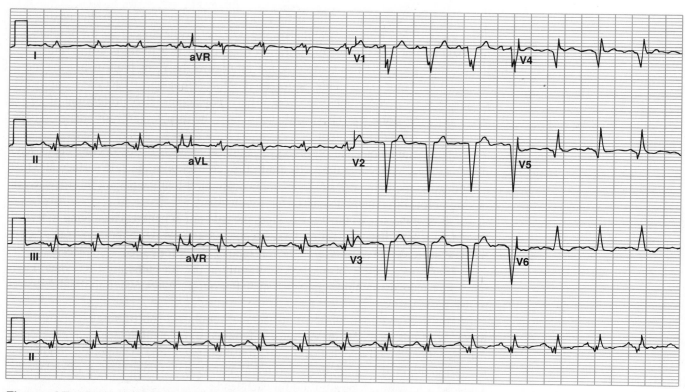

Figure 15.15 A representation of an EKG tracing. The newer computerized machine format prints all twelve leads simultaneously. Note: the machine will also diagnose the EKG by means of an on-board computer.

All EKG paper is formatted with a grid of 5-mm squares that are subdivided into 1-mm squares. This allows measuring the waveform in mm both horizontally and vertically. The significance of an ST elevation or a Q wave can be determined from the measurement. Also, abnormalities on serial tracings can be compared to determine improvement or exacerbation of the condition. In addition to measurement, the horizontal plane of the EKG acts as a time line. At a setting of 25 mm/second (the standard paper speed) each 1-mm square is the equivalent of 0.04 second. With this in mind, the P-R intervals and width of the QRS can be measured, and the presence of AV blocks and bundle branch blocks can be identified (Figure 15.16).

The Holter Monitor

Occasionally a patient complains of symptoms that may be related to cardiac dysrhythmias but cannot be determined during the office exam. Patients may relate periodic episodes of palpitations, dizziness, or syncopal episodes. On exam, the cardiac rhythm is found to be normal, and the symptoms identified are absent.

In these cases, the physician may elect to use a device known as the Holter Monitor. Approximately six inches long, three inches wide, and two inches thick, the monitor weighs approximately one pound and comes in a carrying case with a neck strap for patient convenience. The Holter Monitor is a battery-powered, fully portable continuous EKG recording device, which makes an accurate record of the patient's cardiac rhythm against a time line.

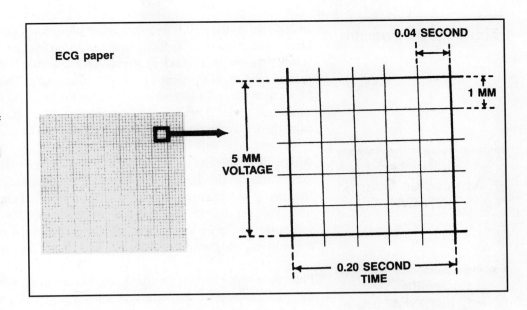

Figure 15.16 EKG paper. Time is measured on the horizontal axis with EKG calipers. Each small square is the equivalent of 0.04 second, the larger squares being 0.2 second at the standard speed of 25 mm/sec. For measurement of size, each square is 1 mm x 1 mm. (Reproduced with permission from Blowers and Sims, *How to Read an ECG*, 4th Ed., Delmar Publishers Inc., 1988)

EKG electrodes are applied to the patient's skin after proper preparation, as outlined earlier in the section on EKG. Lead placement for the monitor differs from that for the EKG leads. Holter monitors record two EKG leads simultaneously and use a five-electrode system. Electrodes are placed as follows: One lead is placed at the top right sternal border; one at the top left sternal border; one at the right sternal border at the level of the fifth rib; one at the left anterior axillary line at the level of the fifth rib; and the last at the lower right rib cage over a bony area. The last electrode serves as a ground for both patterns. Wires from the monitor are connected to the leads, and the monitor is connected to an EKG machine to verify that the tracing is adequate. The clock in the Holter Monitor is set.

The patient is instructed to protect the monitor from moisture and not to bathe or swim while the monitor is in use. The patient is also instructed to keep a detailed log of any symptoms occurring during the monitoring period, along with the exact time of each occurrence and a notation of any activity being performed at that time. In addition, there is an "event" button on the monitor that is to be pressed at the time the symptoms occur. Electric blankets should not be used while the monitor is in use due to the artifact caused by their electrical field. The monitor should be left in its case at all times, and the patient should avoid handling the electrodes.

The patient is instructed to return to have the device removed on completion of the monitoring period, usually twenty-four hours. On occasion, the monitor may be used for longer periods but batteries and recording paper should be changed and fresh EKG electrodes applied to the skin each twenty-four hours. At the completion of the monitoring period, the patient's log and the tracing are compared by a technician, and a report of all symptoms and relevant dysrhythmias is supplied to the physician. With this data in hand, the physician is then able to diagnose the condition and prescribe further treatment.

The convenience of the Holter Monitor allows the patient to continue a daily routine and eliminates the need for costly hospitalization for observation when minor cardiac dysrythmias are suspected.

The Echocardiogram

In addition to the EKG, there are other procedures that aid in differential diagnosis. One of the most popular today is the echocardiogram. This procedure, which uses a state-of-the-art ultrasound, is noninvasive and painless and yields a wealth of information relating to a patient's general cardiac status. The functioning of the valves can be seen on the radar-like screen. Wall thickness of the ventricle can be measured and weakened areas identified. The ejection fraction (the percentage of blood expelled from the left ventricle with each contraction) can be computed.

Multigated Acquisition Scan (MUGA)

Although an invasive procedure, this test is very effective in computing the left ventricular ejection fraction by "tagging" red blood cells with an isotope. The normal fraction is approximately 65%. Less than 50% is indicative of ventricular dysfunction. Patients should be educated for this procedure by explaining the need for venipuncture for the procedure. The danger from the radioactive isotope is virtually nonexistent, and the procedure is painless except for the needle stick.

Cardiac Catheterization

Patients with a history of unstable angina are often sent to an acute care facility for the performance of the cardiac catheterization. A great deal of anxiety is often associated with this procedure. Although this procedure is not performed in the physician's office, scheduling is often done by the office. At the time the appointment is scheduled, you can often place the patient at ease by briefly educating the patient on the procedure.

The procedure involves placing a large-bore catheter in an artery (the femoral is the most common site, though the brachial is sometimes used). It is done in the catheterization laboratory after local anesthetic is applied to the site. The patient should feel small "pin pricks" as the local anesthetic is introduced. From that point on, there will be a sensation of pressure as the catheter is advanced, but there should be no pain. Once the catheter is in position, a **radiopaque**, iodine-based dye is injected, and the coronary arteries are observed by fluoroscopy. Many cardiologists encourage the patient to watch the procedure on a television monitor to observe the travel of the dye through the arteries. At the point that the dye is injected, the patient should feel a sensation of warmth throughout the body similar to a "hot flash." This is normal and is no cause for alarm.

After the procedure, a bulky pressure dressing is applied to the site after the removal of the catheter. The patient returns to their room and lies in bed, where they are kept in a supine position with the operative leg extended for a period of three to six hours. This allows the puncture of the femoral artery to close properly without bleeding into the surrounding tissues. The patient is often kept overnight for observation and discharged the following day.

Pulmonary Function Testing

One of the fastest methods of evaluating pulmonary function is the *arterial blood gas* (ABG). Blood is drawn from an artery by the physician, physician assistant, or RN. Arterial blood draw is never a function of the medical assistant. The blood is run through a battery of measurements performed by a blood gas analyzer. The analyzer is a complex computer that performs a series of tests on the sample. Out of the variety of results received, the most important are pH, PaO_2, $PaCO_2$, HCO_3, and O_2 saturation. Through these values rapid diagnosis of the situation by the physician can be made.

Normal blood gas values are as follows:

pH: 7.35 to 7.45
$PaCo_2$: 35 to 45 mm Hg

PaO_2: 80 to 100 mm Hg
HCO_3: 22 to 26 mEq/L
O_2 sat.: >95%

These values are based on an average person with normal pulmonary function breathing room air (21% O_2). Values of the drawn blood gas are adjusted for supplemental oxygen and body temperature.

The first step in blood gas interpretation involves the pH. If the pH is < 7.35, the patient is in *acidosis*. If the pH is > 7.45, the patient is in *alkalosis*. The remainder of the values reveal the cause of the acidosis or alkalosis. First, the value of $PaCo_2$ is examined. If the value is abnormal, then the patient may have a "respiratory component." Carbon dioxide increases the pH of the blood by combining with water to form carbonic acid ($H_2O + CO_2 = H_2CO_3$). If the pH is low and the CO_2 level is elevated, then the patient is in *respiratory acidosis* and needs more oxygen. *Note*: If the pH is low and the CO_2 is normal or low, then the patient's body is compensating for another condition. If the patient's pH is high and the CO_2 level is low, then the condition is *respiratory alkalosis*, and the patient needs to retain more CO_2 (the patient is hyperventilating). This can be accomplished with a "rebreathing mask" or in an emergency with a simple paper bag. In order to diagnose a respiratory problem, both the pH and the CO_2 levels have to be abnormal and in opposite directions.

If the patient's pH is abnormal and the CO_2 level is not conversely abnormal, then the bicarbonate level (HCO_3) will be examined. Bicarbonate acts as a buffer, binding to hydrogen to form carbonic acid (H_2CO_3). Carbonic acid raises the pH of the blood and depletes the supply of bicarbonate in the circulating blood.

If the patient's pH is low and the HCO_3 level is low, the condition is *metabolic acidosis*. The treatment is to administer bicarbonate to raise the blood level, decrease the blood levels of hydrogen, and raise the pH to a normal level. Usually this is done by administering sodium bicarbonate ($NaHCO_3$) orally or intravenously. Common household baking soda would do the job in a pinch.

If the patient's pH is high and the HCO_3 level is high, the patient is in respiratory alkalosis. This is a most difficult situation to resolve and is usually dealt with by waiting the problem out, allowing the body to correct the situation naturally. In cases of extreme emergency, in an intensive care setting, IV fluids containing ammonium nitrates can in some cases be used, but this therapy is dangerous and used only as a last resort.

The O_2 saturation level is a good quick reference to determine the patient's oxygenation status. Often when the O_2 sat. is low and all other values are within normal parameters, the blood count will indicate a low hemoglobin count. (Hemoglobin is the component of blood responsible for carrying oxygen). In these cases, a blood transfusion may be in order. *Note*: **Hypoxemia** is often accompanied by changes in the level of consciousness (LOC).

SPIROMETRY

Pulmonary function studies involve measurement of lung capacity and compliance and are done by many laboratories and doctors' offices. Compliance is the ability of the lung to expand.

Several measurements are made by having the patient breathe into a device that measures the volume of air expired or inspired. The amount of air that passes in and out of our bodies with normal respiration is termed tidal volume (TV). There is always a certain amount of air that remains in the respiratory system even after full exhalation. This air keeps the alveoli from collapsing and fills the bronchioles and bronchial tubes and is referred to as *residual capacity* (RC). During pulmonary function studies, the tidal volume is measured and the residual capacity is calculated based on the patient's body size.

PROCEDURE FOR SPIROMETRY

The procedure should be explained to the patient. Seat the patient at the spirometer and make as comfortable as possible. Ask the patient to breathe in as deeply as possible and measure and record this volume, inspiratory capacity (IC). Following the maximal inspiration, ask the patient to exhale fully, blowing out as much air as possible. Also measure and record this volume, vital capacity (VC).

Several measurements of these volumes may be performed during a pulmonary function test. As a result of the dizziness that occurs with deep inhalation and exhalation, it is wise to allow the patient resting periods between measurements.

Based on the measurements obtained and computed, the results can be compared to tables that give the normal values for a patient in relation to body size. This comparison yields the percentage of pulmonary function and contributes to the diagnosis of a variety of chronic lung disorders (Figure 15.17).

X-Ray and Other Radiological Studies

Most radiological studies are scheduled and performed in hospital or out-patient radiological laboratories. It is imperative that the medical assistant become familiar with the basic studies and patient preparation required for those studies. The laboratory with which you will be scheduling your patients will be happy to supply you with preparatory information and patient requirements for the studies they will be performing. Many of the studies will require patient preparation that includes taking laxatives and enemas and/or orally ingested dyes prior to the patient arriving for the examination. Some laboratories prefer to provide patient directions themselves and will direct you to send the patient to them for this information. Be sure to provide your patient with verbal and written directions to the laboratory, including the date and time of the appointment and the address and telephone number of the laboratory.

There are a variety of studies available for noninvasive examination of internal body structures. The most well known of these is the X ray, a still image of internal structures.

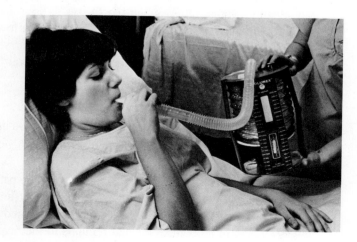

Figure 15.17 Pulmonary function testing (Reproduced with permission from Narrow and Buschle, *Fundamentals of Nursing Practice,* 2nd Ed., John Wiley & Sons, Inc., 1982)

Some physician offices have X-ray equipment that will allow the physician's office to perform limited radiological studies. Performance of these studies by the medical assistant requires a limited radiologic technician certificate, which can be obtained only after an appropriate course of study and testing. Due to the need for this limited certification, we discuss in this chapter only the various uses for radiology testing and the need for adequate explanation and preparation of the patient prior to the examination.

The most well-known application of X rays is in the diagnosis of bone fractures. Views commonly used in the diagnosis of a fracture include anteroposterior (AP), posteroanterior (PA), lateral, and oblique. These examinations may be done with the limited radiological certification.

Chest X rays are used in the differential diagnosis of pneumonia, cancer, tuberculosis, and pulmonary edema caused by congestive heart failure. The chest X ray can also detect pneumothorax and hemothorax. The most common group of chest X rays are anterior-posterior (AP) and lateral. This group gives a clear, concise picture of the entire lung field. These examinations may be performed under the limited radiological certificate.

Radiological examinations are not limited to still pictures. Scans are done of the soft tissue area and bone when a large area of coverage is required. The pendulum-like mechanism of the machine is often frightening to patients, but there is no danger or pain involved in the procedure. As with all facets of the delivery of medical care, a thorough explanation of the procedure telling the patient what is being done and what to expect relieves a great deal of anxiety. Preparing the patient makes everyone's job much easier.

Fluoroscopy, often described as a motion picture X ray, projects the image on a cathode ray tube (TV screen) and is used for a variety of soft tissue studies. The patient is placed on the examination table, and the head of the machine is positioned over the area to be studied. The fluoroscope yields a continuous moving picture of the area. Angiograms and cardiac catheterization are done under fluoroscopy (Figure 15.18). Radiopaque dyes are sometimes used during the procedure (see below on CT scans for prep information).

The most widely used scan today is computerized axial tomography (CAT or CT scan). CT scans are used for the brain and other soft tissue areas. The machine has a "space-age" appearance—a large "doughnut" at the end of a motorized table upon which the patient is placed. The CT scan takes a series of X ray images at various levels throughout the subject area that are like slices of the organ being studied. This enables the location of small tumors otherwise hidden from the conventional X ray or the identification of small areas of hemorrhage deep within the brain. CT scans can be performed with or without contrast media.

When a contrast media is used, a radiopaque, iodine-based dye is introduced intravenously. This is one area in which discussing the procedure with the patient is paramount. People who have an allergy to iodine or shellfish can have severe **anaphylactic** reactions to the dye that may even result in death. Questions about these allergies before the procedure are a must. Even those not allergic will usually experience a sensation of heat similar to "hot flashes" experienced during menopause. This can be quite alarming to the unsuspecting patient and is easily explained during the procedure if the patient has been well prepared in advance. If the patient has not been well prepared, panic may set in, and the technician is left to undo the damage (Figure 15.19).

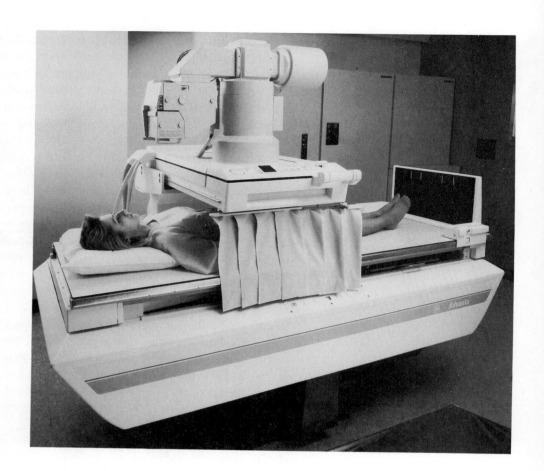

Figure 15.18
Flouroscopy during angiography (Courtesy GE Medical Systems)

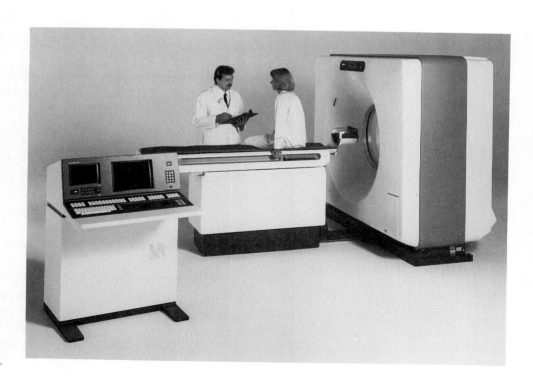

Figure 15.19
Computerized axial tomography (Courtesy GE Medical Systems)

Nonradiological Studies

MAGNETIC RESONANCE IMAGING (MRI)

Magnetic resonance imaging (MRI) is closely related to the CT scan and performs basically the same function with a few additional benefits. The primary advantage of the MRI is that there is no exposure to radiation. The MRI uses magnetic fields to outline areas of the body. The procedure is very safe, completely painless, but can be disconcerting if you're claustrophobic. The patient is again placed on a motorized table and travels inside a long tube with very little room to spare. The procedure takes approximately forty-five minutes, and when the machine is running, there are intermittent loud noises that have been compared to machine gun fire. If the patient is uncomfortable in close quarters, the procedure will be absolute agony for them. If this is the case, the physician often will premedicate the patient with an antianxiety agent (Valium, Xanax) before the procedure. Sometimes this helps, but it is not unusual to have an hysterical patient on your hands. Question the patient about prior claustrophobic incidents and inform the physician if they exist (Figure 15.20).

The MRI does pose a danger to anything susceptible to magnetic fields. Proximity to the machine when it is running can erase credit cards, ruin a wristwatch, or cause the wearer of metallic objects to experience some strange phenomena. Encourage the patient and others in the area to remove these items and place them in a secure area away from the procedure prior to beginning the scan.

ULTRASOUND

Ultrasound studies are another way to study soft tissue areas without radiation. The ultrasound uses sound waves to outline organs and other structures. Gel is applied to the area, and the head of the handset is moved over the target area until a picture is obtained. This procedure is painless, but the gel and the head of the handset are almost always cold, causing slight discomfort to the patient. A conscientious technician will warm the instrument and the gel prior to the procedure. The procedure is very safe and is used routinely to observe the unborn fetus in the womb (Figure 15.21).

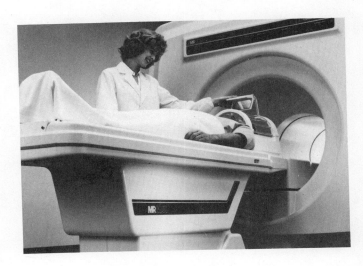

Figure 15.20
Magnetic resonance imaging (MRI) (Reproduced with permission from Keir, Wise, and Krebs-Shannon, *Medical Assisting,* 2nd Ed., Delmar Publishers Inc., 1989)

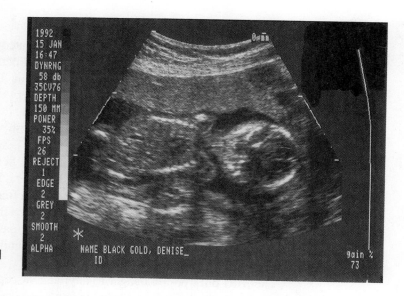

Figure 15.21 Ultrasound image

1. Trace the path of blood as it circulates through the heart.

2. What is the function of the sinus node?

3. What causes artifact?

4. How are electrodes placed for a standard EKG?

5. Name two life-threatening dysrhythmias and describe them.

6. What preparation should be made to the skin prior to performing an EKG?

7. How might artifact be corrected?

8. How many leads are mounted for an EKG tracing?

9. What is the purpose of conduction gel?

10. What is the purpose of an implanted pacemaker?

11. Why are Holter Monitors used?

12. What diagnostic information is gained by the cardiac catheterization?

13. Name two types of pulmonary function tests.

14. Explain the difference between the CT scan and the MRI scan.

15. What is the function of ultrasound?

16. What is fluoroscopy?

17. What does the term radiopaque mean?

18. What should be removed prior to an MRI scan?

19. What differentiates the CT scan from a standard X ray?

20. Who in the physician's office may draw arterial blood for arterial blood gases?

21. What type of certification is required of the medical assistant who is to perform radiological studies in a medical office?

CHAPTER 16

Treatment Modalities

On completion of this chapter, you will be able to:
- Demonstrate the principles of teaching crutch walking.
- Demonstrate the principles of sound body mechanics.
- Discuss the rationale for the application of heat and cold and cite the various situations when use is appropriate.
- Define the uses of hydrotherapy.
- Discuss the principles of range of motion therapy.
- Discuss the principles of diathermy and ultrasound therapy.
- Discuss the objectives and indications of casting and splinting.

Vocabulary— Glossary of Terms

Atrophy	The loss of normal size or mass, usually referring to musculature.
Bursitis	Inflammation of the fluid-filled sac or sac-like cavity where friction of tissues would normally occur at a joint.
Contracture	The shortening of tendons and musculature through lack of use, so that an extremity is in a permanent condition of flexion.
Cryotherapy	The application of cold for therapeutic response.
Debridement	The removal of necrotic tissue by various means to allow healing of the living tissue underneath.
Decubitus Ulcer	A breakdown of soft tissue to various degrees as a result of pressure and immobility. Usually noted over areas of bony prominence in the elderly and chronically ill patient.
Extension	Movement in which the ends of a jointed extremity are moved farther apart.
Febrile	Having a temperature above normal range.
Flexion	Movement in which the ends of a jointed extremity are moved closed together.
Hydrotherapy	Immersion of part or all of the body in water of varying temperature, with or without whirlpool action, for the purpose of increasing motion, circulation, and healing.

Hypothermia Blanket	A device that may be placed under and/or on top of the patient to reduce body temperature by pumping chilled water through the plastic blanket from a control unit. Applications for warming the patient are also available.
Necrotic	Area of dead tissue, due to lack of circulation.
Rheumatoid Arthritis	A particularly crippling form of degeneration and inflammation of joint tissues.
Tendonitis	Inflammation of the tendon, tendon sheath, or tendon–muscle attachments.
Thermotherapy	Application of heat for therapeutic response.

T here are a variety of therapies used to promote healing, relieve pain, reduce swelling, and restore mobility to an afflicted area. This chapter covers a sampling of those therapies and the rationale behind them.

The basic principles of physical therapy have the objective of restoring *optimal* use, not necessarily maximal use, to the affected part, based on the ability of the patient. The goal in physical therapy is to improve the patient's condition to the best of the patient's ability, not force the patient to exceed their capability. It is sometimes difficult to judge what amount of motivation is required, for there is a very fine line between motivation and cruelty where an injured patient is concerned. In this area, no text can replace good sound clinical experience, but we can take a lesson from the Latin phrase *primam non nocere* (first, do no harm) as a sound guideline for practice.

Application of Heat and Cold

The application of heat (**thermotherapy**) must be performed with the protection of the patient's skin in mind. Those who are elderly and those with certain diseases (e.g., diabetes) are extremely sensitive to application of heat or cold as a result of the normal aging process or peripheral neuropathy. Therefore, it is the responsibility of the therapist to control the procedure, guaranteeing the patient's safety.

The application of heat falls into two categories, dry and moist. Dry heat takes the form of light, hot water bottles, and electric heating pads. It always presents the danger of a burn to the patient and should be monitored closely. The goal of dry heat is to promote healing by increasing circulation to an area through dilation of capillary beds.

Heat lamps are often applied to promote healing by drying areas with infrared radiation (as in the case of the **decubitus ulcer**) and at the same time increasing circulation to the affected area. Most heat lamps consist of a simple gooseneck fixture with a small (less than 40-watt) bulb. When a heat lamp is used, the area to be treated should be clean and free of ointment or cream. The patient should be positioned in a way to provide access to the area to be treated and still provide comfort for the patient, who should be draped to provide privacy. The lamp should be positioned to shine on the desired area and should be between eighteen and thirty-six inches from the skin surface, depending on the type of lamp and the patient's tolerance. The duration of the treatment is short, usually fifteen to twenty minutes (Figure 16.1).

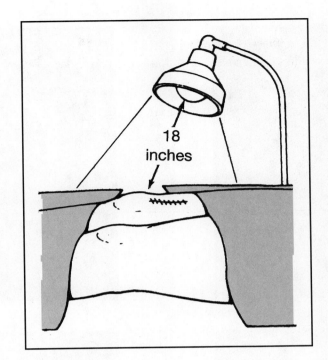

Figure 16.1 Gooseneck heating lamp therapy. Note the placement of the lamp in relation to skin surface and draping of patient to allow privacy. (Adapted with permission from Hegner and Caldwell, *Nursing Assistant, A Nursing Process Approach,* 6th Ed., Delmar Publishers Inc., 1992)

Ultraviolet light is used frequently for dermatological treatment and is applied in the same manner as with the heat lamp. Ultraviolet light not only provides heat but also has the capability to kill some skin bacteria. Treatments of very short duration are used. The duration varies, usually starting with thirty seconds or less and increasing to several minutes, based on the patient's tolerance. Several hours after the treatment the patient's skin becomes slightly reddened as in the case of a mild sunburn; this is normal. Care should be taken to protect the patient's eyes during therapy.

Hot water bottles are used for the application of dry heat, often over moist dressings to keep them warm. Before filling a hot water bottle, measure the temperature of the water with a thermometer. An acceptable temperature range for adults is 115 to 125 degrees Fahrenheit. The temperature should be slightly less for infants and the elderly. When filling a hot water bottle, fill halfway, then squeeze out the air before capping. This technique decreases weight and allows the bottle to conform to body contours more readily. Always cover a hot water bottle with a pillow slip or towel to prevent direct contact with the skin surface (Figure 16.2).

Electric heating pads are often used to provide a source of dry heat. The selector switch should be set to low or medium, as designated by the physician. Lower settings are used for children and the elderly. The heating pad should always be covered with a pillow slip or towel to prevent direct contact with the skin surface and should be placed on top of the patient. Lying on top of the pad should be discouraged due to the risk of burns. The duration of treatment is established by the physician.

The application of moist heat can be accomplished by soaking in hot water, hot compresses, or hot packs. Moist heat penetrates deeper into the musculature, providing relief for injuries that are embedded farther from the surface. The principle remains the same, increasing circulation to the affected area by dilation of the vasculature.

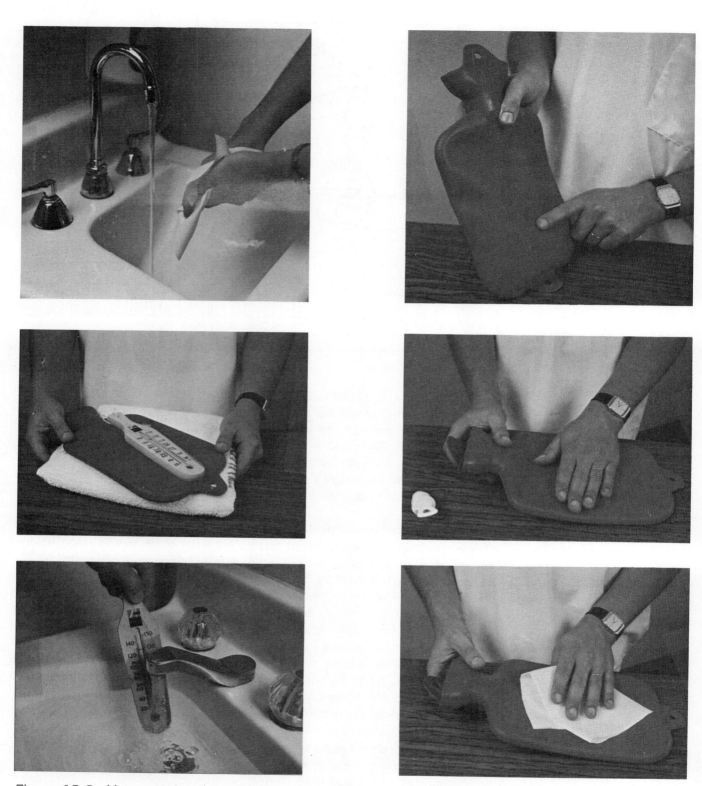

Figure 16.2 Hot water bottle application. Expel air from bottle before capping and apply a protective cover to prevent burns. (Reproduced with permission from Hegner and Caldwell, *Nursing Assistant, A Nursing Process Approach,* 6th Ed., Delmar Publishers Inc., 1992)

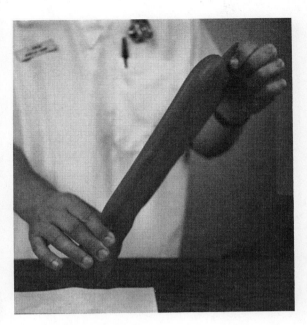

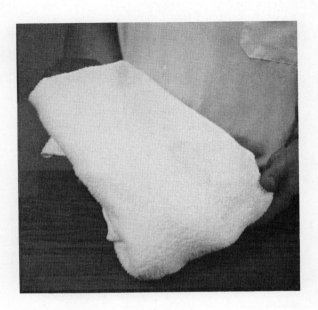

Figure 16.2 continued

Soaking body parts can be accomplished with a basin and warm water if the affected area is an extremity. Soaks can also involve medicated solutions, but when an open wound is involved aseptic technique must be observed to prevent infection. With open wounds, a sterile basin and solution are necessary. If larger body areas are involved, a Sitz bath or Hubbard tank may be used (**hydrotherapy**). Solution temperatures should range between 105 and 110 degrees Fahrenheit, based on patient tolerance.

The patient should be allowed to immerse the body part gradually, as they are able to tolerate, at the beginning of therapy. You may add warm solution during the procedure, taking care to avoid pouring directly onto the patient's body part and to mix the added solution into the existing bath to prevent burns. Duration of therapy is usually fifteen to twenty minutes (Figure 16.3).

To apply a hot, moist compress to a body part, soak a towel or washcloth in warm water and after wringing out the excess, place directly on the affected area. Compresses are generally used for small areas. Hot packs share the same principle but are generally used for larger body areas. Commercial hot packs contain a silicone gel and are heated in a hot water bath, then wrapped in towels prior to placing on the patient. The compress or pack should be introduced gradually to the patient to allow time for adjustment. Frequent checks of the skin surface should be made to avoid burns.

Another method of introducing heat for patients with complaints of **rheumatoid arthritis** is the paraffin bath. Paraffin is kept in a liquid state in a warmer. After checking to make sure no moisture is present on the part to be treated (usually hands or fingers; moist areas conduct heat more readily and severe burns can result), immerse the patient's hand in the paraffin bath. As the hand is removed from the bath the paraffin becomes solid, coating the entire skin surface with gentle warmth. This

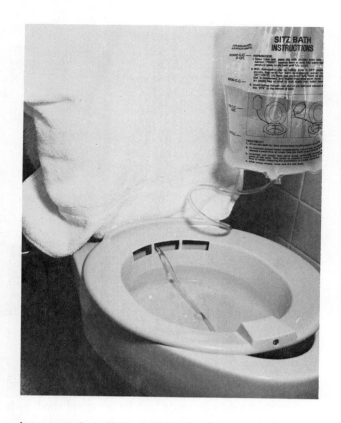

Figure 16.3 Portable Sitz bath (Reproduced with permission from Simmers, *Diversified Health Occupations*, 2nd Ed., Delmar Publishers Inc., 1988)

is repeated until the hand is coated with a substantial layer of wax. The hand is then wrapped in a towel for a period of fifteen to twenty minutes to hold the heat. After the completion of the treatment, the wax may be peeled off and returned to the bath. Increased circulation and joint mobility usually are enjoyed for up to three hours after this therapy, which is an excellent time for range of motion exercises (Figure 16.4).

The application of cold (**cryotherapy**) is used to reduce edema and constrict the capillary beds. As with heat, cold applications can be either dry or moist.

Dry cold is applied by either ice packs or ice collars. They involve the same principle but have a different configuration. Ice packs are designed to be placed upon an area of the body. They are filled a little more than half full with crushed ice to minimize air spaces. The air is squeezed out and the cap placed on the bag. Be sure to check for leaks. They are then placed in a protective cover to prevent direct contact with the skin surface. An ice collar follows the same principle but can be wrapped around a body part. With both the ice pack and the ice collar the treatment usually lasts thirty minutes to an hour. If continuous treatment is ordered, the pack/collar should be removed for approximately thirty minutes after one hour of therapy and then resumed to appreciate the full effect of the therapy and to avoid discomfort. The skin surface should be checked frequently during therapy to prevent damage to tissue (Figure 16.5).

Moist cold is applied by means of cold compresses or packs, ice massage, and alcohol baths. Cold compresses are applied in the same manner as hot compresses. Immerse a washcloth or towel in a bath of ice and water, wring out thoroughly, and apply to the designated area for a period of twenty to thirty minutes. Check skin surface frequently to prevent injury. Repeat treatment every two hours, or as ordered by the physician.

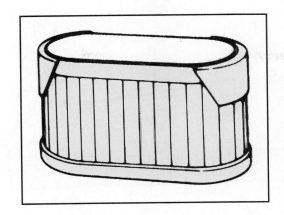

Figure 16.4 The paraffin hand bath is common for patients suffering from rheumatoid arthritis

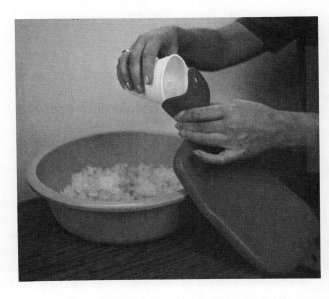

Figure 16.5 Ice bag/ice collar; note that excess air is removed before closure (Reproduced with permission from Hegner and Caldwell, *Nursing Assistant, A Nursing Process Approach*, 6th Ed., Delmar Publishers Inc., 1992)

Ice massage is accomplished by gently rubbing the area with a large piece of ice. This is usually used on a recent injury to prevent swelling. The period of therapy is usually five minutes or less.

In the past alcohol sponge baths were used to rapidly reduce a high fever and are still used in homes today for **febrile** patients. A bath with half tepid water and half alcohol is prepared, and the patient's body is sponged with the mixture. Because alcohol evaporates rapidly, the body temperature is reduced dramatically in a short period of time. Areas of the body should be covered with a light blanket while not being sponged, and care should be taken to prevent the patient from shivering. Shivering actually elevates body temperature and is counterproductive to this therapy. With the advent of the **hypothermia blanket**, there is little need for alcohol sponge baths in medical facilities. An elevation of temperature can be corrected easily and safely with the hypothermia blanket without the drying of the skin encountered with alcohol sponge baths (Figure 16.6).

Hydrotherapy

As mentioned in the section on moist heat, hydrotherapy involves soaking larger areas of the body in warm or cool water, as directed. The modalities vary based on the body part involved. The benefits of hydrotherapy include increased circulation and ease of exercise and hydromassage. Whirlpool tanks are available to accommo-

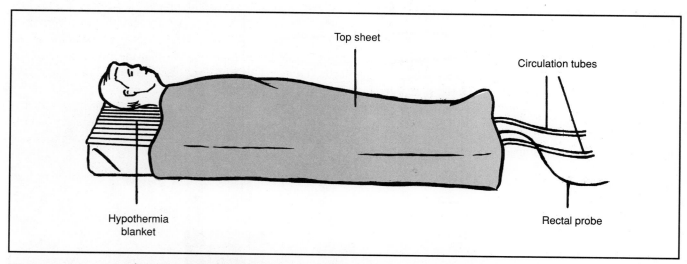

Figure 16.6 Hypothermia blanket (Reproduced with permission from Gomez and Hord, *Fundamentals of Clinical Nursing Skills*, John Wiley & Sons, Inc., 1988)

date an extremity and are used to promote healing and increase range of motion in muscle and joint injuries. Hubbard tanks are used when the entire body needs to be immersed and are used frequently for **debridement** of burn patients.

Debridement is a painful but very necessary aspect of helping burn patients heal properly. Tissue areas that are **necrotic** as a result of burns must be removed to allow oxygen and circulation to reach the area of new granulating tissue. This can be accomplished by applying wet dressings to the area, allowing them to dry, and then removing them along with the necrotic tissue. Debridement can also be accomplished with a sterile wire brush. Most humane of all methods is the Hubbard tank, where the warmth of the water and the whirlpool action accompanied by gentle massage washes away the necrotic tissue, as well as increasing circulation to the healing tissue underneath. This is not to imply that debridement by Hubbard tank is painless, but it is said to be less painful than the alternative methods. Recovery from major burns is, without a doubt, one of the most painful of all therapies. Pain is not felt only by the patient but also in the hearts of the very special people who have chosen this area of specialty.

Active and Passive Range of Motion (ROM)

After an injury or insult to a joint or extremity, the goal of physical therapy is to restore as much use as possible or to restore optimal use of the affected part. Please note the use of the terminology *affected part* throughout the text. This term is preferred over "good leg/bad leg" when working with patients. Remember, the patient is dealing with enough body image changes without the negative reinforcement invoked by the terms good vs. bad.

When we are injured and lose the use of a limb, our musculature deteriorates very rapidly. Muscles **atrophy** at the rate of approximately 3% per day when not used. Over the long term that can account for a substantial loss in muscle tone. Joints become less flexible, and movement translates into pain.

The goal of physical therapy is to restore use. It is a slow process requiring a great deal of patience on the part of both the patient and the therapist. To rush the process is to cause injury, possibly permanent injury.

First, we need to define terms to fully understand range of motion. Using your own arm as an example, stretch the arm out until it is fully straightened, forming a straight line; that is **extension**. If you are able to extend your arm past the point of 180 degrees, that is *hyperextension*. Now bend the elbow so that the distal point of the extremity, the hand, approaches the proximal, the shoulder; this is **flexion**. Forcing the extremity to go even farther toward the shoulder is *hyperflexion* (Figure 16.7).

Range of motion is simply causing flexion and extension by means of moving the extremity. At the end of each motion, the extremity is moved gently a little farther to stretch tendons and muscles and increase the range. When conditions of

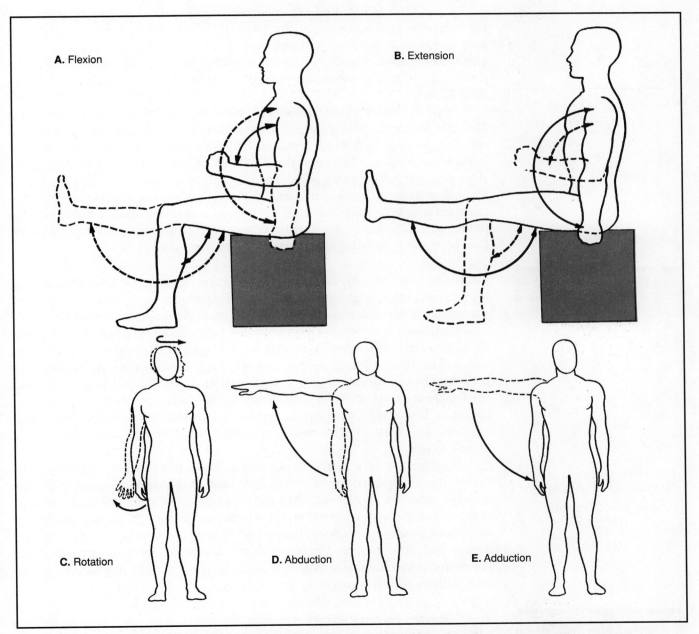

Figure 16.7   Joint extension/flexion (Reproduced with permission from Hegner and Caldwell, *Nursing Assistant, A Nursing Process Approach,* 6th Ed., Delmar Publishers Inc., 1992)

hyperextension and flexion are reached, the range of motion is complete. Again, this must be a slow, gradual process to prevent injury. Often, several sessions must be spent to increase the range only a slight amount. By not rushing the process, the patient will be more cooperative, experience less pain, and progress more rapidly in therapy.

When performing range of motion exercises (ROM) with a patient, the first step is to explain the goals and procedures involved in therapy. Through explanation and reassurance a trust is developed between patient and therapist. The second step is never to violate that trust. The third step is to encourage the patient to try harder and give praise when appropriate.

Active range of motion refers to movement that the patient can perform unassisted. Encourage the patient to move a joint through as much of the full range of extension and flexion as is possible until resistance is met. At the point of resistance the extension or flexion should be continued gently but not to the point of pain. This should be repeated; over time the point of resistance will change, and mobility will be increased.

Passive range of motion is used when the extremity will not function unassisted. This can be the result of paralysis, **contracture**, or severe joint injury. It is then necessary to assist with range of motion. The same principles apply. Move the joint through extension and flexion gently to the point of resistance and very gently apply slight pressure, but not to the point of pain. Continue to repeat this therapy and teach the patient to do the same. Encourage the patient to use the unaffected arm/leg to move the affected arm/leg. Although this process is slow and often very discouraging to the patient, the results are usually positive. Encourage the patient, not by giving false hope, but by pointing out the positive gains made (Figure 16.8).

Ultrasound and Diathermy

Ultrasound and diathermy are both used for treatment of muscle spasm, **tendonitis, bursitis**, and other deep tissue injuries. Both techniques create heat in deep tissue structures. The mechanisms are somewhat different, but the principles are the same.

Ultrasound is performed by introducing high frequency sound waves to deep tissue areas to produce heat. Conduction gel is applied to the skin over the target area, and the head of the instrument is moved slowly around on the skin surface. The head must be kept moving to prevent burns to deep tissue. The patient generally does not feel heat during the treatment, which usually lasts ten minutes or less. Care should be taken when treatment is applied to areas in which patients have metal implants. The metal may become heated due to the vibration, which may loosen some implants.

Diathermy is very similar to ultrasound, but in this instance, electromagnetic current instead of sound waves provides the heat. In diathermy the head of the unit does not come into contact with the patient, so conduction gel is not used. The head of the unit is held approximately one inch from the skin surface. The patient may not wear metal jewelry and must be on wooden furniture, or severe burns can result. This therapy cannot be used on a patient with metal implants. In diathermy, the patient should feel a comfortable sensation of warmth. The treatment should last approximately fifteen to twenty minutes.

Body Mechanics

There are often instances when the medical assistant is called upon to assist a patient who is unable to move or transfer without help. In addition, the day-to-day stresses of the job take a physical toll on the medical assistant. Thus, it is essential that you

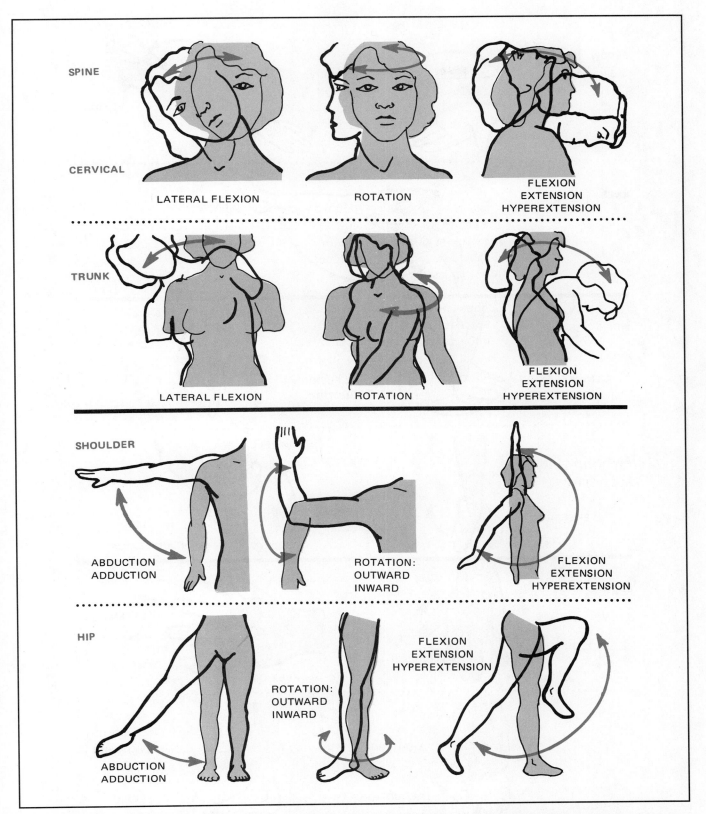

Figure 16.8 Assisting the patient with passive range of motion (Reproduced with permission from Keir, Wise, and Krebs-Shannon, *Medical Assisting,* 2nd Ed., Delmar Publishers Inc., 1989)

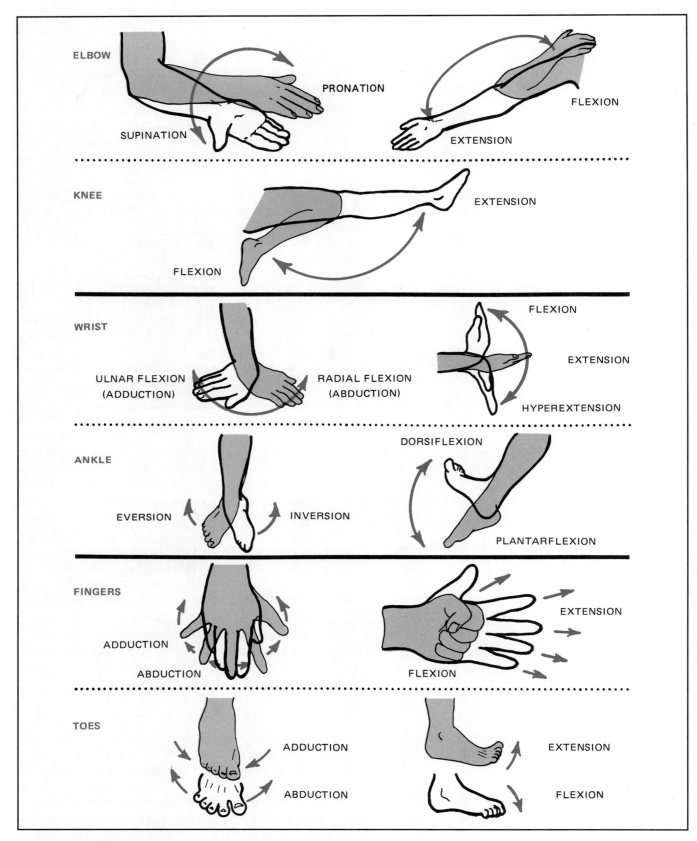

Figure 16.8 continued

be familiar with the principles of body mechanics for the protection of yourself and your patient.

Wear sensible shoes with a no-slip sole that provide adequate support. Keep in mind that a large part of your day will be spent on your feet. For females, support hose can give a little extra to help you go a little further at the end of the day.

Back injuries are one of the most common causes of lost time in the medical industry. You not only can lose time from work with a back injury, but you also can discover pain and physical therapy from the patient's point of view. Most lower back injuries occur in the lumbar region L_3 through L_5.

The rules for protecting your lower back are simple:

1. Keep your back straight at all times.
2. Never bend your back when you can bend your knees.
3. Allow your leg muscles to do the work.
4. Keep your feet spread shoulders-width apart for a wide base of support.
5. Avoid twisting movements.
6. When lifting, keep the load close to your body and below your center of gravity.
7. If you don't think you can do it alone, *get help*.

Before moving a patient, size up the situation, plan your actions, and share that plan with the patient. Determine how you intend to move, reduce the distance of the move as much as possible, and don't exceed your capability.

When transferring a patient from a chair to a high exam table, have a footstool available. Position the patient at a right angle to the table. If the patient has an affected side, keep it away from the table and allow the patient to pivot on the unaffected leg. Explain what you are going to do before you start and enlist the patient's help. Grab the patient firmly beneath the scapula, bend your knees to lower your center of gravity, and rock your body backward slowly. This will bring the patient to their feet. When the patient reaches a standing position, block the knee of the affected leg with your knee to prevent the leg from collapsing. Pivot the patient slowly and return them to a sitting position by leaning slightly backward, bending your knees, and rocking forward. Talk to the patient during transfer, giving encouragement and remaining calm. To return the patient to the chair, simply reverse the procedure (Figure 16.9).

Should a patient start to fall during transfer, call for help immediately. If you are unable to prevent the fall, lower the patient to the floor gently in order to prevent serious injury. When help arrives, get the patient up to a chair or examining table.

Casting and Splinting

Application of casts and splints itself requires a course of instruction. In this section we will cover the basic tenents of the procedure. Medical assistants in orthopedic settings frequently are called upon to assist the physician in the application of casts or splints.

In the event of a fracture, after the initial swelling has decreased, the physician may choose to apply a cast. Although plaster of paris casts are still used, the most common casts today are of fiberglass construction. Fiberglass is much lighter in weight and far stronger than plaster of paris.

To prepare for the application of a cast, the medical assistant should assemble the casting material (usually in foil-covered rolls), felt for lining the cast, scissors, clean latex gloves, a cover gown for the physician, and a pail of warm water.

Position the patient for comfort and ease of access to the fracture site. The physician will position the fractured area when it is to be casted. The medical assistant should support the extremity to maintain that position. The physician will

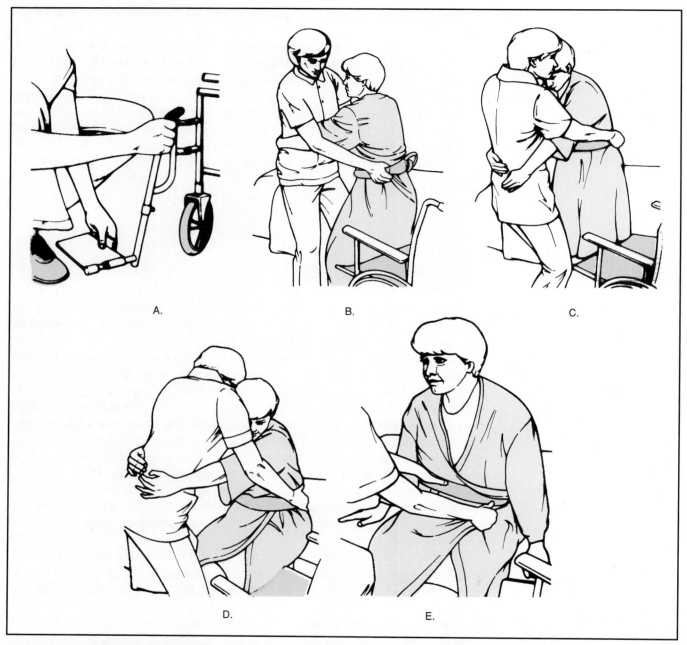

A.

B.

C.

D.

E.

Figure 16.9 Transfer of patient from chair to table. Note the position of the medical assistant's back and the relationship to the patient. Patient is positioned so as to be moved a minimal distance.

wrap the extremity in felt. Open the rolls of casting material and place the first in the pail of warm water. After soaking for a short period, the roll of casting material is removed from the water and the excess liquid wrung out. The extremity is then wrapped by the physician in a similar way to the application of an ace bandage. Areas requiring extra support will receive additional layers.

Once the cast is applied, the patient should experience a sensation of warmth in the casted area. This is a normal result of the chemical action of the compounds in the casting material and should subside in approximately thirty minutes. The patient should be instructed to keep the affected area elevated as much as possible over the next forty-eight hours. The physician usually will instruct the patient on weight bearing and bathing during the course of healing; this should be reinforced by the medical assistant. The patient should be instructed that if the cast becomes wet, it should be thoroughly dried (blow dryers used for hair are good for this). The patient should also be cautioned against putting foreign objects inside the cast in an attempt to scratch the affected extremity. This practice poses considerable danger of infection over the course of treatment. It is also unwise to put talcum powder inside a cast.

The patient will need a follow-up visit, usually within fourteen days after the cast is applied, to check their progress and make any necessary adjustments. Instruct the patient to notify the physician if swelling of the distal extremity, loss of sensation in the distal extremity, or discoloration of the distal extremity occurs. Before the patient leaves the office, check the distal pulses of the casted extremity and compare to those of the noncasted extremity. Document the character of the pulses.

Splints are used for more stable fractures that do not bear any weight and for severe sprains. The extremity is immobilized by means of casting material or a metal splinting device. Fiberglass preformed splints and immobilizers are also used.

Position the extremity prior to application of the splint. Apply the splinting material and wrap the extremity with an ace elastic bandage. Check pulses to ensure adequate circulation, and give the patient instructions similar to those for cast care. The physician may allow the patient to remove the splint at various times. It then becomes the responsibility of the medical assistant to teach the patient the proper methods of applying the splint and checking for proper neurological and circulatory function.

Preformed fiberglass splints and immobilizers usually have Velcro tabs to make application and adjustment easier. These devices are a great convenience to the patient learning to remove and apply the splint. It is still important that the medical assistant go over the procedure with the patient before the patient leaves the office. What may seem quite routine for those in the medical field can often be quite confusing to the patient or family (Figure 16.10).

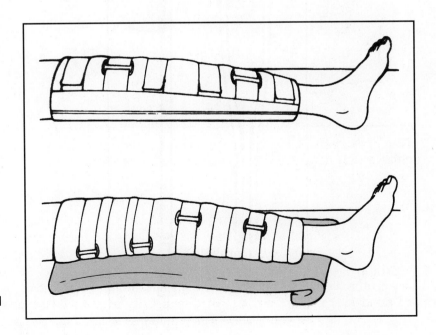

Figure 16.10 Preformed splint: knee immobilizer

Crutch Walking

The first step in teaching the patient to use crutches is to ensure that the adjustment of the crutches is correct for the patient. The most common crutch type is the axillary crutch. The crutch head should never touch the axillary area with the patient standing upright. There should be between one and two inches of space between the crutch head and the axillary area. The palms of the hands should rest easily on the handgrips with the arms bent slightly. The legs of the crutch and the handgrips of the crutch can be moved up or down as necessary to fit the patient. Less commonly used for temporary support is the forearm or Canadian crutch, which is a common choice of paraplegics (Figure 16.11).

Based on the type of injury, the physician will order partial weight bearing or no weight bearing for the patient. The medical assistant should proceed to teach the patient a crutch walking technique to meet the needs of the order.

First, have the patient stand with the crutches and check the adjustment. Instruct the patient to support weight with the hands not the axillary area. Severe and sometimes irreversible neurological damage can result from prolonged pressure on the axillary area. Once the patient has become accustomed to standing with the crutches, you may proceed to teach the proper gait based on weight-bearing requirements.

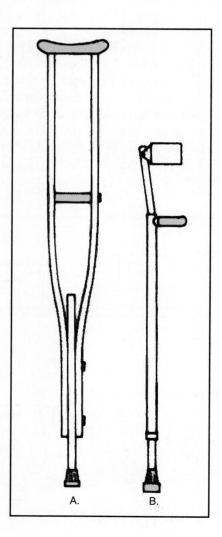

A.   B.

Figure 16.11　Crutch types: (A) Axillary crutch. (B) Forearm or Canadian crutch.

PARTIAL WEIGHT BEARING

Three-point gait (used when one leg is weaker than the other). Place both crutches out in front of the patient, step with the affected leg, then step with the unaffected leg using the crutches for support. Repeat the procedure (Figure 16.12).

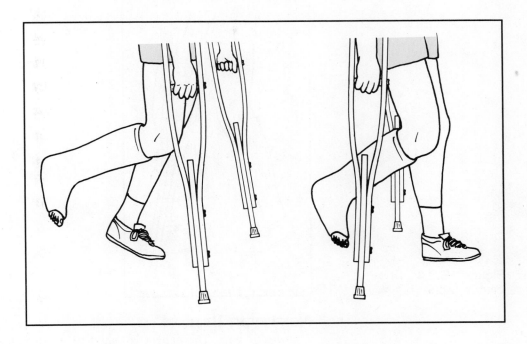

Figure 16.12 Three-point crutch gait

Four-point gait (used when both legs are affected). Place the left crutch forward, step with the right foot even with the left crutch, place the right crutch forward, step with the left foot even with the right crutch. Repeat the cycle (Figure 16.13).

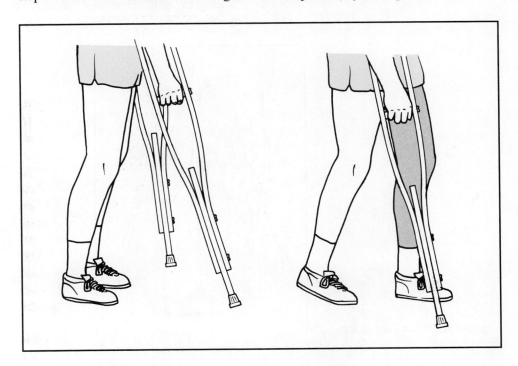

Figure 16.13 Four-point crutch gait

One-crutch or cane gait. Always position a single crutch or cane on the side opposite the injury. Advance the crutch or cane with the injured leg, then step through with the unaffected leg (Figure 16.14).

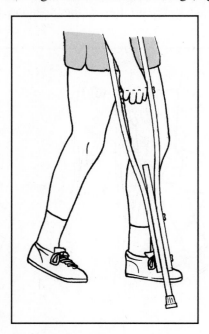

Figure 16.14 One-crutch/cane gait

NONWEIGHT BEARING

Two-point gait. The patient is taught to stand on the unaffected leg and hold the affected leg up from the floor. Both crutches are then placed in front of the patient, and the patient is taught to hop forward landing on the unaffected leg. The patient may choose to use a "swing through" technique, passing the feet of the crutches, or may use a "swing to" gait, advancing the unaffected leg to a point even with the position of the crutch feet (Figure 16.15).

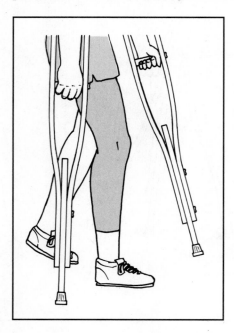

Figure 16.15 Two-point crutch gait

It takes time to master the rhythm and technique of crutch walking. Encourage the patient to proceed slowly until they become more proficient. Some facilities have stairsteps on which patients may practice their skills. The technique for stairs varies with the individual and type of crutch walking used. Be sure to caution the patient against trying to hurry in navigating stairs. The slow and systematic method is the safest in this case.

1. Define the goal of physical therapy.

2. To what danger is the patient exposed with the application of heat?

3. How does the application of heat improve healing?

4. Describe two types of heat therapy and give an example of each.

5. What is the therapeutic purpose of application of cold?

6. To what dangers are the patient exposed with the application of cold?

7. What should you do to protect the patient during the application of cold?

8. What is hydrotherapy? List two purposes of its use.

9. What is the purpose of range of motion exercise?

10. What is the difference between active and passive range of motion?

11. What are the differences between ultrasound and diathermy?

12. List three principles of good body mechanics that help to protect your lower back when working with patients.

13. What should you do if a patient starts to fall during a transfer?

14. What are the differences between a cast and a splint?

15. How should crutches be adjusted to fit the individual patient?

16. Name three crutch gaits and explain their use.

CHAPTER 17

Emergencies

On completion of this chapter, you will be able to:
- Demonstrate methods of preventing accidents.
- Demonstrate methods of dealing with phone emergencies.
- Demonstrate methods of handling various emergencies.
- List the supplies and equipment necessary for handling office emergencies.
- Identify the types of agencies that provide emergency services in the community.
- Explain the role of the medical assistant in an emergency.

Vocabulary— Glossary of Terms

Aphasia
: A condition in which the patient loses the ability to express or understand speech or written language.
  A. *Expressive Aphasia*—inability to speak and/or write in a manner that can be understood.
  B. *Receptive Aphasia*—inability to understand spoken and/or written word.

Coma
: A state in which the patient is unable to respond to verbal or noxious stimuli.

Conscious
: A state in which the patient is able to show a response to verbal and or tactile/noxious stimuli.

Emergency
: Any situation that demands immediate attention.

Fracture
: The interruption of the integrity of a bone.

Irrigation
: The introduction of a fluid into a cavity, allowing the solution to run out.

Ischemia
: Loss of oxygen to tissue.

Postictal
: The period immediately following a seizure.

Trauma
: An injury.

I n the office setting, as in all other areas of clinical practice, both minor and major **emergencies** may arise. The well-prepared medical assistant should perform as directed by office policy, making efficient use of time and resources available.

Supplies and Equipment

One function of the orientation period for a new employee in a medical office should be to familiarize the new employee with the location of both daily and emergency supplies and equipment. The new employee should become thoroughly familiar with the office emergency procedures. There should be available in every office, if not in each examination or procedure room, a "crash cart." The crash cart should contain emergency drugs recommended by the American Heart Association, resuscitation equipment, supplies needed to obtain venous access and administer intravenous fluids, and a selection of needles and syringes. Crash carts often resemble a mechanic's rolling tool box with several drawers located on the front (Figure 17.1). These carts have a flat top, which can hold a portable defibrillator/cardiac monitor (Figure 17.2). The medical assistant is responsible for checking the cart periodically to make sure that expiration dates on medications have not passed; if they have, replace them. Equipment and supplies should be checked to make sure they are in good working order and, if sterile, that packaging has not been perforated or otherwise damaged.

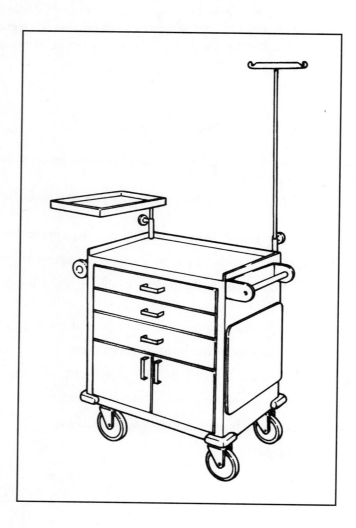

Figure 17.1 Typical crash cart

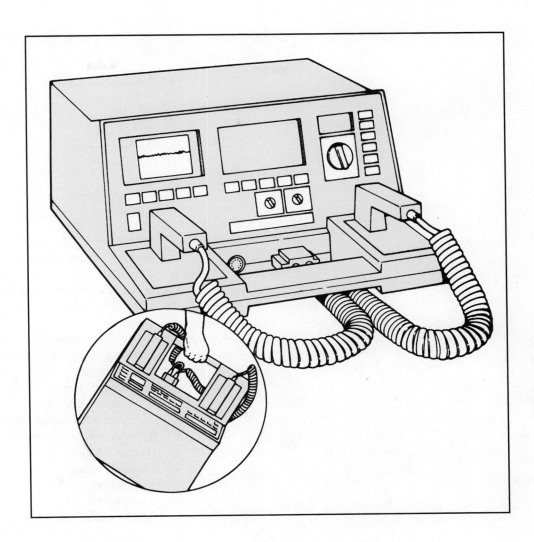

Figure 17.2
Defibrillator/portable
cardiac monitor

SAMPLE CRASH CART

Drawer #1		*Emergency drugs*	Quantity
	a.	Atropine 1 mg/10 cc	2
	b.	Bretyllium 500 mg/10 cc	4
	c.	Calcium chloride 100 mg/10 cc	1
	d.	Dilantin 100 mg/2 cc	2
	e.	Epinepherine 10 mg/10 cc	2
	f.	Isuprel 1 mg/10 cc	2
	g.	Lidocaine 100 mg/10 cc	2
	h.	Nitroprusside 50 mg/2 cc	1
	i.	Procainamide 1 gram/10 cc	2
	j.	Sodium bicarbonate 50 mEq/50 cc	2
	k.	Tridil 50 mg/10 cc	1
	l.	Valium 10 mg/2 cc	2
	m.	Verapamil 5 mg/2 cc	2

Drawer #1	*Intravenous Supplies*	Quantity

    a.   Intravenous catheters
       1.   18 gauge
       2.   20 gauge
       3.   22 gauge
    b.   Alcohol wipes
    c.   Tourniquet
    d.   Tape
    e.   Dressing supplies
    f.   Assorted syringes and needles

Drawer #2   *Resuscitation Supplies*

    a.   Airways (assorted sizes)
    b.   Bite blocks
    c.   Blood pressure cuff
    d.   Conduction gel
    e.   Doppler
    f.   Endotracheal tubes (assorted sizes)
    g.   Extension tubing for suction with connectors
    h.   Laryngoscope
       1.   Straight blade
       2.   Curved blade
       3.   Spare bulbs and batteries
    i.   Nasogastric tubes (assorted sizes)
    j.   Oxygen tubing
    k.   Suction catheters
    l.   Stethoscope
    m. Tonsilar suction
    n.   Water-soluble lubricant

Drawer #3   *Intravenous Fluids*

    a.   5% dextrose and water (D_5W)
       1.   500 cc
       2.   250 cc
    b.   Normal saline (0.9%)
       1.   1000 cc
    c.   Premixed drug infusions
       1.   Dopamine 200 mg/250 cc D_5W
       2.   Lidocaine 2 grams/500 cc D_5W

Additional Equipment:

    a.   AMBU bag with oxygen tubing (Figure 17.3)
    b.   Cardiac monitor/defibrillator
    c.   CPR board
    d.   Portable oxygen tank

In addition to the crash cart, there should be readily available a supply of bandages and dressing materials, splints, disposable ice packs, blankets, and ammonia ampules or smelling salts.

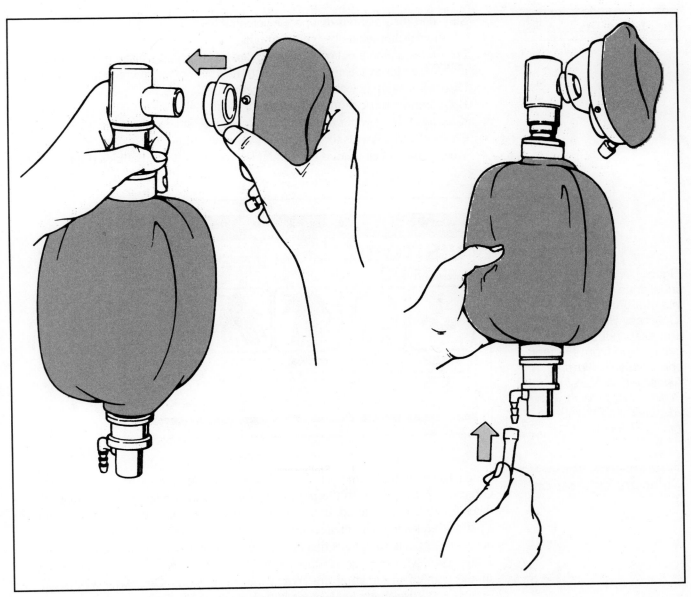

Figure 17.3   AMBU bag

Emergency Services Available in the Community

The medical assistant should be aware of the area agency that handles medical emergencies. These services are provided by the fire or police department in some areas and by private ambulance services that maintain a paramedic force in other areas.

Each office or clinic should display the telephone numbers for the nearest poison control center in a prominent place for easy access in an emergency. The means of contacting emergency agencies should also be known before the need arises so that action becomes automatic. Many communities use the universal emergency number 911. Once contact is made with the appropriate agency, remain calm, state the emergency, state the address, and remain on the line until all information is confirmed and you have been assured that help is on the way.

Accident Prevention

- Stay alert for situations that pose a potential hazard.
- Clean spills immediately to prevent falls.
- Position equipment out of the mainstream and especially away from escape routes used for evacuation in the event of a fire or other emergency.
- Dispose of sharp objects in the proper container.
- Use common sense with electrical equipment.
- Keep away from water and inflammable liquids and gases.
- Check electrical cords for fraying or exposed wiring.
- Wear gloves when there is a potential for contact with body fluids (Figure 17.4).

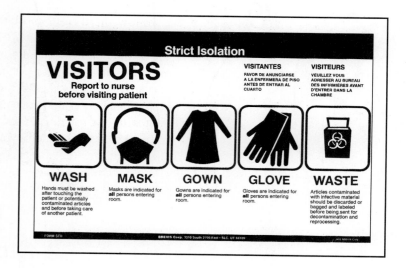

Figure 17.4 Body substance isolation using international symbols (Courtesy Brevis Corporation. Reproduced with permission from Hegner and Caldwell, *Nursing Assistant, A Nursing Process Approach*, 6th Ed., Delmar Publishers Inc., 1992)

Patient Education

When faced with an emergency situation, we all seek help from another source. Often our patients turn to the physician, someone they respect as a source of help when they are ill or injured. In practice, you may find yourself answering a call from a patient requesting help in an emergency situation. These can be difficult times. It is never easy to make a "phone diagnosis," particularly when the facts are coming from a layperson who may be on the verge of hysteria. The office procedure manual should contain information on "When the Physician Is Out of the Office and an Emergency Arises." Act in accordance with established office procedure.

If there is no established office procedure, remember that the scope of your abilities can be your greatest asset. Remember basic first aid and common sense, and realize that the ability to recognize when the situation is beyond your scope is the key to helping the person on the other end of the line. Your best bet, in most circumstances, is to advise the patient to get trained help at the scene. Confirm the location of the patient and secure a telephone number. Advise the caller to hang up the phone, telling them that you will contact emergency assistance for them, and then call back to let them know that help is on the way. In some cases, however, basic common sense and the sound of a familiar voice are the only tools required. In the sections that follow under "Types of Emergencies" are suggested approaches to the "phone-in emergency." The most important advice you can give in an emergency is "Get Help." If the patient is being referred to an acute-care facility, the physician or on-call replacement should be advised as to the patient's name, nature of the emergency, emergency assistance contacted, and the facility to which the patient is being taken.

The Role of the Medical Assistant

When faced with an emergency situation the first duty of a medical assistant is to call for help. After the type of emergency has been identified and help called for, support the patient as appropriate for the type of situation. When help arrives, assist the physician or nurse as necessary, get emergency equipment and supplies prepared, and make notes of the times and actions taken to assist the patient to recovery. Above all, remain calm.

Types of Emergencies

The following guidelines are designed to make the medical assistant aware of the general procedures for dealing with various types of emergency situations. Usually each office or clinical area also has guidelines for dealing with emergency situations, which may or may not be similar to the actions outlined in the following sections. When in doubt, follow the directions of the facility by which you are employed.

There should never be a situation in which the medical assistant is left to face an emergency situation without assistance. Your first action should always be to get appropriate help. Once help arrives, follow the instructions of the physician, nurse, or other emergency medical personnel on the scene, doing those tasks delegated to you and avoiding interfering with other medical personnel in the completion of the tasks that they are performing. Above all, maintain your composure and reassure the patient and family members present. In some instances, that may be the most important action you can take. Take frequent measurements of vital signs (blood pressure, pulse, and respiration) and record them to document the patient's condition during the emergency situation.

REASSURANCE

Throughout the following sections, the medical assistant repeatedly is encouraged to offer the patient and family reassurance in the face of an emergency. Never confuse offering reassurance with telling a patient or their family members a lie. They will appreciate your ability to be forthright and honest. You should be honest, but never blunt. Diplomacy plays an important role in dealing with patients and families.

When beginning procedures, explain your intent in simple and understandable terms, maintain honesty, but avoid frightening the patient or family members. If a procedure is going to be uncomfortable or painful, warn the patient and explain the rationale for the procedure and the possible alternatives to the procedure. Allow yourself a degree of empathy for the patient by considering what you would be feeling in their place, but only to the point of being understanding. Do not, under any circumstances, allow yourself to perform a less than acceptable procedure because you empathize with the patient. You owe your patients the best of your ability; never compromise on that. You also owe them reassurance, and often that is the most important function you perform.

CARDIAC/RESPIRATORY ARREST

Phone Emergency: Advise the caller to activate the local EMS (Emergency Services System) by dialing 911 and to initiate CPR if able.

Assess the patient immediately upon discovering the patient to be unresponsive. Quickly try to arouse the patient by shouting their name and asking if they are all right. Check for a pulse and respiration while calling loudly for help. If no pulses or respiration are noted, begin CPR (cardiopulmonary resuscitation) immediately. Remember the ABCs of CPR and follow them.

A. AIRWAY: Establish a patent airway. Tilt the patient's head backward and open the mouth using the jaw thrust by placing your fingers at the hinge of the mandible and pulling forward to open the jaws. Check the mouth and throat for foreign objects that could obstruct the airway. Take care in placing your fingers in the mouth of an unconscious or semiconscious patient. Use a pair of hemostats rather than your fingers to remove a foreign object. Insert an airway, placing the curved end in the mouth facing upward, then turning the curve downward as the airway is advanced (Figure 17.5).

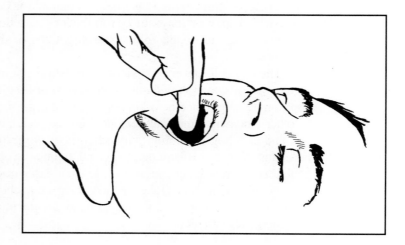

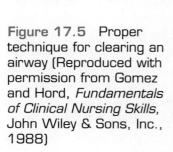

Figure 17.5 Proper technique for clearing an airway (Reproduced with permission from Gomez and Hord, *Fundamentals of Clinical Nursing Skills,* John Wiley & Sons, Inc., 1988)

B. BREATHING: Listen for respiration. If none is detected, begin giving the patient respiratory support. The most desirable method is via an AMBU bag and 100 percent oxygen. Attach the AMBU bag to the oxygen tubing and turn the flow up to 10 to 15 liters/minute. Place the mask of the bag over the patient's mouth and nose, press tightly for a good seal, and squeeze the bag. Observe the patient's chest for rise and fall as the bag is compressed. If the chest moves with the air flow, then give a second breath after allowing the patient to exhale. If there is no movement of the chest, check the seal of the mask on the patient's face or reevaluate the airway, clearing obstructions as necessary. In the absence of an AMBU bag, it may be necessary to perform mouth-to-mouth resuscitation. There are one-way valves on the market that can be placed over the patient's mouth to prevent direct mouth-to-mouth contact. Once the valve is in place, pinch the patient's nostrils closed with the fingers of your hand, press your mouth tightly against the seal, and blow firmly into the patient's mouth. Observe for the rise of the chest. If the chest rises, give a second breath, and proceed to check the pulse. If the chest does not rise, check the airway for obstruction (Figure 17.6).

C. CIRCULATION: After two successful breaths are delivered to the patient, check for a pulse. The carotid artery on the side of the neck just below the angle of the jaw is the best bet for finding a pulse. If a pulse is felt, continue to support the patient's respiration with the AMBU bag until they are able to breathe on their own. If no pulse is felt, begin cardiac compression at the rate of eighty per minute. The patient should be on a firm surface; if necessary, place a board under the patient's back. Find the xiphoid process of the sternum by following the line of the lowest rib to the midline. Place two fingers on the

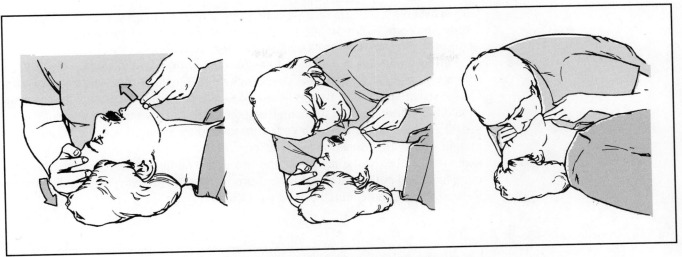

Figure 17.6 Proper ventilation technique

xiphoid process to mark the location of proper hand placement; place the heel of your hand on the sternum just above your fingers, and move your other hand to a position on top of the hand on the sternum, interlocking your fingers. Compress the chest 1½ inches on an adult at the rate of eighty times per minute. Use the cadence "one and two and three and four...". Deliver fifteen compressions and stop; check the carotid pulse. If no pulse can be felt, deliver two quick breaths and resume compressions. Continue this cycle until the pulse is felt or until the physician tells you to stop (Figure 17.7).

Figure 17.7 Proper hand placement for cardiac compression (Reproduced with permission from Hegner and Caldwell, *Nursing Assistant, A Nursing Process Approach*, 6th Ed., Delmar Publishers Inc., 1992)

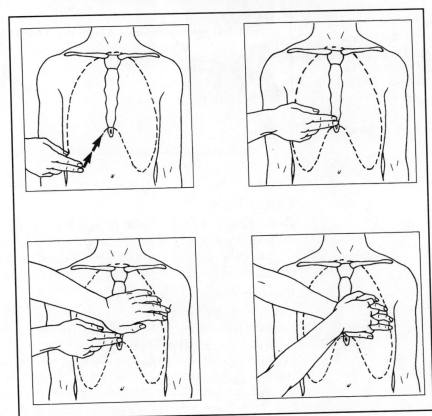

CHOKING

Phone Emergency: Advise the caller to activate EMS system by dialing 911 and to perform the Heimlich maneuver if patient is unable to speak.

In the event that a patient is thought to be choking, immediately ask them if they are all right. If the patient is able to talk or cough, no further action is necessary. On the other hand, if the patient is unable to talk or cough, the Heimlich maneuver should be performed. Call for help. Bring the patient to a standing position. Position yourself behind the patient with your arms around the patient's waist. Find the lower margin of the ribs, make a fist with one hand, and place it against the patient's abdomen just below the margin of the ribs at the midline. Grasp the fist with your other hand and pull upward and inward firmly, compressing the patient's diaphragm. Repeat this procedure until the airway is cleared (Figure 17.8).

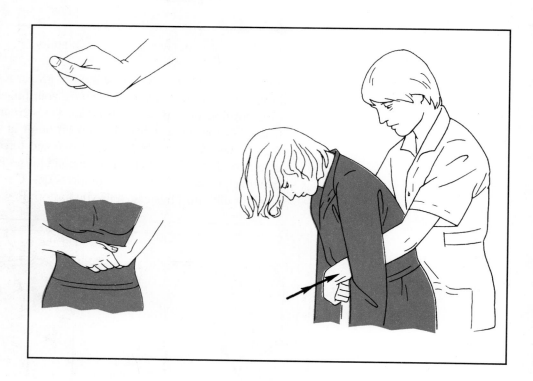

Figure 17.8 Correct technique for performing the Heimlich maneuver (Reproduced with permission from Hegner and Caldwell, *Nursing Assistant, A Nursing Process Approach*, 6th Ed., Delmar Publishers Inc., 1992)

CHEST PAIN

Phone Emergency: Advise caller to activate EMS system by dialing 911, to monitor the patient for cardiopulmonary arrest, and to initiate CPR if necessary.

In the event that a patient complains of chest pain, immediately assist them to lie down and elevate their head at least fifteen degrees. Ask them about the pain:

Is it sharp or dull?
Where is the pain located?
Does the pain radiate to the arms, neck, or jaw?
Have they had this type of pain before?
Do they use sublingual nitroglycerin?
Are they nauseated?
Are they diaphoretic?

If the patient uses sublingual nitroglycerin, have them take a dose, then record their blood pressure. Apply oxygen at 2 liters per minute by nasal cannula or mask. Stay with the patient and call for help. Repeat the blood pressure at two-minute intervals until the pain subsides. Check pulse for rate and regularity. Reassure the patient.

SHOCK

Phone Emergency: Advise caller to activate EMS system by dialing 911, to keep patient supine and warm until help arrives.

A patient in shock generally has marked pallor, complains of nausea and dizziness, and has a feeling of impending doom. The patient in shock should be assisted to a lying position with feet elevated above the level of the heart (Trendelenburg position) and should be kept warm. Call for help. Vital signs should be taken and repeated every two minutes until the condition of the patient improves. Reassure the patient (Figure 17.9).

HEMORRHAGE

Phone Emergency: Advise caller to activate EMS system by dialing 911, and to apply direct pressure to the site of bleeding until help arrives.

In a case of hemorrhage the patient should be assisted to a lying position. Identify the type of bleeding. Venous bleeds have a continuous flow of dark blood, whereas arterial bleeds spurt blood that is a much brighter red and are often more difficult to control. If the hemorrhage is from an external wound, put on gloves, place a dry, sterile 4 × 4 gauze over the bleeding area and apply firm direct pressure to the wound for three to five minutes. Call for help. If the bleeding does not stop with direct pressure, locate an artery proximal to the wound and apply pressure to the artery as well as direct pressure to the wound for three to five minutes.

In cases of internal hemorrhage, treat the patient for shock and call for help. Reassure the patient.

UNCONSCIOUSNESS

Phone Emergency: Advise caller to activate the EMS system by dialing 911, to stay with patient until help arrives, to observe for signs of cardiopulmonary arrest, and to initiate CPR if necessary.

When a patient is found un**conscious**, you must first verify that they are breathing and that there is a strong pulse. Call for help. Assist them to a lying position.

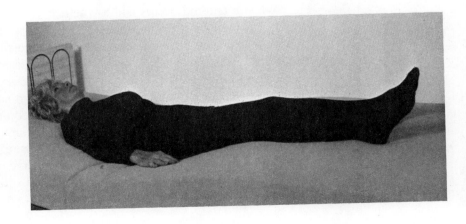

Figure 17.9 Patient in Trendelenburg position (Reproduced with permission from Hegner and Caldwell, *Nursing Assistant, A Nursing Process Approach*, 6th Ed., Delmar Publishers Inc., 1992)

Keep the patient warm in a side-lying position (in case of vomiting). Take vital signs and repeat every two minutes until the condition is resolved. Examine the patient's head for lacerations or bumps that may be the result of a fall.

Whenever a patient is found unconscious, a diabetic **coma** or insulin reaction should be suspected. In these cases, always give sugar to the patient, as brain damage occurs with hypoglycemic states. If the patient's blood sugar is elevated, insulin can be given after blood is drawn for laboratory tests. If the patient's blood sugar is low and insulin is given, death may result.

Sugar may be given to the patient by the physician or registered nurse by intravenous injection if the patient is unconscious. If the patient is arousable and able to drink liquids, two teaspoons of sugar in a twelve-ounce glass of orange juice may be given.

SEIZURES

Phone Emergency: Advise caller to activate the EMS system by dialing 911, to note the length of time of the seizure, to protect the patient from injury, and to keep the patient supine in a side-lying position to protect airway until help arrives.

If a patient is observed having a seizure, call for help immediately. Note the time of the onset of the seizure and the duration. Make note of the characteristics of the seizure, in terms of which body parts are involved:

Is the seizure affecting only a specific area?
Is only one side of the body involved?

Do not try to prevent the patient from moving during the seizure. Protect the patient from injury by moving away objects that could cause injury and by padding objects that cannot be moved. *Never* try to prevent the seizure. Allow it to run its course. *Never* place your fingers in or near a patient's mouth during a seizure. When the seizure is over, note the time, duration, and other information in the patient's medical record. Assist the patient to a side-lying position in case of vomiting and keep the patient warm. Patients are often unresponsive for a short period during the **postictal** phase. Avoid shining bright lights in the patient's eyes immediately after the seizure; stimulation can often initiate another seizure. When the patient begins to regain consciousness, reassure the patient.

FRACTURES

Phone Emergency: Advise caller to immobilize the suspected fracture using a magazine roll, piece of wood, or other rigid material, and to transport the patient to the nearest emergency facility, or activate the EMS system by dialing 911.

When a **trauma** occurs and a **fracture** is suspected, the area should be supported and immobilized immediately. There are a variety of easy-to-use splinting materials available. In the absence of a commercially manufactured splint, wood, cardboard, a roll of magazines, or any other firm material may be attached to the area by means of gauze, elastic bandages, or rags if necessary (Figure 17.10). If possible, the area should be elevated to reduce swelling and an ice pack applied. Pulses and sensation should be checked distal to the suspected injury. When an obvious deformity is noted, as in the case of a separated fracture, no effort should be made to change the contour or straighten the extremity (Figure 17.11). It should be splinted in the position in which it is found, as the risk of nerve or circulatory damage is great; manipulation of the fracture should be left to an orthopedist. Treat the patient for shock and offer reassurance.

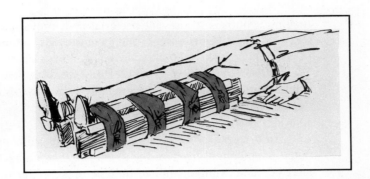

Figure 17.10 Proper splinting technique (Reproduced with permission from Simmers, *Diversified Health Occupations*, 2nd Ed., Delmar Publishers Inc., 1988)

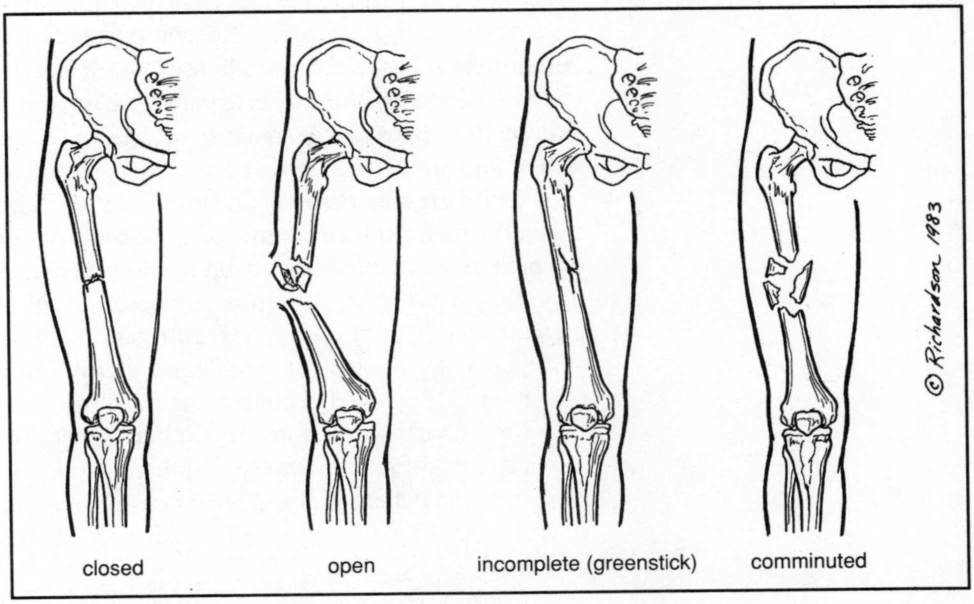

Figure 17.11 Types of fractures (Reproduced with permission from Fong, Ferris, and Skelley, *Body Structures and Functions*, 7th Ed., Delmar Publishers Inc., 1989)

closed   open   incomplete (greenstick)   comminuted

© Richardson 1983

POISONING

Phone Emergency: Advise the caller to activate the EMS system by dialing 911 and to send container with patient to emergency facility.

If poisoning is suspected, the item ingested must be determined. The label of the container is invaluable in the treatment of suspected poisoning. Read the label of the container and make note of the ingredients. Contact the nearest poison control center, inform them of the item(s) ingested and the information obtained from the label, so they may determine the appropriate action for the given substance. Do not assume that inducing vomiting is the answer for all substances. Caustic chemicals usually must be neutralized and will cause additional harm to the digestive tract if vomiting is induced. Keep the patient warm, treat for shock, and monitor vital signs. Observe for changes in level of consciousness and for possible cardiac or respiratory arrest.

BURNS

Phone Emergency: Advise caller to flood affected area with cold water, apply a cool wet dressing and transport the patient to the nearest emergency services facility.

Burns are categorized according to the amount of damage to the layers of tissue. In all cases, burns are painful and willing sites for infection. The goal in treating a burn is to prevent bacterial contamination and to reduce the amount of damage to underlying tissues. The greatest risk to a burn patient is from infection.

Classification of Burns. Burns are classified by the amount of damage to the tissue and underlying structures. The severity of the injury increases with each degree of burn, and the prognosis becomes less.

First-Degree Burn. First-degree burns, although painful, damage only the outer or epidermal layer of the skin. They are characterized by a reddening of the affected area without an interruption of skin integrity. A sunburn is the classic example of the first-degree burn. There is no damage to underlying structures.

Second-Degree Burn. Second-degree burns damage the fatty layer of tissue beneath the skin surface, the adipose layer. These burns are painful and are characterized by reddening of the affected area and the formation of vesicles or blisters on the skin surface. Because the integrity of the skin surface is interrupted, there is a greater risk of infection.

Third-Degree Burn. The third-degree burn affects the underlying muscle tissue and structures beneath the skin. Because of damage to nerve structures, there is no pain from a third-degree burn. However, due to the physiology of the burn process, each degree of burn is composed of all lesser degrees as well. That is, an area affected by a third-degree burn is surrounded by an area of second-degree burn surrounded by an area of first-degree burn. The areas of the wound that may be classified as first- and second-degree will account for a considerable sensation of pain for the victim of a third-degree burn. There is a large danger of infection due to the deep area of tissue damage and the massive interruption of skin integrity. Dehydration of the patient is also a great consideration in this type of burn. Characteristics of the third-degree burn include a severely charred appearance of the flesh in the main body of the wound.

Fourth-Degree Burn. When a patient is the victim of intense flame of extremely caustic chemicals, the burn may be so severe as to damage the skeletal structure. In these cases, the flesh and bone are charred. This is a fourth-degree burn. Most of the time, fourth-degree burns are ultimately fatal. In the period prior to death the patient is at risk for severe infection and suffers from severe dehydration. The characteristics of this burn are severely charred appearances of the flesh with possible exposure of the skeletal structure.

Body Surface Area. In addition to evaluating the severity of the burn, it is important to estimate the percentage of the body surface area affected by the burn. This is accomplished by using a simple formula commonly referred to as "The Rule of Nines." This formula divides the body area into areas representing 9% of total area for the purpose of determining the percentage of burn area in relation to the total body surface area (Figure 17.12).

The areas are as follows:

Head (anterior and posterior surface)	9%
Left arm (anterior and posterior surface):	9%
Right arm (anterior and posterior surface):	9%
Anterior thorax:	9%
Posterior thorax:	9%
Anterior right leg:	9%
Posterior right leg:	9%

Anterior left leg:	9%
Posterior left leg:	9%
Genital Area:	1%
TOTAL	100%

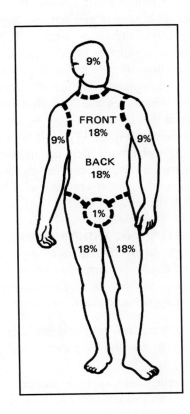

Figure 17.12   The Rule of Nines (Reproduced with permission from Keir, Wise, and Krebs-Shannon, *Medical Assisting,* 2nd Ed., Delmar Publishers Inc., 1989)

By estimating the degree of severity and percentage of body surface area damaged, one can communicate the severity of the injury to other health-care personnel during the emergency.

Initial treatment of the burn victim is a very important aspect of care, and understanding the physiology of the burn is paramount. Damage to tissue continues after the source of the burn is removed, making time a large factor in treatment.

It is important to cover the burned area with a clean, if not sterile, material and saturate that material with cool, *sterile* saline solution. If you are able to remove clothing from the wound surface without damage to the underlying tissues, do so carefully. Synthetic materials often melt during a fire and become imbedded in the tissues. *Do not* attempt to remove materials imbedded in the wound, as the chance of increasing damage to tissues is too great. The covering and the saline keep the wound moist and slow dehydration of the tissue. The sterile solution reduces the danger of further contamination of the wound. The cool liquid reduces the heat contained in the wound and slows tissue damage. *Do not* cover the wound with greasy or oily substances (e.g., butter or other home remedies); this only holds heat in the wound area, increases damage to the tissues, and supplies a medium for bacteria.

Treat the patient for shock and get help immediately. The greater the severity of the burn, the less time there is before major complications occur as a result of hypothermia and shock.

DYSPNEA

Phone Emergency: Advise the caller to activate the EMS system by dialing 911 and to keep the patient in an upright sitting position to assist respiratory effort.

When a patient has difficulty breathing, the first reaction is panic. It is important that the medical assistant remain calm, reassure the patient, and call for help. Check the patient for an occluded airway and remove any obstructions, being extremely careful to keep fingers out of the patient's mouth by using forceps or similar instruments. Sit the patient as upright as practical to allow full movement of the diaphragm, and apply low-flow oxygen by nasal cannula at 2 liters per minute. If the patient is breathing predominantly through the mouth, attempt to teach them to breathe in through the nose and exhale through pursed lips. If you are unable to get the patient to breathe in this manner, it may be necessary to apply a face mask to deliver supplemental oxygen (Figure 17.13). It is important to avoid giving oxygen at higher flow rates (greater than 2 liters per minute) to patients with a history of chronic obstructive pulmonary disease, particularly those with emphysema. The physiology of the disease alters the patient's regulation of breathing, and high flow oxygen can in some cases result in apnea.

LACERATIONS, CONTUSIONS, AND ABRASIONS

Phone Emergency: Advise the caller to apply a dressing to lacerations with direct pressure to stop bleeding. Cleanse abrasions with soap and water and apply a dressing. Apply ice packs to contusions. Transport the patient to the nearest emergency services facility for evaluation and treatment.

Lacerations. A laceration, simply defined, is a cut with uneven edges. The first order of treatment is to reassure the patient and stop active bleeding.

1. Apply gloves.
2. Using a piece of sterile gauze, apply direct pressure to the wound.
3. Once the bleeding has subsided, observe the wound for foreign objects and remove them with sterile forceps.
4. Clean the wound with a mixture of sterile saline and betadine or similar antimicrobial solution.
5. Apply a loose, moist dressing to keep the tissue from dehydrating and elevate the wound if possible.
6. Wait for further instructions.

Contusions. A contusion, simply defined, is a bruise. Reassure the patient, clean the area gently with warm water and soap, apply an ice pack after protecting the skin surface with a towel, and elevate the affected part if possible. Wait for further instructions.

Abrasions. An abrasion, simply defined, is a scrape. Wear gloves. Reassure the patient, cleanse the area with warm water and soap, apply betadine or similar antimicrobial agent to the skin surface, and cover with a dry, sterile dressing. Wait for further instructions.

CEREBROVASCULAR ACCIDENTS

Phone Emergency: Advise the caller to activate the EMS system by dialing 911 and to stay with patient until help arrives.

The cerebrovascular accident (CVA), commonly referred to as stroke, follows one of two mechanisms of physiologic damage to the structures of the brain. The

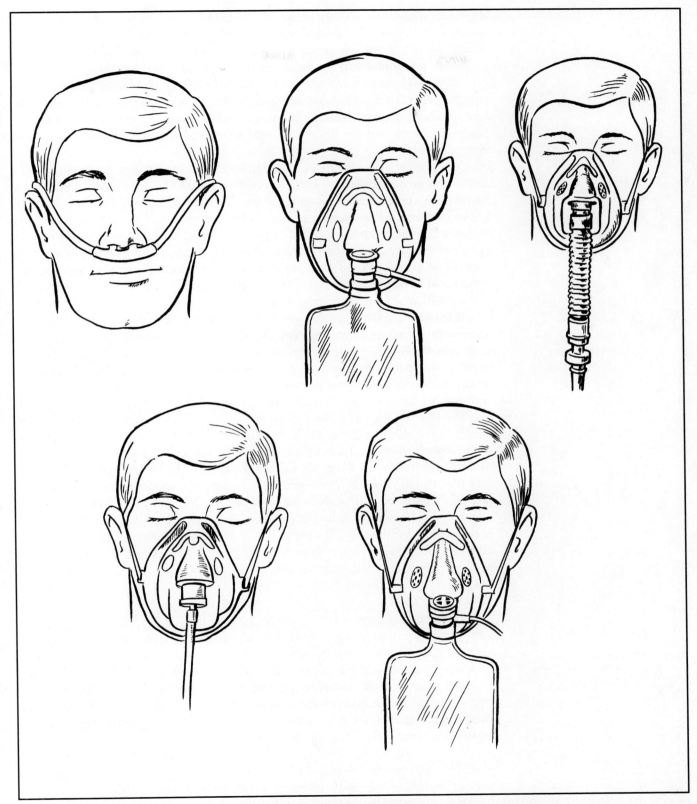

Figure 17.13 Supplemental oxygen devices (Reproduced with permission from Gomez and Hord, *Fundamentals of Clinical Nursing Skills,* John Wiley & Sons, Inc., 1988)

rupture of a blood vessel may cause a hemorrhagic infarct causing pressure on brain tissues or structures. The *occlusion* of a blood vessel may cause the interruption of circulation to brain tissue or structures, causing anoxic damage. In either case, the symptoms are similar, and the assessment techniques are the same.

Cerebrovascular accidents can be characterized by alterations in the level of consciousness, from mild variations such as forgetfulness to the point of coma; by loss of motor function in one or more areas of the body; by impairment of speech, hearing or sight; by impairment of vital functions; or any combination of these symptoms.

Onset is usually quite rapid, although a series of small CVAs commonly known as transient **ischemic** attacks (TIA), sometimes called little strokes, may contribute to a long-standing deterioration over a period of time. CVAs are usually associated with the elderly but are not limited to that group and have been known to affect even children and young adults.

The primary goal of treatment is to collect as much of the history prior to the incident as possible in an effort to rule out other possible causes. Support of the patient and family is paramount. Observe the patient for respiratory embarrassment, cardiac difficulties, and changes in neurological function.

Changes in motor function generally affect, but are not limited to, one hemisphere of the body, leading to hemiplegia, hemiparesis, or paresthesia. Assessment of sensory and motor function comparing bilateral extremities should be made. Assessment of pupillary function should be made and documented. Observe for facial asymmetry evidenced by facial droop on the affected side. Assess speech patterns and observe for slurring or various forms of **aphasia.** Keep in mind that a patient may develop expressive aphasia, a condition in which the patient is able to think clearly but unable to express themselves through spoken or written word. Be patient with these patients, at all times remembering how frustrating it must feel to be able to think coherently but being able to speak only in garbled or nonsense language. Patients that fall victim to CVA often are very slow in response because their thought process is impaired. Allow them adequate time to respond to each question; avoid confusion by requiring rapid-fire response to a series of questions. Patients often become repetitive and will try the patience of medical personnel. Remember, it is your obligation to the patient to be understanding during times like this; causing the patient unnecessary frustration borders on cruelty.

HEAD INJURIES

Phone Emergency: Advise caller to activate the EMS system by dialing 911 if loss of consciousness, seizure, or neck injury is suspected. In other cases, transport the patient to the nearest emergency services facility for evaluation and treatment.

Head injuries as the result of trauma often can appear benign at the onset but are often insidious, with symptoms appearing as long as two weeks post injury. The type of injury varies from concussions to contusions to intracerebral hemorrhage. Head injuries should never be taken lightly; this should be stressed to the family of the patient, particularly where children are concerned.

As with all emergencies, it is important to obtain as much information as possible regarding the mechanism of injury and the patient's medical history. As always, the patient and family members should be given reassurance.

If loss of consciousness occurred, the length of time that the patient was unconscious should be noted. A thorough neurological assessment should be performed.

The family of the patient should be instructed to assess the patient's level of consciousness each hour through the night and to report immediately any changes to the physician. Another significant factor is the appearance of nausea or vomiting, particularly projectile vomiting.

Ice packs generally can be applied to any visible contusions or abrasions. The patient should be observed for respiratory depression or seizure activity. If seizure activity occurs, the length of time of the seizure should be noted as well as how much of the body was involved. The seizures may be focal (or Jacksonian) in nature and involve only a particular area of the body with tremors or twitching, or thay may be as severe as a grand mal seizure, in which the entire body convulses. Any abnormality or suspected abnormality should be reported to a physician without delay.

During the recuperative period the patient should get plenty of rest and keep activity to a minimum. Strenuous exercise is prohibited. The patient's neurological status should be assessed hourly for the first twenty-four to forty-eight hours after the injury occurs.

EYE AND EAR INJURIES

Phone Emergency: Advise the caller to transport the patient to the nearest emergency services facility for evaluation and treatment. Do not attempt to remove foreign bodies from the eye or ear. Flush eyes with cool water if caustic substance has entered the eye.

Eye injuries are both painful and frightening. After reassuring the patient, examine the eye for foreign particles. Keep the lights dim in the examination room for patient comfort. *Never* attempt to remove a foreign body from the eye by means other than **irrigation** with a sterile ophthalmic solution under the direction of a physician. Removal of foreign particles that cannot be dislodged by irrigation should be left to a trained ophthalmic professional. Discourage the patient from rubbing the eye. Placing a gauze pad over both eyes, keeping them closed, will often lessen discomfort. Because of the physiology of the eye, both eyes move in unison. If only the injured eye is covered, movement of the unaffected eye will cause movement of the affected eye and could contribute to further injury.

PROCEDURE FOR IRRIGATION OF THE EYE
1. **Assemble the necessary supplies.**
   a. sterile ophthalmic irrigant
   b. towel
   c. small basin
   d. gauze pads
   e. latex gloves
2. **Explain the procedure to the patient.**
3. **Position the patient in a sitting position** with head tilted slightly back.
4. **Wash and dry hands. Put on latex gloves.**
5. **Cover the patient's chest with a towel** to protect clothing.
6. **Ask the patient to look upward.** Take the vial of irrigant between the thumb and forefinger of your hand with the dropper pointed downward. Use the middle finger of the same hand to **gently pull the patient's cheek downward to expose the lower canthus of the eye.**

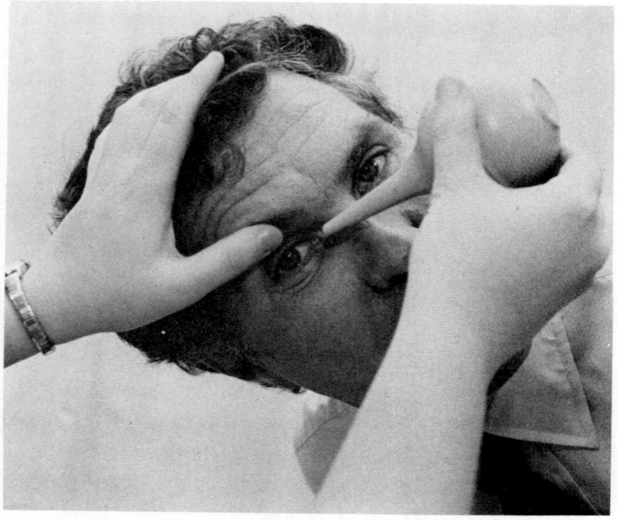

Figure 17.14 Proper eye irrigation technique (Reproduced with permission from Simmers, *Diversified Health Occupations*, 2nd Ed., Delmar Publishers Inc., 1988)

7. Holding the dropper above the midpoint of the lower canthus, **allow the drops to fall into the conjunctival sac.** Ask the patient to hold the basin or a gauze pad next to the cheek below the eye to catch the irrigant as it flows out of the eye.
8. **Irrigate as directed by the physician's order.**
9. **When the procedure is completed, return items to their proper area, clean soiled equipment, remove gloves, and wash and dry your hands** (Figure 17.14).
10. **Record the date and time of the procedure, the type of irrigant, and the outcome of the procedure in the patient's medical record.**

There will be occasions when you will be required to irrigate the ear under a physician's order. The technique varies between adults and children because of the orientation of the ear canal.

PROCEDURE FOR IRRIGATION OF THE EAR

1. **Assemble necessary equipment.**
    a. bulb syringe
    b. irrigating solution warmed to approximately 100 degrees.
    c. basin
    d. towel
    e. gauze pads
    f. latex gloves
2. **Wash and dry hands and put on latex gloves.**
3. **Explain the procedure to the patient.**
4. **Position the patient so the affected ear may be turned slightly downward.**
5. **Place a towel over the patient's shoulder** to protect clothing from moisture.
6. **Place the basin directly beneath the affected ear.**
7. **Draw the warm solution into the bulb syringe, check the temperature by allowing a drop or two to drip to your forearm** (similar to the technique for checking temperature of baby formula). The solution should feel pleasantly warm; if it burns the forearm, it is too hot.

8. **On an adult, grasp the ear pinna with the thumb and forefinger and pull gently upward and backward to align the ear canal. On a child, pull downward and backward.**

9. While holding the ear pinna in position, **gently insert the tip of the syringe into the ear canal,** being careful to avoid occluding the canal with the syringe.

10. **Gently compress the bulb of the syringe, introducing a gentle flow of irrigant into the ear canal.** Allow the flow of irrigant to flow out of the ear into the basin. If there is no return flow, check the placement of the tip of the syringe to ensure that the canal is not occluded. If pressure builds in the ear canal, the tympanic membrane can rupture.

11. **Continue irrigating as ordered,** refilling the syringe as necessary.

12. **At the completion of the procedure, dry the patient with the gauze pads, clean up the basin, place materials in the proper area, remove gloves, and wash and dry your hands** (Figure 17.15).

13. **Record the date, time, type of procedure, irrigant used, and the outcome of the procedure in the patient's medical record.**

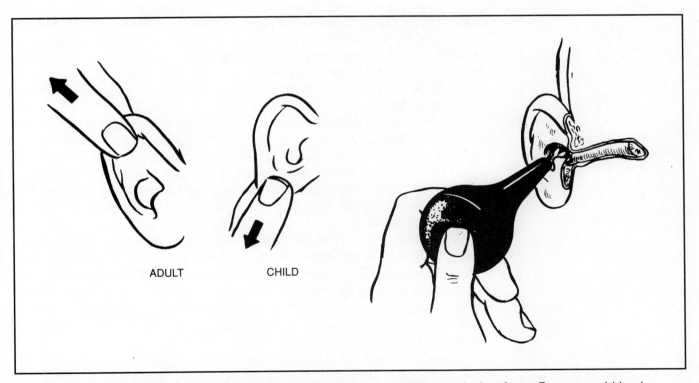

ADULT   CHILD

Figure 17.15   Proper ear irrigation technique (Reproduced with permission from Gomez and Hord, *Fundamentals of Clinical Nursing Skills,* John Wiley & Sons, Inc., 1988)

ABDOMINAL PAIN

Phone Emergency: Advise the caller to transport the patient to the nearest emergency services facility for evaluation and treatment.

Abdominal pain can be due to gastric distress or can be the precursor of very serious conditions. Obtain a complete history of the present condition as well as the patient's previous medical history. Reassure the patient and family members. Question the patient about items ingested over the last twenty-four hours and make a list for the patient's chart. Determine if the patient has had nausea, vomiting, constipation, or diarrhea prior to the onset of pain. Question the patient about possible changes in stool color or consistency and note the time of the last bowel movement. Ask the patient if they have recently used laxatives or cathartics and how often they use such products.

Assess the patient's abdomen, listening for bowel sounds with the diaphragm of the stethoscope for at least one full minute in each abdominal quadrant. Palpate the abdomen for tenderness and/or rigidity. A normal abdomen should be soft to the touch and free of pain with palpation. Do not allow the patient to eat or drink liquids. Place them in a comfortable position and keep them warm. Report the findings of your assessment to the physician and record in the patient's chart.

BITES AND STINGS

Phone Emergency: Advise caller to apply ice to insect bites and stings. Apply a dressing to animal bites. Transport the patient to the nearest emergency services facility for evaluation and treatment.

Animal bites and insect stings can be very frightening and painful, particularly to the pediatric patient. Reassure the patient and family members. Obtain details of the injury. If the injury involves an animal bite, are the whereabouts of the animal known? Obtain the patient's medical history. Questions involving insect bites should include a history of allergies to bee stings. Patients with a history of allergy to bee stings can develop anaphylactic shock, which can lead to death without prompt medical attention.

While obtaining the medical history for a patient with an animal bite, cleanse the wound with soap and warm water, apply an antimicrobial solution such as betadine, and place a dry, sterile dressing over the injured area. In cases of animal bites in children, the patient should be assessed thoroughly for additional sites of injury. Children often focus on the most serious injury as a result of shock. So there may be multiple injuries that would be overlooked without thorough assessment.

If the injury involves an insect bite, apply ice to slow the spread of toxins through the system. If the offender was a bee, the wound should be examined for the barb of the stinger left in the wound. Under the direction of a physician, the barb may be removed using forceps. When doing this procedure, use magnification. Before attempting removal, observe the proximal end of the barb for a small sac, which contains the toxins. Avoid compressing the sac with the forceps during removal to prevent introducing additional toxins to the wound.

Apply ice to snake bites as well. Avoid tourniquets and the technique of cutting parallel slits to the muscle and "sucking out the venom." This is rarely appropriate in the office or clinic, and experience has proven that if the rescuer has a cut in the oral mucosa he or she will very likely become the next patient.

Elevate the limb where appropriate to decrease swelling and keep the patient warm and comfortable.

ABUSE

Phone Emergency: Advise caller to transport the patient to the nearest emergency services facility for evaluation and treatment. Encourage the responsible party to file a police report concerning the incident.

The area of office emergencies cannot be covered adequately without mention of suspected physical abuse. People most often consider abuse in relation to children, but this is not the only group affected by abuse. Abuse also affects spouses, both male and female, the elderly, and others.

Often the party guilty of the abuse is the same party who brings the victim in for treatment. Usually the explanation for the injury sounds reasonable enough, but in many cases the excuse is not believable even given the most unlikely circumstances.

Be alert for the party who overexplains the injury or who changes the events with the retelling of the incident. Observe the patient's reaction to the account of the accident and the patient's reaction to the party giving the account. Observe the patient's prior medical history for a pattern of repeated traumatic injury. This often may be indicative of a clumsy toddler, but it may very well establish a pattern of abuse.

The best guideline in these circumstances is "when in doubt, report the suspected abuse to the proper authority." Most if not all states protect the party reporting abuse from repercussions as a result of making the report. This is especially true when child abuse is suspected. The action takes only a simple phone call; describe the facts observed and the parties involved. You may need to repeat this information in writing on the appropriate agency form at a later time. Be sure to document in the medical record the date, time, and all of your findings, including the agency to whom the report was made and the name of the person taking the report.

If you suspect abuse during the examination, it is your moral duty to report those suspicions to the authorities. Waiting for someone else to take action may be too late. If abuse is occurring, statistics prove that it will continue and usually get progressively worse until the abusing party receives professional help.

Documentation

When dealing with office emergencies, it is most important to document the events accurately and completely. The following list of suggested topics to cover in charting is intended as a guideline for recording the events and interventions for emergency situations.

1. List the initial symptoms that made you aware of the emergency situation and the time that these symptoms were observed.
2. Chart a baseline set of vital signs (blood pressure, pulse, and respiration) and record vital signs every five minutes while the emergency is in progress.
3. Document your call for help, the time and to whom the call was made.
4. List all interventions made on the patient's behalf, the time that they were initiated, and the results of those interventions.
5. Document the final outcome of the emergency.
6. Document any information regarding the accident obtained from the patient or person accompanying the patient. Use quotation marks whenever possible.

Be brief but accurate in charting. List the facts as they occurred and remember to sign all entries. The following is an example of charting for an emergency situation.

Mrs. Johnson carries her four-year-old son into the office and states that the child was injured in a fall from a bookcase approximately thirty minutes ago. The child struck his head on the staircase and reportedly lost consciousness for approximately five minutes. You take the child into the examination room and allow the mother to be present while you conduct your examination.

Oct 10, 1989

10:30 am Alert, awake and oriented x3. Skin warm and dry. PERRLA at 3mm with active consensual reflex, moves extremities to command x4. Contusion noted at left temporal area approximately 5 cm. in diameter with small abrasion noted on left cheek below eye. BP=110/68, HR=138, Resp=24. Mother states "I think he was knocked out for about five minutes." Mother denies seizure activity or history of previous falls. No previous medical history available.

10:35 am Ice pack applied to L temporal area, abrasion at L cheek cleansed with soap and warm water. Remains alert and oriented. BP=104/70, HR=128, Resp=22. Notified Mary Smith, R.N., of patient's status.

10:40 am Examined by Dr. Phillips. Instruction for care of head injuries explained to mother along with printed instructions. Discharged ambulatory accompanied by mother after bandaid applied to abrasion at left cheek. BP=114/62, HR=110, Resp= 18. Follow-up appointment made for Oct 12, 1989, at 10:00 am.

Jane Jones, CMA

REVIEW/ SELF-EXAMINATION

1. Define the role of the medical assistant in an emergency.

2. Why is it important to be familiar with the emergency services available in the community?

3. What is a crash cart?

4. If a person is thought to be choking, what should your first action be?

5. What is the greatest danger to a burn patient?

6. What do the ABCs of cardiopulmonary resuscitation stand for?

7. When is the Heimlich maneuver used?

8. What should you do when a patient has a seizure?

9. Name three household items that can be used as a splint.

10. What is the most important piece of information when poisoning is suspected?

11. Explain the difference between a laceration and a contusion.

12. What is the first duty of a medical assistant in an emergency?

13. What should the parents of a child with a head injury be instructed to observe?

14. Who should be called if poisoning is suspected?

15. What is meant by expressive aphasia?

16. When should the medical assistant wear gloves?

17. What is the best position for a patient with dyspnea? Why?

18. Describe Trendelenburg position. When is it used?

19. How do you irrigate the ear of a child?

20. What is the "Rule of Nines"?

21. How are burns classified?

CHAPTER 18

Health Maintenance

**Vocabulary—
Glossary of Terms**

Amblyopia	Dimness of vision.
Anorexia	Loss of appetite.
Ascites	Accumulation of fluid in the peritoneal cavity.
Beriberi	A disease caused by a deficiency of vitamin B_1 and characterized by inflammation of nerves, edema, and cardiac pathology.
Bradycardia	Slow heart rate; normally less than 60 beats per minute.
Cachectic	Extreme state of malnutrition.
Ceroid	An insoluble, acid-fast, lipid pigment found in the liver, nervous system, and muscle.
Cheilosis	A condition characteristic of riboflavin deficiency with fissuring and scaling of the lips and corners of the mouth.
Collagen	The protein substance of connective tissue.
Dermatitis	Inflammation of the skin.
Diet	The food and drink consumed daily by individuals.
Ecchymoses	Bruises.

Flaccid	Weak, lax, and soft.
Glossitis	Inflammation of the tongue.
Keratomalacia	Softening of the cornea.
Legumes	The pod or fruit of a plant such as beans and peas.
Megadose	Excessively large dose as compared to normal.
Nutrition	The total process of ingesting, assimilating, and utilizing nutrients.
Osteomalacia	Softening of bone, usually due to impaired mineralization or vitamin D deficiency.
Palpation	The act or process of feeling with the hand.
Pancytopenia	Deficiency of all blood cell elements.
Pellagra	A condition produced by deficient niacin and characterized by dermatitis, diarrhea, inflammation of mucous membranes, and psychic symptoms.
Petechiae	Pinpoint hemorrhages in the derma or mucous membrane.
Polydipsia	Excessive thirst.
Polyuria	Excessive urination.
Pruritis	Itching.
Rickets	A condition of vitamin D deficiency associated with osteodystrophy.
Stomatitis	Inflammation of the mouth.
Tetany	Muscle spasm.
Xerophthalmos	Dryness of the conjunctivae and cornea associated with vitamin A deficiency.

Diet

While food and water are essential for survival, humans do not eat for sustenance of the physical body alone. Food helps to meet a number of personal, social, and cultural needs and is therefore related to both physical and emotional health.

It is essential for the professional medical assistant to become well versed in **diet** therapy since this area of treatment modality involves a great deal of patient education. While the physician will prescribe the diet and exercise plan for the patient, usually it is the responsibility of the medical assistant to educate the patient in sensible diet planning to meet their nutritional needs.

The medical assistant must develop a sound basic working knowledge of **nutrition** and the individual patient's personal life style and situation. The principles of nutrition education must be applied in every situation to improve the individual's nutritional status, combat malnutrition, and motivate the individual to change eating habits.

Good food habits based on moderation and variety will help build and maintain sound, healthy bodies. A variety of foods from the four basic food groups—milk and dairy products, meats, vegetables and fruits, and bread and cereals—will provide the normal nutrient requirements of most individuals. Refined sugar, fat, saturated fat, and cholesterol should be eliminated or minimized. Complex carbohydrate foods (starches) are better sources of energy and will also help to increase dietary fiber. Too much sodium (salt) should be avoided. Salt substitutes and other spices may be used as replacements. Alcohol, if ingested at all, should be taken in moderation, as it provides no nutrients and is high in empty calories.

The medical assistant must recognize that meal patterns will vary with individual living situations and energy demands, but a well-balanced meal at the beginning of the day, and a fairly even eating pattern throughout the remainder of the day can work more efficiently and sustain a more even energy supply. Providing patients with sound nutritional information in a manner that meets their individual needs will provide the basis for building sound eating habits.

Human nutritional needs usually are based on age, stress factors that depend on individual life situations, health status (the individual's degree of health or disease, both real and perceived), and basic human needs required for physiologic survival, such as food and water, safety and comfort. Since these needs are variable, the nutritional needs of the patient are also variable. Pregnant and lactating females have increased nutritional considerations. Babies require more protein per pound of body weight for growth and development than adults. Geriatric dietary planning needs to take into account chewing difficulties, which can result in protein deficiency as well as frequent intolerance of fat. Physical activity among the elderly is often diminished, affecting caloric requirements. Obesity in this age group is often a problem, as some individuals will eat to excess out of boredom, loneliness, or anxiety. The addition of cooked fruits to the diet will add bulk to prevent constipation, and the addition of fiber will stimulate peristaltic activity.

ADEQUATE NUTRITION

Dietetics is the science of diet and nutrition and their effects on the body. Nutrition refers to the sum of the processes involved in ingesting nutrients, assimilating them, and then using them to meet human needs. Good nutrition is evidenced by a well-developed body of ideal weight for body size and by good muscles. The skin is smooth and clear. Hair is glossy, and the eyes are bright and clear. Appetite, digestion, elimination, and posture are good, and facial expression is alert. People who are well-nourished are more likely to be alert mentally and physically and to have a happier outlook on life. In addition, good nutrition can extend the period of their normal activity for more years.

Individuals with adequate nutrition will have enough nutrients to provide energy sources, build tissue, and to regulate the metabolic processes, which are the total of all body processes that sustain life.

An adequate diet will contain enough fuel for heat and energy, which are provided primarily by carbohydrate and fat and secondarily by part of the protein consumed in the diet. Protein provides building units or amino acids needed to build and repair body tissues necessary for growth and maintenance of a strong body structure.

Regulation and control of the multiple chemical processes in the body must be maintained as a smooth, balanced operation. The control agents that help to maintain this state of balance within the body are vitamins, minerals, water, and fiber.

Vitamins are micronutrient organic substances found in foods and are essential, in small quantities, for growth, health, and preserving life itself. They serve as coenzymes in enzymatic reactions and are required only in trace quantities since they are not consumed in the metabolic reactions. Recommended daily dietary allowances (RDAs) have been established by the Food and Nutrition Board of the National Research Council. Vitamins are designated by the letters A, C, D, E, and K and the term B-complex. The B vitamins and vitamin C are water soluble. The remainder of the vitamins are fat soluble and are not absorbed unless the digestion and absorption of fats in the body is normal.

Vitamin A is found principally in dairy products, fish liver oils, liver, and egg yolk, as well as green leafy or yellow vegetables. It acts on the photoreceptor mechanism of the retina and maintains integrity of epithelia, lysosome stability, and glycoprotein synthesis. Deficiency of this vitamin demonstrates itself in night blindness, **xerophthalmos**, and **keratomalacia**. Toxicity may result from hypervitaminosis (excess of the vitamin) and may result in headache, **pruritis**, peeling of the skin, enlargement of the spleen, and thickening of bone.

Vitamin B_1 (thiamine) is found in dried yeast, whole grains and cereal products, meats (especially pork and liver), nuts, **legumes**, and potatoes. The function of thiamine is on carbohydrate metabolism and peripheral nerve cell and myocardial function. Deficiency of this vitamin can result in **anorexia**, certain types of neuritis, and in severe cases **beriberi**.

Vitamin B_2 (riboflavin) is found in dairy products, liver, meat, eggs, and enriched cereal products. Function is concerned with oxidation-reduction reactions and metabolism of carbohydrates. Deficiency of this vitamin is believed to be one of the most common vitamin deficiencies in the United States and can result in **cheilosis, stomatitis**, corneal vascularization, **amblyopia**, and sebaceous dermatosis.

Niacin (nicotinic acid) is a B vitamin found in dried yeast, liver, meat, fish, legumes, and whole-grain-enriched cereal products. It is involved in energy production, protein metabolism, and maintaining the integrity of mucous membranes. Deficiency of this vitamin can result in **pellagra**, which manifests itself in **dermatosis, glossitis**, and gastrointestinal and central nervous system dysfunction.

The vitamins in the B_6 group include vitamin B_6 (pyridoxine), biotin, folic acid, pantothenic acid, choline, inositol, and para-aminobenzoic acid and are found in dried yeast, liver, organ meats, fish, legumes, and whole-grain cereals. These vitamins are involved in the metabolism of nitrogen and linoleic acid. Folic acid is essential to the maturation of red blood cells and synthesis of purines and pyrimidines. Biotin is essential to the metabolism of amino acid and fatty acid. Deficiency of these vitamins is associated with anemias, neuropathy, convulsions in infancy, dependency states, **pancytopenia**, megaloblastosis, dermatitis, and glossitis.

Vitamin B_{12} (cyanocobalamin) is found in liver, meat, organ meats, eggs, and dairy products. It is essential to DNA synthesis as well as methionine and acetate synthesis, neural function, and maturation of red blood cells. Deficiency of this vitamin is manifested in sprue, dependency states, nutritional amblyopia, anemias, and some psychiatric syndromes. When a substance called *intrinsic factor* is missing from the normal secretions of the stomach, inability to absorb vitamin B_{12} in the small intestine occurs, which results in pernicious anemia.

Vitamin C (ascorbic acid) is found in citrus fruits, tomatoes, cabbage, green peppers, and potatoes and is essential to the development of osteoid tissue, **collagen** formation, vascular function, tissue repair, and wound healing. Cooking and storage destroy much of the vitamin C content of foods. Deficiency of this vitamin results in gingivitis, loose teeth, hemorrhages, and scurvy.

Vitamin D is found in fortified milk, fish liver oils, dairy products, and ultraviolet radiation. It is essential to calcium and phosphorus absorption, resorption, mineralization, and collagen maturation of bone. Deficiency of this vitamin is sometimes associated with **tetany** and is seen in **osteomalacia** and **rickets**. Toxicity may demonstrate in anorexia, renal failure, and metastatic calcification.

Vitamin E is found in vegetable oils, wheat germ, leafy vegetables, egg yolk, margarine, and legumes. While the role of this vitamin is not entirely certain, it does appear to be essential as an intracellular antioxidant and for the stability of biologic membranes. In many species, it is a dietary necessity for normal reproduction, muscular development, and normal resistance of red blood cells to hemolysis. Individuals with erythrocyte hemolysis, creatinuria, and **ceroid** deposition in muscle tissue demonstrate deficiency of Vitamin E.

Vitamins K, K_1 (phytonadione), and K_2 (menaquinone) are found in leafy vegetables, vegetable oils, pork, and liver. These vitamins are essential to prothrombin formation and normal coagulation of blood. Deficiency of these vitamins may result in hemorrhage from deficient prothrombin. Toxicity generally demonstrates as kernicterus.

Minerals are naturally occurring, nonorganic, homogeneous solid substances and are supplied by a diet of varied or mixed animal and vegetable products. Recommended daily requirements have been established by the Food and Nutrition Board of the National Research Council for only calcium and iron, which along with iodine are the three elements most often missing from the diet. Minerals that are most often involved in metabolic disturbances are copper, iron, magnesium, potassium, and zinc (Figure 18.1).

FOOD AND NUTRITION BOARD, NATIONAL ACADEMY OF SCIENCES—NATIONAL RESEARCH COUNCIL
RECOMMENDED DIETARY ALLOWANCES.[a] Revised 1989
Designed for maintenance of good nutrition of practically all healthy people in the United States

Category	Age (years) or Condition	Weight[b] (kg)	(lb)	Height[b] (cm)	(in)	Protein (g)	Fat-Soluble Vitamins — Vitamin A (µg RE)[c]	Vitamin D (µg)[d]	Vitamin E (mg α-TE)[e]	Water-Soluble Vitamins — Vitamin K (µg)	Vitamin C (mg)	Thiamin (mg)	Riboflavin (mg)	Niacin (mg NE)[f]	Vitamin B6 (mg)	Folate (µg)	Vitamin B12 (µg)	Minerals — Calcium (mg)	Phosphorus (mg)	Magnesium (mg)	Iron (mg)	Zinc (mg)	Iodine (µg)	Selenium (µg)
Infants	0.0–0.5	6	13	60	24	13	375	7.5	3	5	30	0.3	0.4	5	0.3	25	0.3	400	300	40	6	5	40	10
	0.5–1.0	9	20	71	28	14	375	10	4	10	35	0.4	0.5	6	0.6	35	0.5	600	500	60	10	5	50	15
Children	1–3	13	29	90	35	16	400	10	6	15	40	0.7	0.8	9	1.0	50	0.7	800	800	80	10	10	70	20
	4–6	20	44	112	44	24	500	10	7	20	45	0.9	1.1	12	1.1	75	1.0	800	800	120	10	10	90	20
	7–10	28	62	132	52	28	700	10	7	30	45	1.0	1.2	13	1.4	100	1.4	800	800	170	10	10	120	30
Males	11–14	45	99	157	62	45	1,000	10	10	45	50	1.3	1.5	17	1.7	150	2.0	1,200	1,200	270	12	15	150	40
	15–18	66	145	176	69	59	1,000	10	10	65	60	1.5	1.8	20	2.0	200	2.0	1,200	1,200	400	12	15	150	50
	19–24	72	160	177	70	58	1,000	10	10	70	60	1.5	1.7	19	2.0	200	2.0	1,200	1,200	350	10	15	150	70
	25–50	79	174	176	70	63	1,000	5	10	80	60	1.5	1.7	19	2.0	200	2.0	800	800	350	10	15	150	70
	51+	77	170	173	68	63	1,000	5	10	80	60	1.2	1.4	15	2.0	200	2.0	800	800	350	10	15	150	70
Females	11–14	46	101	157	62	46	800	10	8	45	50	1.1	1.3	15	1.4	150	2.0	1,200	1,200	280	15	12	150	45
	15–18	55	120	163	64	44	800	10	8	55	60	1.1	1.3	15	1.5	180	2.0	1,200	1,200	300	15	12	150	50
	19–24	58	128	164	65	46	800	10	8	60	60	1.1	1.3	15	1.6	180	2.0	1,200	1,200	280	15	12	150	55
	25–50	63	138	163	64	50	800	5	8	65	60	1.1	1.3	15	1.6	180	2.0	800	800	280	15	12	150	55
	51+	65	143	160	63	50	800	5	8	65	60	1.0	1.2	13	1.6	180	2.0	800	800	280	10	12	150	55
Pregnant						60	800	10	10	65	70	1.5	1.6	17	2.2	400	2.2	1,200	1,200	320	30	15	175	65
Lactating	1st 6 months					65	1,300	10	12	65	95	1.6	1.8	20	2.1	280	2.6	1,200	1,200	355	15	19	200	75
	2nd 6 months					62	1,200	10	11	65	90	1.6	1.7	20	2.1	260	2.6	1,200	1,200	340	15	16	200	75

[a] The allowances, expressed as average daily intakes over time, are intended to provide for individual variations among most normal persons as they live in the United States under usual environmental stresses. Diets should be based on a variety of common foods in order to provide other nutrients for which human requirements have been less well defined. See text for detailed discussion of allowances and of nutrients not tabulated.

[b] Weights and heights of Reference Adults are actual medians for the U.S. population of the designated age, as reported by NHANES II. The median weights and heights of those under 19 years of age were taken from Hamill et al. (1979) (see pages 16–17). The use of these figures does not imply that the height-to-weight ratios are ideal.

[c] Retinol equivalents. 1 retinol equivalent = 1 µg retinol or 6 µg β-carotene. See text for calculation of vitamin A activity of diets as retinol equivalents.

[d] As cholecalciferol. 10 µg cholecalciferol = 400 IU of vitamin D.

[e] α-Tocopherol equivalents. 1 mg d-α tocopherol = 1 α-TE. See text for variation in allowances and calculation of vitamin E activity of the diet as α-tocopherol equivalents.

[f] 1 NE (niacin equivalent) is equal to 1 mg of niacin or 60 mg of dietary tryptophan.

Figure 18.1 Current RDA table (Reproduced with permission from *Recommended Dietary Allowances,* © 1989, by the National Academy of Sciences, National Academy Press, Washington, D.C.)

SUMMARY TABLE Estimated Safe and Adequate Daily Dietary Intakes of Selected Vitamins and Minerals[a]			
		Vitamins	
Category	Age (years)	Biotin (µg)	Pantothenic Acid (mg)
Infants	0–0.5	10	2
	0.5–1	15	3
Children and adolescents	1–3	20	3
	4–6	25	3–4
	7–10	30	4–5
	11+	30–100	4–7
Adults		30–100	4–7

		Trace Elements[b]				
Category	Age (years)	Copper (mg)	Manganese (mg)	Fluoride (mg)	Chromium (µg)	Molybdenum (µg)
Infants	0–0.5	0.4–0.6	0.3–0.6	0.1–0.5	10–40	15–30
	0.5–1	0.6–0.7	0.6–1.0	0.2–1.0	20–60	20–40
Children and adolescents	1–3	0.7–1.0	1.0–1.5	0.5–1.5	20–80	25–50
	4–6	1.0–1.5	1.5–2.0	1.0–2.5	30–120	30–75
	7–10	1.0–2.0	2.0–3.0	1.5–2.5	50–200	50–150
	11+	1.5–2.5	2.0–5.0	1.5–2.5	50–200	75–250
Adults		1.5–3.0	2.0–5.0	1.5–4.0	50–200	75–250

[a] Because there is less information on which to base allowances, these figures are not given in the main table of RDA and are provided here in the form of ranges of recommended intakes.

[b] Since the toxic levels for many trace elements may be only several times usual intakes, the upper levels for the trace elements given in this table should not be habitually exceeded.

Figure 18.1 continued

INADEQUATE NUTRITION

Poor nutritional status frequently is evidenced by a listless, apathetic, or **cachectic** appearance. The hair may become stringy, dull, brittle, or dry or show evidence of depigmentation. Eyes may become dry with increased vascularity and a glassy appearance. Conjunctivae may become thickened, and there may be evidence of infection.

The mouth may evidence absent teeth or wearing of the surfaces, mottling, marginal redness, or swelling of the gums, or they may become spongy and begin to recede. The tongue may demonstrate papillary atrophy and a smooth appearance or glossitis.

The skin may become rough, dry, and scaly as well as pigmented with evidence of **petechiae** and **ecchymoses.** The abdomen is generally swollen, with evidence of **ascites** in cases of severe malnutrition.

The musculoskeletal system may demonstrate bowlegs, knock-knees, beaded ribs, prominent scapulae, and deformity of the chest at the diaphragm. Muscles may be underdeveloped and tender or **flaccid** with poor tone. Posture may be poor, with sagging shoulder, a sunken chest, and a humped back.

Individuals who are malnourished generally will be inattentive, irritable, and easily fatigued due to lack of energy. They will also appear apathetic and frequently will complain of anorexia, indigestion, constipation, or diarrhea.

VITAMIN AND MINERAL SUPPLEMENTS

Dietary surveys show that approximately one third of the population of the United States is living on a diet below optimum level. While this does not mean that one third of Americans are undernourished since some persons can maintain good health on somewhat less than optimal amounts of various nutrients, it does mean that these individuals have a greater risk of physical illness than persons receiving proper amounts.

Americans have been bombarded for years now by supplement merchants with information indicating the need for supplemental vitamins and minerals or **megadose** vitamin and minerals. In fact, the vitamin and mineral supplement business has grown to a multibillion dollar industry.

As noted previously in the chart showing recommended dietary allowances, the individuals who do indeed eat a well-balanced diet with representation from the four basic food groups should easily meet or exceed their daily vitamin and mineral requirements. This is especially true now that many of the foods we eat are vitamin fortified.

Vitamin and mineral supplements were never intended as a replacement for proper nutrition. Claims that dietary supplements or megadosing can prevent or cure a long list of disorders should be viewed with skepticism. In fact, there is strong evidence to support the idea that megadosing can be harmful.

Daily megadoses of vitamin C (above 500 mg) frequently result in nausea, vomiting, and diarrhea and may also cause increased acidity of the urine, leading to the formation of cystine kidney stones in individuals predisposed to this type of medical problem.

Megadosing with the B vitamins has been shown to obscure anemia due to vitamin B_{12} deficiency, and megadoses of nicotinic acid have resulted in itching and flushing, arrhythmia of the heart, and gastrointestinal distress.

Fat-soluble vitamins pose even more of a problem that the water-soluble vitamins, as they are not excreted from the body in urine and are normally stored in the body in considerable amounts. In well-nourished adults it may take from several months to more than two years for deficiency symptoms to develop after withdrawal of one or more of the fat-soluble vitamins from the diet.

Hypervitaminosis A is a toxic condition that can result from excessive intake of vitamin A; it produces acute symptoms, including violent headache, nausea, vomiting, sluggishness, dizziness, and peeling of the skin. Symptoms of chronic toxicity include dryness, itching and peeling of the skin, loss of hair, bone and joint pain, headache, enlargement of the liver, anorexia, fatigue and weakness, cessation of menses, and an increase in cerebrospinal pressure. Carotenes, unlike vitamin A, are not toxic, but ingested in large amounts will sometimes turn the skin yellow. This phenomenon frequently is seen in individuals on the so-called "carrot diet" and in children who go on carrot-eating binges. Cessation of this dietary over indulging will alleviate the condition.

Continuing megadoses of vitamin D has been reported to delay growth in infants and cause high concentrations of calcium in the blood, in both adults and children, that eventually result in calcifications of soft tissue such as the kidneys and blood vessels, resulting in death or irreversible damage. Other symptoms of toxicity are anorexia, nausea and vomiting, **polyuria** and **polydipsia**, constipation, pruritis, **bradycardia**, and other arrhythmias of the heart.

PATIENT EDUCATION

In order to effectively educate patients in meeting nutritional goals established by the physician, it is essential that the medical assistant determine the life situation of the patient in terms of food habits and dietary history, as well as food purchasing and preparation planning and methods.

It is frequently helpful to have the patient keep a food record for twenty-four hours, three days, one week, or even longer to help in identifying food preferences. If possible, this record should include quantity, preparation methods including seasonings, and snacking habits. It may also be of some use to identify the time of day that the recorded foods are ingested. This will help establish the dietary patterns of the patient.

After the patient's food habits have been analyzed, you may be able to help in developing a menu and meal plans. The patient may also need help with shopping, economical buying, and suggestions for preparation of specific foods.

The average American family spends approximately twenty percent or more of its income on food. Much of this amount is spent on fast food, prepackaged convenience foods, expensive cuts of meat, out-of-season fruits and vegetables, and delicatessen items. Low-income and fixed-income families frequently need counseling to help maximize the purchasing power of their available food dollars. Other considerations in patient education include the food likes and dislikes of family members, special dietary needs of any family member, number of family members, and whether any of the family food is produced or preserved at home by canning or freezing. Time available for food preparation and available transportation for shopping may also have a real bearing on the dietary habits of the patients. You should also know the value placed on food by the family, as well as the number of meals normally eaten out, the amount and kinds of entertaining done by the family, and the food storage and cooking facilities at home.

Baking and broiling are alternatives to help eliminate frying, reducing the amount of fat in the diet. Restricting or eliminating use of salt and by using other spices or salt substitutes will reduce the amount of sodium in the diet. Nonfat milk, evaporated milk, and buttermilk are less expensive and just as nutritious as the more expensive whole milk. Ice milk and frozen yogurt are usually better bargains than ice cream. Good and standard grades as well as less tender cuts of meat are a better bargain than the more expensive prime and choice grades and tender cuts. Whole broiler-frying chickens and large turkeys are a better dollar value than chicken parts and small turkeys.

Fresh fruits and vegetables in season are always a good buy. Canned fruits and vegetables are normally much more economical than their frozen counterparts. Breads and rolls made at home are usually less expensive than ready-made but may have a higher fat content. Enriched pasta and brown or converted rice are usually a better buy than their unenriched, frozen, quick-cooking, or canned counterparts.

Patients should be encouraged to eat three or more well-balanced meals each day, dividing their nutrient requirements over the total number of meals. They should be encouraged to read labels on packaged foods, seeking those with the lowest sugar, sodium, and fat contents. Food portions at meals should be accurately weighed or measured when portion size or caloric count is a consideration. There are a number of good, inexpensive scales available for this purpose.

Patients may also be referred to the local home adviser of the county agricultural extension service for food preparation and purchasing materials. Home economists employed by the electric and gas companies are also valuable sources of information, as are dieticians employed by the local hospitals.

The public library can also provide information on nutrition, special diets, food preparation, etc., and even television can be a source of information on food preparation and purchasing (Figure 18.2).

MENU PLAN

BREAKFAST

Fruit rich in vitamin C.
Grain cereal, muffin, toast or roll.
Butter or fortified margarine prefer low-fat, low
   cholesterol.
Milk prefer low-fat or skim for cereal or beverage.
Egg serve one; no more than twice weekly.
Beverage tea or coffee; preferably decaffinated.

LUNCH

Main Dish should contain cheese, eggs, fish, meat or
   poultry (could be soup, salad, sandwich or a
   casserole dish); 1 egg, or 2-4 ounces of fish,
   meat or poultry per person.
Vegetable preferably raw.
Grain muffin, bread or roll.
Fruit rich in vitamin C.
Beverage low-fat or skim milk; decaffinated tea or
   coffee.

DINNER

Meat, poultry or fish 2-6 ounces per person.
Vegetables (2) at least 1 green leafy; the other may
   be yellow or potatoe.
Salad may be vegetable or fruit.
Dessert 1/2 cup custard, gelatin, ice cream or yogurt.
Beverage low-fat or skim milk; decaffinated tea or
   coffee.

Figure 18.2 Menu plan

Exercise

Good health, vitality, and longevity are desirable goals, but they are not achieved without effort. A positive attitude toward personal health and well being requires that physical fitness be an essential part of daily living.

Exercise helps control weight and prevent insomnia, and there is impressive evidence that people who exercise frequently and correctly are less prone to heart problems, strokes, and other life-threatening conditions and generally have increased longevity over their sedentary counterparts.

Exercise helps you look and feel your best. Aerobic exercise is the most effective type of exercise since it increases the efficiency of the lungs and heart and blood circulation by increasing oxygen consumption and utilization.

A warming up and cooling down period should be an integral part of any type of exercise or sport, particularly aerobics, as it is dangerous and inefficient to go from rest to maximum activity. These warming up and cooling down exercises may consist of a series of flexion and extension movements involving various body parts and the body as a whole.

Aerobic exercise programs include walking, jogging, running, swimming, and bicycle riding. They can be alternated with or substituted for aerobic dancing, skipping rope, and skiing.

Before beginning any aerobic program, it is essential to have a medical checkup to ensure that the particular program you have chosen is appropriate for you. The physician may also suggest or recommend some combination of activities that will better suit your individual needs.

PATIENT EDUCATION

Patients need to be advised that the purpose of a good aerobic program is to help them look and feel their best. Involving all of the family members in the program will make it easier for the patient and assist the remainder of the family in achieving a healthier and more productive lifestyle.

Exercise will provide many benefits, including stress reduction, weight loss and control, relief of pain, such as backache and menstrual pain, relief from depression, improved muscle tone, reduced risk of heart and arterial disease, improved sleep, increased strength and stamina, and improved ability to concentrate, enabling better performance at work and at home. It will also help patients who are trying to quit smoking and help prevent those who have stopped from starting again.

Whatever aerobic activity or program is decided upon it must become a habit, like brushing your teeth. The ultimate goal is to exercise for at least twenty minutes each day, three times a week. Each program will have three variables—frequency, duration, and intensity. Manipulation of these factors will allow the patient to build endurance and progress to higher levels of fitness.

Exercise should be at a time of day convenient to the patient's schedule, but preferably two or more hours after a meal. Never exercise when feeling ill and never exercise to the point of pain or exhaustion.

The patient should be taught how to take both a carotid and a radial pulse. They will need to be able to determine resting heart rate (pulse rate at the lowest level of activity, usually on awakening). It is also essential that the patient be able to determine their target heart rate, i.e., the most effective rate for maximum cardiovascular benefit; beginning exercisers will generally use sixty percent, and regular exercisers will use seventy percent. This is the rate at which most exercise will be conducted. The recovery rate is the pulse rate that occurs during the cooling down period.

To determine target heart rate is relatively easy once the patient knows how to take a radial or carotid pulse. The patient should make the calculation using the following directions and write them down on a piece of paper for future reference

To Determine Target Heart Rate

1. Everyone starts from a base of 220, so record 220 as the baseline.
2. Subtract the patient's age from 220.
3. Subtract the patient's resting heart rate.
4. Multiply by the target zone, which will usually be sixty percent or seventy percent.
5. Add the patient's resting heart rate.

Since it is extremely difficult to take a pulse rate, either radial or carotid, for a full minute while exercising, divide the target rate by six so that the patient can take the pulse for only ten seconds while exercising.

Remember that the above formula is merely a guide. The medical assistant will need to check with the physician prior to patient teaching to see if there are any modifications that need to be made (Figure 18.3).

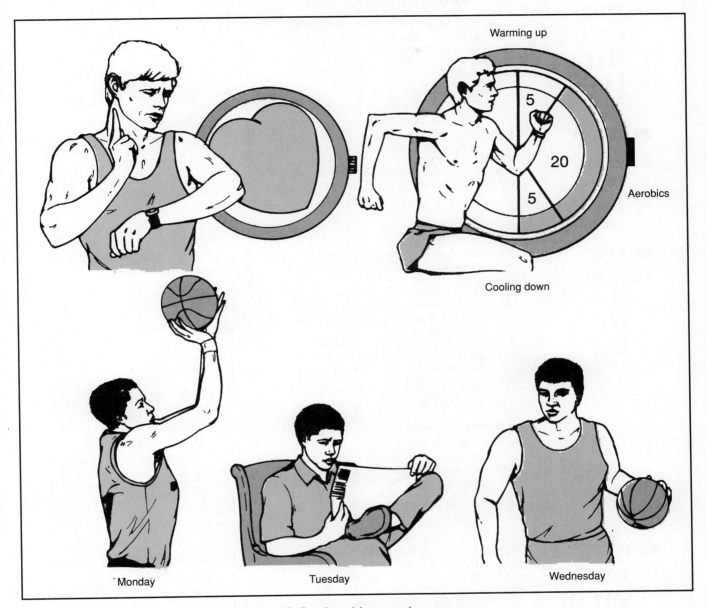

Figure 18.3   Aerobic exercise program

Self-Examination

Health awareness means body awareness. In order to determine whether the body is trying to tell you that something needs attention, you should examine it on a regular basis. Stand in front of a full-length mirror and check for skin lesions, bruises, or other abnormalities. Have moles (nevi) grown larger or changed color? Do you notice anything else unusual or that needs attention or bears watching?

When you bathe or shower, palpate your axillae (armpits) for lumps. If you are a male, palpate your testes for lumps or other abnormalities that may need to be checked by a physician.

■ WHY DO THE BREAST-SELF EXAM?

*T*HERE ARE MANY GOOD REASONS FOR DOING THE BREAST SELF-EXAM (BSE) EACH MONTH. ONE REASON IS THAT BREAST CANCER IS MOST EASILY TREATED AND CURED WHEN IT IS FOUND EARLY. ANOTHER IS THAT IF YOU DO BSE EVERY MONTH, IT WILL INCREASE YOUR SKILL AND CONFIDENCE WHEN DOING THE EXAM. WHEN YOU GET TO KNOW HOW YOUR BREASTS NORMALLY FEEL, YOU WILL QUICKLY BE ABLE TO FEEL ANY CHANGE. ANOTHER REASON, IT IS EASY TO DO.

REMEMBER: BSE COULD SAVE YOUR BREAST— AND SAVE YOUR LIFE. MOST BREAST LUMPS ARE FOUND BY WOMEN THEMSELVES, BUT, IN FACT, MOST LUMPS IN THE BREAST ARE NOT CANCER. BE SAFE, BE SURE.

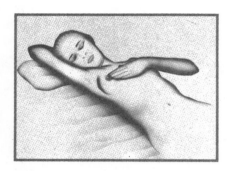

■ WHEN TO DO BSE

*T*HE BEST TIME TO DO BSE IS ABOUT A WEEK AFTER YOUR PERIOD, WHEN BREASTS ARE NOT TENDER OR SWOLLEN. IF YOU DO NOT HAVE REGULAR PERIODS OR SOMETIMES SKIP A MONTH, DO BSE ON THE SAME DAY EVERY MONTH.

■ NOW, HOW TO DO BSE

1. LIE DOWN AND PUT A PILLOW UNDER YOUR RIGHT SHOULDER. PLACE YOUR RIGHT ARM BEHIND YOUR HEAD.

2. USE THE FINGER PADS OF YOUR THREE MIDDLE FINGERS ON YOUR LEFT HAND TO FEEL FOR LUMPS OR THICKENING. YOUR FINGER PADS ARE THE TOP THIRD OF EACH FINGER.

3. PRESS FIRMLY ENOUGH TO KNOW HOW YOUR BREAST FEELS. IF YOU'RE NOT SURE HOW HARD TO PRESS, ASK YOUR HEALTH CARE PROVIDER. OR TRY TO COPY THE WAY YOUR HEALTH CARE PROVIDER USES THE FINGER PADS DURING A BREAST EXAM. LEARN WHAT YOUR BREAST FEELS LIKE MOST OF THE TIME. A FIRM RIDGE IN THE LOWER CURVE OF EACH BREAST IS NORMAL.

4. MOVE AROUND THE BREAST IN A SET WAY. YOU CAN CHOOSE EITHER THE CIRCLE (A), THE UP AND DOWN LINE (B), OR THE WEDGE (C). DO IT THE SAME WAY EVERY TIME. IT WILL HELP YOU TO MAKE SURE THAT YOU'VE GONE OVER THE ENTIRE BREAST AREA, AND TO REMEMBER HOW YOUR BREAST FEELS EACH MONTH.

5. NOW EXAMINE YOUR LEFT BREAST USING RIGHT HAND FINGER PADS.

6. IF YOU FIND ANY CHANGES, SEE YOUR DOCTOR RIGHT AWAY.

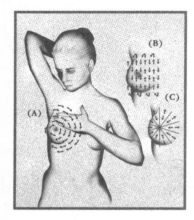

■ FOR ADDED SAFETY:

*Y*OU MIGHT WANT TO CHECK YOUR BREASTS WHILE STANDING IN FRONT OF A MIRROR RIGHT AFTER YOU DO YOUR BSE EACH MONTH. SEE IF THERE ARE ANY CHANGES IN THE WAY YOUR BREASTS LOOK: DIMPLING OF THE SKIN, OR CHANGES IN THE NIPPLE, REDNESS OR SWELLING. YOU MIGHT ALSO WANT TO DO AN EXTRA BSE WHILE YOU'RE IN THE SHOWER. YOUR SOAPY HANDS WILL GLIDE OVER THE WET SKIN MAKING IT EASY TO CHECK HOW YOUR BREASTS FEEL.

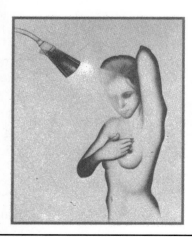

Figure 18.4 Breast self-examination (BSE) procedure (Courtesy American Cancer Society)

BREAST SELF-EXAMINATION (BSE)

Men as well as women may get breast cancer, so everyone from high school on should learn and practice self-examination of their breasts on a routine basis. Make this part of good health practices, just like eating well-balanced meals and exercising. Doing a routine BSE will help you become familiar with your breasts and locate changes early.

The American Cancer Society recommends that you examine your breasts monthly. Have your doctor examine your breasts at least every three years, and if you are a female between the ages of 35 and 39 you should have a baseline mammogram. If you are female and over age 40, you should have a mammogram at least every two years.

Schedule a routine time each month for your BSE. If you are still having menstrual periods, wait until one week after the beginning of your menstrual period. If you are breast-feeding an infant, do the BSE as soon as you have finished nursing. Men should do a BSE on the same date each month (Figure 18.4).

The patient should be instructed to contact the physician should any of the following be found on a BSE:

1. Lump or thickening in the breast or underarm.
2. Puckering, dimpling, or rash on the breast or nipple.
3. Change in nipple direction or a discharge from the nipple in nonlactating women or men.
4. Change in the shape or contour of the breast.

If any of the above changes are found, don't panic. Remember, most changes that occur in the breast are not cancerous, but only the physician can tell for sure after the appropriate examination and testing.

Men should also perform a testicular self-examination (TSE) on a monthly basis. After a warm shower or bath, the patient should **palpate** and roll each testical between the fingers to locate any abnormalities such as nodules. The scrotum should be examined for signs of swelling or tenderness and the penis for lesions, discharge, or other abnormalities (Figure 18.5).

The local chapter of the American Cancer Society will be happy to supply your office with pamphlets on BSE and TSE to distribute to your patients.

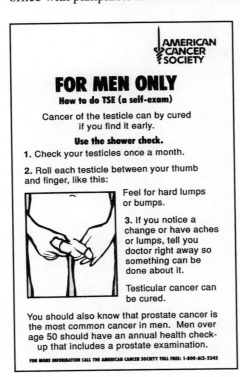

Figure 18.5 Testicle self-examination (TSE) procedure (Courtesy American Cancer Society)

**REVIEW/
SELF-EXAMINATION**

1. What factors affect an individual's nutritional needs?

2. List the four basic human needs.

3. List some special nutritional considerations of the elderly.

4. How is good nutrition evidenced?

5. What is the function of protein in the diet?

6. Why do we need vitamins and minerals?

7. What are vitamins?

8. List at least one disease associated with deficiency of each of the vitamins.

9. List the primary food sources of each of the vitamins.

10. What are minerals?

11. What minerals are frequently involved in metabolic disturbances?

12. Are vitamins capable of producing toxic effects?

13. Which vitamins are water soluble?

14. Which vitamins are fat soluble?

15. Can megadosing vitamins be harmful? Why?

16. If a patient is having difficulty with menu planning, food purchasing, and food preparation, to whom might you refer them for assistance?

17. List the benefits of exercise.

18. Why should all exercise include a warming up and cooling down period?

19. What is meant by aerobic exercise?

20. How is target heart rate determined?

21. Why perform self-examination?

22. List the steps in BSE.

23. Who needs to do self-examination?

24. At what age should a woman have her first mammogram?

25. Develop a one-day menu plan for yourself.

26. Develop an exercise program for yourself.

CHAPTER 19

Professionalism

OBJECTIVES

On completion of this chapter, you will be able to:
- Write a cover letter.
- Produce an error-free resume.
- Complete a neat and error-free job application.
- Identify job opportunities for the medical assistant.
- Discuss the interview process.
- Demonstrate interview readiness.
- Discuss the need for participation in professional organizations and continuing education.

Seeking the Right Position

As a professional medical assistant you will be performing a multitude of functions in the medical office that require a sound background in medical terminology, secretarial skills, administrative skills, and a knowledge of pharmacology, diagnostic procedures, laboratory procedures, asepsis, and surgical procedures. You must possess a genuine liking for people and such personal traits as intelligence, integrity, dependability, and enthusiasm. A high degree of patience, accuracy, and a motivation to serve humanity are also necessary.

Job opportunities for the medical assistant are available in medical clinics, hospitals, medical offices, public health facilities, research institutions, laboratories, pharmaceutical firms, government-related health service agencies, and insurance agencies.

Answering the following questions will help you focus on the jobs that hold the most appeal for you and to which you would bring the optimum in skills and enthusiasm.

1. In what type of facility would you like to work?
2. Would you prefer a solo medical practice over a larger one?
3. Would you prefer family practice over a specialty?
4. What hours do you prefer to work? Would working overtime be a problem?
5. Are you able to relocate if necessary?
6. How far are you willing to travel to work?
7. If applicable, do you have adequate childcare arrangements?
8. What if your child becomes ill?
9. How can you get to work if your car is in the repair shop?

10. What salary do you anticipate?
11. What benefits interest you the most?
12. Are you prepared to purchase uniforms if they are required?
13. What skills do you bring to the potential employer?
14. Do you hesitate to accept responsibility?
15. Are you willing to help out where needed?

Some medical facilities are open twenty-four hours a day and require staffing for all of those hours. Even in the so-called "8 to 5" jobs, it is unlikely that you will be able to leave exactly by 5:00 pm every work day.

Prior to beginning your job search, you should do some research on the types of positions that most interest you. Discuss with working medical assistants how many hours they work per week, what those hours are, pay ranges, benefits, etc. This can arm you with valuable information to use during the interview process. For example, if the starting medical assisting salaries in your area are $5.00–$6.00 per hour, it would be foolish for you to ask for a starting salary of $8.00 per hour.

WRITING A RESUME

The most important thing you can do in preparing to seek employment as a medical assistant is to develop, write, and produce a neat, concise, accurately spelled and attractively designed resume. It must contain all the basic information that a prospective employer may desire and will frequently act as your introduction to a potential employer. Therefore, it is imperative that you present yourself in the best possible fashion. Your resume should tell the employer:

1. Who you are.
2. What education you have had.
3. What skills you possess.
4. Any special training that qualifies you for the employment you are seeking.
5. Any previous employment history.
6. References from past employers, teachers, or people who know you well, other than relatives.

There are many styles of resumes and you will need to develop the style most suited to your needs. Resumes may be in outline form or in a narrative style and should reflect your personality. Whatever style you choose, remember that you are writing a document that will act as a marketing tool, and the item being marketed is *you*. Your resume should be typewritten on a good-quality, plain bond paper. Black ink on white bond is still the standard, but a light, buff-colored bond makes for an attractive resume as well (Figure 19.1).

In accordance with the Civil Rights Act of 1964, there is some information that you do not need to provide on a resume or job application. This includes your date of birth, social security number, marital status, ethnic background, dependent information, previous job duties, previous salary information, and particular skills. I would remind you, however, that when you are preparing your resume, you are preparing a marketing tool and to market yourself in the best light, the more information you supply, the better marketing tool you have. Think of it as putting together an advertisement.

Now that your resume has been prepared, you are ready to begin your job search. Your local newspaper's classified section is an obvious source of potential jobs. State and private employment agencies are also excellent sources of jobs since

RESUME

Mary J. Smith
15 West 10th Avenue
Your Town, US 00000
(123) 456-7890

Date of Birth: May 4, 1957
Social Security #:   066-21-8817
Marital Status: Single

WORK EXPERIENCE

1988–1989   Peter M. Kern, M.D.
                   28 East 5th Street
                   Your Town, US 00000

                   File Clerk and relief receptionist

EDUCATION

1987–1989   A.S. Degree, Your Town College,
                   Medical Assisting Certificate,
                   Your Town College

SKILLS

                   Typing 70 wpm. Word Processing-
                   WordPerfect, WordStar and
                   Displaywrite. Fluent in Spanish.

ACTIVITIES

                   Student member American Association
                   of Medical Assistants, Inc.
                   Local Chapter–Student President

REFERENCES

                   Furnished on request

Figure 19.1a Sample resumes

MARY JANE SMITH
15 West 10th Avenue
YOUR TOWN, US 00000
(123) 456-7890

CAREER OBJECTIVE

Administrative Medical Assistant

EDUCATION

1988–1990	Your Town Community College Expect to graduate in June with certificate in Medical Assisting.
1984–1988	Your Town High School Diploma

WORK EXPERIENCE

1988–1990	Peter M. Kern, M.D. 28 East 5th Street Your Town, US 00000 Externship Program and part-time file clerk.
1987–1988	Mary M. Clark, M.D. 15 West River Drive Your Town, US 00000 Part-time file clerk.

REFERENCES

Provided on request

Figure 19.1b   Sample resumes

many employers would prefer an outside agency to screen applicants and do any required testing to minimize the number of interviews the employer must conduct and ensure that they are interviewing only the most qualified applicants for the position. While state employment agencies normally charge no fee, private employment agencies do charge a fee to the job applicant for service. This fee varies but may be as high as one-month's salary. Many times the agency fee will be paid by the employer or is negotiable. Before signing a legally binding contract, you need to know who is responsible for the fee. *Do not sign any contract for payment of agency fee until you have read it thoroughly and agree to the stipulations contained therein.*

Your job search should also include visiting the personnel offices of hospitals, medical clinics, medical offices, insurance companies, etc. It is a good idea to take a copy of your resume with you since many of these offices will keep a copy on file even if they do not have current openings. When openings do occur, they will go through the resumes on file and attempt to fill openings without having to advertise.

Some job seekers use the telephone directory to advantage, using the yellow pages for names and addresses of potential employers. Should you decide to do this, you will need to send an accompanying cover letter with a copy of your resume. If you live in a small town, you may wish to saturate the market with copies of your resume. Keep in mind that if you send too few resumes, you may receive no replies. Send enough to allow you to be selective. Remember, you are seeking the right job for you, not just any job.

THE APPLICATION

For some of you, your first introduction to the prospective employer will be through a job application form. The information requested on the form is usually more comprehensive than that supplied on a resume. Fill out the job application form in black or blue ink and be careful to avoid errors. Applicants frequently find it convenient to carry a portfolio with them that contains the information that will be needed on the job application form (Figures 19.2 and 19.3).

There are various job application forms but all require more or less the same basic information. For your convenience, the following instructions are included for filling out the employment application form:

1. *Be prepared*—carry two ballpoint pens with the same shade of ink and have your portfolio with the necessary information readily available.
2. *Name*—use your legal name. It should be the same name that appears on your social security card. Be sure to have your social security card with you in case the employer wishes to see it.
3. *Address and telephone*—your residence address is usually required here. If your mailing address is different from your residence, such as a post office box, be sure to provide it. If you do not have a telephone, arrange for someone to take messages for you. Indicate in the appropriate space on the application whether the telephone number is your own or a message number.
4. *Birth record and/or naturalization*—it is desirable to have a photostat of your birth certificate available to show on request. This can be secured from the Bureau of Vital Statistics located in the capital of the state in which you were born, if you were born in the United States. If you were born outside the United States, you may be asked to furnish a Certificate of Derivative Citizenship, even if both parents are United States citizens by birth. This certificate may be obtained from the United States Immigration and Naturalization Service.

EMPLOYMENT APPLICATION   Date _____

Name
in Full (print) _____

Social
Security No. _____

Street
Address _____ City _____

Own Phone: _____ Neighbor _____

Do you have any physical condition which may limit your ability to perform the job(s) applied for? _____
_____

Kind of work desired _____ Wages expected _____

In case of emergency or accident, notify _____ Phone _____

Address _____ City _____ State _____
(Zip)

PREVIOUS EMPLOYERS (Address and Tel. No.)   TYPE OF WORK   FROM   TO   REASON FOR LEAVING

SIGNATURE: (For reference see reverse side)

REFERENCES (other than immediate family):

EDUCATION: High School Graduate _____ Yes or No

College _____ Yes or No

Other: _____

REMARKS:

Figure 19.2 Short-form application

5. *Physical characteristics*—list eye and hair color by natural color such as blue, green, black, or brown. You may also be asked for distinguishing marks such as scars, and you may be asked questions regarding your state of health and whether you would be willing to have a physical examination.

6. *Military*—complete as required.

7. *Person to be notified in case of an accident*—this is usually a spouse or parent, but may be anyone of your choice. Be sure to provide the correct address and telephone number.

Riverside Community College District
4800 Magnolia Avenue
Riverside, CA 92506

Classified Personnel Application
Affirmative Action/Equal Employment
  Opportunity Employer   M/F/H

For Office Use Only

Position(s) applying for _____   Date _____

Type or print all information in ink

Name_____

Last   First   Middle

Address_____

Number   Street   Apt

City   State   Zip Code   Soc. Sec No. _____

Home   (   ) _____
Phone: Work   (   ) _____
Message   (   ) _____

EDUCATION: Check appropriate box if you possess one of the following:
High School Diploma ☐   G.E.D. Certificate ☐   California High School Proficiency Certificate ☐
Give Highest Grade or Educational Level Achieved _____

Names of colleges/universities attended	Dates Attended	Course of Study/Major	Units Completed Semester Quarter	Type Degree	Date Degree Requirements Completed
A)					
B)					

Other schools/training completed: Course Studied/Hours Completed   Certificate Awarded
C) _____
D) _____

SKILLS:
Typing _____ wpm   Shorthand _____ wpm   Word Processing _____
                                                              Type of Equipment

Office Machines _____
Other Equipment _____

List the languages you speak, read and write fluently_____

Fingerprinting will be required if employed.
Have you ever been convicted of a misdemeanor which resulted in imprisonment or a felony (other than traffic violations)?
      Yes_____ No_____.
      If yes, the interviewer will discuss the offense with you. A conviction will not necessarily disqualify you from employment. Can you, after employment, submit verification of your legal right to work in the U.S.?_____

PHYSICAL CHARACTERISTICS: (Note: A pre-employment physical may be given at our expense. Freedom from tuberculosis is required for employment. Test will be given at district expense. The job relatedness of any handicap shall be determined by the college and no person shall be denied employment because of a handicap not related to the work to be performed.)
If you have any physical condition or handicap which may limit your ability to perform the job applied for, what can be done to accommodate your limitation? _____ Are you 18 years or older? Yes____ No____.

Any application, resume, or other materials submitted, either solicited or unsolicited, for employment at Riverside Community College District will become the property of Riverside Community College District and will not be returned to the applicant.
The Riverside Community College District does not discriminate in the educational programs or activities operated by the district or in the employment procedures and practices of the district. The policies of the district implementing Title IX as developed to date are available for inspection during normal business hours at the district's office at 4800 Magnolia Avenue, Riverside, CA 92506. Any complaints or questions may be referred to the Deputy Superintendent at the district office or to the Director of the Office for Civil Rights of the Department of Health, Education, and Welfare.

NAME _____

RIVERSIDE COMMUNITY
  COLLEGE DISTRICT
  PERSONNEL OFFICE

This information is only for statistical purposes with regard to affirmative action. Your cooperation in providing the requested information is appreciated. This information will be kept separate and confidential and will not be used in any way to make any employment decisions.

Please complete the following:

....
Position Applied For

....
Date

MO	DAY	YR

Birthdate

(CHECK APPROPRIATE BOXES)
☐ Male   ☐ Female

☐ White

☐ Black-Negro, Afro-American

☐ Hispanic: Spanish-Surname, Mexican American, Puerto Rican, Latin American

☐ Asian-American, Oriental

☐ Filipino

☐ American Indian or Alaskan Native

Figure 19.3a Long-form application

List your work history below. Begin with your **present** or most **recent** job and list in reverse order. This section must be completed even though a resume is attached. If more space is needed, ask for supplemental sheet.

Dates of Work	Exact job title:	Name of company or employer
From:_____ *Mo./Yr.* To: _____ *Mo./Yr.* Full time? ☐ *(40 hrs./wk.)* Part time? ☐ If part time, # of hours per week _____ Last Salary $ _____ ☐ yearly ☐ weekly ☐ monthly ☐ hourly	Describe your duties fully:	Company address
		Company phone number
		Your supervisor's name and job title
		Reason for leaving
Dates of Work	Exact job title:	Name of company or employer
From:_____ *Mo./Yr.* To: _____ *Mo./Yr.* Full time? ☐ *(40 hrs./wk.)* Part time? ☐ If part time, # of hours per week _____ Last Salary $ _____ ☐ yearly ☐ weekly ☐ monthly ☐ hourly	Describe your duties fully:	Company address
		Company phone number
		Your supervisor's name and job title
		Reason for leaving
Dates of Work	Exact job title:	Name of company or employer
From:_____ *Mo./Yr.* To: _____ *Mo./Yr.* Full time? ☐ *(40 hrs./wk.)* Part time? ☐ If part time, # of hours per week _____ Last Salary $ _____ ☐ yearly ☐ weekly ☐ monthly ☐ hourly	Describe your duties fully:	Company address
		Company phone number
		Your supervisor's name and job title
		Reason for leaving
Dates of Work	Exact job title:	Name of company or employer
From:_____ *Mo./Yr.* To: _____ *Mo./Yr.* Full time? ☐ *(40 hrs./wk.)* Part time? ☐ If part time, # of hours per week _____ Last Salary $ _____ ☐ yearly ☐ weekly ☐ monthly ☐ hourly	Describe your duties fully:	Company address
		Company phone number
		Your supervisor's name and job title
		Reason for leaving

Would contacting your employer in the preliminary selection process jeopardize your employment? ☐ Yes ☐ No
Please be reminded that if selected as a **finalist,** your employer will be contacted.
COMMENT:

CERTIFICATE OF APPLICANT (Read before signing)
I hereby declare that the statements in this application are true and complete to the best of my knowledge, and I authorize investigation of all statements contained herein. I hereby release from liability all persons and organizations furnishing such information. I understand that any misstatements or omissions of material facts in this application may be cause for disqualification or dismissal.
X Not valid unless signature appears here _____ Date:_____

PLEASE INDICATE IF ANY OF THE FOLLOWING DEFINITIONS APPLY TO YOU	PLEASE COMPLETE THE FOLLOWING:
☐ **VIETNAM ERA VETERAN.** A person who (1) served on active duty for a period of more than 180 days any part of which occurred between 8/5/64 and 5/7/75, and was discharged or released therefrom with other than a dishonorable discharge, or (2) was discharged or released from active duty for service-connected disability if any part of such active duty was performed between 8/5/64 and 5/7/75. ☐ **DISABLED VETERAN.** A person entitled to disability compensation under laws administered by the Veteran's Administration for disability rated at 30 per centum or more or a person whose discharge or release from active duty was for a disability incurred or aggravated in the line of duty. ☐ **HANDICAPPED INDIVIDUAL.** A person who (1) has a physical or mental impairment which substantially limits one or more such person's major life activities, (2) has a record of such impairment or (3) is regarded as having such an impairment.	How did you find out about this job? (Check one or more) ☐ District Personnel Office ☐ From a job flyer or bulletin ☐ From a District Employee ☐ EDD ☐ From a friend or relative Specify Location ☐ Newspaper (Name)_____ ☐ Trade or professional publication (Name) _____ ☐ Community organization Specify ☐ Other_____

Figure 19.3b Long-form application

8. *Marital status*—enter your status as single, married, divorced, separated, or widowed in the appropriate space.
9. *Employment record*—fill in in chronological order, with current or most recent employment listed first.
10. *Special qualifications/skills*—develop a brief statement of your special qualifications and skills for quick reference.
11. *Organizations*—list professional organizations of which you are a member. Be sure to include any officer positions or committee chairs you hold or have held.
12. *Additional information*—include community activities or information that an employer may consider relevant.

While the above information may be requested on the application, I again remind you that in accordance with the Civil Rights Act of 1964 responses related to height, weight, date of birth, marital status, social security number, and physical condition may be excluded.

THE COVER LETTER

If you are responding to an advertisement in the newspaper or professional journal that requires you to send a copy of your resume, you will need to write an accompanying *cover letter*. This letter, like your resume, should be concise, error free, and typewritten on good-quality bond paper. Your cover letter is an application letter and should be written to attract the reader's interest as quickly as possible, preferably in the first twenty to thirty words. It should state your qualifications, why you would like to work in that particular facility and how you learned about the position. Your career objectives should be mentioned, and the concluding sentence should pave the way for an interview by including your telephone number (Figure 19.4).

Before mailing your cover letter and resume, give them a final check for errors.

INTERVIEWING

Once the potential employer has determined from screening resumes and application forms which candidates appear to meet the qualifications of the position, interviews are arranged. The personal interview is the time when the prospective employer and the candidates for the position have the opportunity to meet face to face, talk about the requirements of the position, and discuss any questions about the position, benefits, etc. In a manner of speaking, both parties are conducting an interview. The employer is attempting to determine if the candidate meets the qualifications for the position and will fit in compatibly with the rest of the staff. The candidate is attempting to determine if the position will meet their needs.

Many interviews are now conducted by a panel of two or more employees and the office manager or physician employer. This type of interview allows the candidate the advantage of meeting some or all of the staff and being able to ask more questions and expect realistic answers. The average physician may have the overall picture of how the office is managed but is usually not able to answer some of the job-specific questions you may ask.

Arrive promptly for the interview. When possible, greet the interviewer by name. Always wait to be seated until instructed to do so. Listen attentively to all questions asked, and do not be afraid to ask for clarification if needed. Think before you respond. There is no hurry. Speak confidently and maintain reasonable eye contact with the party asking the question. When discussing past employers, remember to be discreet. Be calm and as relaxed as possible. This will allow you to do a

Mary J. Smith
15 West 10th Avenue
Your Town, US 00000
July 1, 1989

Robert D. Baker, M.D.
Your Town Medical Clinic
28 Riverside Avenue
Your Town, US 00000

Dear Dr. Baker:

As you will see from the enclosed resume, my training and experience qualify me for the position you advertised in Your Town Press on June 30, 1989.

You may reach me by telephoning (123) 456-7890 any day after 1:00 PM. May I have the privilege of a personal interview at your convenience?

Sincerely yours,

cc.
encl. Resume

Mary Jane Smith
15 West 10th Avenue
Your Town, US 00000
May 31, 1989

Robert D. Baker, M.D.
Your Town Medical Clinic
28 Riverside Avenue
Your Town, US 00000

Dear Dr. Baker:

I will be receiving my Medical Assisting certificate from Your Town Community College in June and have one year of experience in a medical office.

Mr. Robertson, the placement officer at Your Town Community College informed me that you have an opening for a medical assistant. I am enclosing a resume and hope that you will be willing to schedule a personal interview for the position.

You can reach me any day after 3:30 PM by telephoning (123) 456-7890.

Yours truly,

cc.
encl. Resume

Figure 19.4 Two sample cover letters

better job of selling yourself and your skills. Whether your interview is one-to-one or a panel interview, you will no doubt be evaluated on the following items:

1. *Appearance*—are you clean, well-groomed, and appropriately attired? Moderation is the key. Do not wear trendy clothing or excessive make-up or jewelry. While a pant-suit is considered acceptable, a dress or suit is still preferred.
2. *Maturity*—are you consistent, accurate, and tactful in your answers to questions? Are you direct and to the point? Does your temperament appear consistent with the position applied for and amenable to patients and staff alike?
3. *Enthusiasm*—is your presentation open and friendly, sincere and yet persuasive?
4. *Preparation*—is your knowledge of the position adequate? Has your education and/or previous employment prepared you for the minimum requirements of the position?

As previously indicated, the interview is also a time for you to interview the prospective employer and to attempt to determine whether you will find satisfaction with the position. The following checklist may serve as a guide:

1. Is the job of a type you will enjoy?
2. Are the hours satisfactory?
3. Do you feel qualified to perform the work expected?
4. Will there be transportation problems in getting to and from the job?
5. Does the staff appear satisfied?
6. Do the surroundings appear conducive to on-the-job efficiency?
7. Are the fringe benefits adequate for your needs?
8. Who will be your immediate supervisor? Does this appear to be someone of whom you would not hesitate to ask a question?
9. Is the beginning salary sufficient?
10. Is there a chance for advancement?

FOLLOWUP

Since there are normally several applicants who are interviewed for a position, a job offer is seldom made at the time of the interview. Most employers will, however, provide the applicant with a time frame in which they intend to make their decision. It is considered both appropriate and in good taste for the applicant to send a letter of thanks to the employer for the interview and a reminder that you are interested in the position (Figure 19.5).

Changing Jobs

There are times when, for a variety of reasons, a medical assistant will change jobs. When this becomes necessary:

1. Notify your employer in writing, giving your termination date. It is customary to provide your current employer with two weeks' notice.
2. Ask your employer for a letter of reference giving the dates you were employed, your job duties, and any personal comments they may wish to make.
3. Be sure to remove any personal belongings prior to your termination date.

Professional Organizations

Once the job has been secured, even though you are new and have a great deal to learn, you are now a professional medical assistant. As a professional medical assistant, you will want to actively participate in one of the national organizations introduced in Chapter 1.

Mary J. Smith
15 West 10th Avenue
Your Town, US 00000

July 15, 1989

Robert D. Baker, M.D.
Your Town Medical Clinic
28 Riverside Avenue
Your Town, US 00000

Dear Dr. Baker:

Thank you for granting me an interview on July 13, 1989, for the Medical Assisting position.

I am very much interested in the position and feel that I can perform to your satisfaction. If you require additional information to assist you in arriving at a decision regarding my qualifications for the position, I can be contacted at (123) 456-7890, weekdays after 1:00 PM.

Yours truly,

cc.

Figure 19.5 Follow-up letter

Certification

Both of the professional organizations offer certification examinations and revalidation procedures. Information can be obtained by writing to the organization directly.

Continuing Education

Continuing education is a vital function of your professional organization. There will be workshops and seminars offered at local, state, and national levels in which you can actively participate.

Many two-year colleges offer vocational programs for medical assistants that lead to an associate of arts or associate in science degree. Independent study programs are also available through AAMA for preparation for the certification examination, continuing education units, and upgrading of skills.

For those who are interested, your local colleges and universities offer extension programs that can lead to various related certifications, such as in the field of insurance and workman's compensation. They also offer vocational education programs and baccalaureate and master's degrees in related health programs for the individual who wishes to pursue a higher degree.

1. List seven job skills a medical assistant must possess.

2. List three personal traits a medical assistant must possess.

3. What is the purpose of a resume?

4. In accordance with the Civil Rights Act of 1964, what information does not need to be provided on a resume or job application?

5. What information is usually requested on a job application?

6. What is the purpose of a cover letter?

7. What two organizations offer certification examinations for medical assistants?

8. Who is entitled to use CMA after their name?

9. Why concern oneself with continuing education?

10. Give the date, location, and time of your local professional association meetings.

APPENDIX

Correlation of 1990 Dacum Guidelines to Chapters

1.0   DISPLAY PROFESSIONALISM

1.1   Project a Positive Attitude
- A.   Chapter 1 Introduction to Clinical Medical Assisting
- B.   Chapter 19 Professionalism

1.2   Perform Within Ethical Boundaries
- A.   Chapter 1 Introduction to Clinical Medical Assisting
- B.   Chapter 4 Data Collection

1.3   Practice Within the Scope of Education Training and Personal Capabilities
- A.   Chapter 1 Introduction to Clinical Medical Assisting

1.4   Maintain Confidentiality
- A.   Chapter 1 Introduction to Clinical Medical Assisting
- B.   Chapter 4 Data Collection

1.5   Work as a Team Member
- A.   All chapters

1.6   Conduct Oneself in a Courteous and Diplomatic Manner
- A.   All chapters

1.7   Adapt to Change
- A.   All chapters

1.8   Show Initiative and Responsibility
- A.   All chapters

1.9   Promote the Profession
- A.   Chapter 1 Introduction to Clinical Medical Assisting
- B.   Chapter 19 Professionalism

2.0 COMMUNICATE

2.1 Listen and Observe
    A.   Chapter 4 Data Collection
    B.   Chapter 5 Vital Signs
    C.   Chapter 6 Assisting with the Physical Examination
    D.   Chapter 7 Bandages and Dressings
    E.   Chapter 9 Office Surgery
    F.   Chapter 10 The Healing Process
    G.   Chapter 11 Pharmacology
    H.   Chapter 12 Administration of Medications
    I.   Chapter 13 Specimen Collection
    J.   Chapter 14 Laboratory Examinations
    K.   Chapter 15 Other Diagnostic Tests
    L.   Chapter 16 Treatment Modalities
    M.   Chapter 17 Emergencies
    N.   Chapter 18 Health Maintenance

2.2 Treat All Patients with Empathy and Impartiality
    A.   Chapter 4 Data Collection
    B.   Chapter 5 Vital Signs
    C.   Chapter 6 Assisting with the Physical Examination
    D.   Chapter 7 Bandages and Dressings
    E.   Chapter 9 Office Surgery
    F.   Chapter 10 The Healing Process
    G.   Chapter 11 Pharmacology
    H.   Chapter 12 Administration of Medications
    I.   Chapter 14 Laboratory Examinations
    J.   Chapter 15 Other Diagnostic Tests
    K.   Chapter 16 Treatment Modalities
    L.   Chapter 17 Emergencies
    M.   Chapter 18 Health Maintenance

2.3 Adapt Communication to Individuals' Abilities to Understand
    A.   Chapter 1 Introduction to Clinical Medical Assisting
    B.   Chapter 4 Data Collection
    C.   Chapter 18 Health Maintenance

2.4 Recognize and Respond to Verbal and Nonverbal Communication
    A.   Chapter 4 Data Collection
    B.   Chapter 5 Vital Signs
    C.   Chapter 6 Assisting with the Physical Examination
    D.   Chapter 9 Office Surgery
    E.   Chapter 15 Other Diagnostic Tests
    F.   Chapter 16 Treatment Modalities
    G.   Chapter 17 Emergencies
    H.   Chapter 18 Health Maintenance

2.5 Serve as Liaison Between Physician and Others
    A.   Chapter 1 Introduction to Clinical Medical Assisting
    B.   Chapter 19 Professionalism

2.9   Interview Effectively
    A.   Chapter 4 Data Collection
    B.   Chapter 19 Professionalism

2.10 Use Medical Terminology Appropriately
    A.   Chapter 2 Agents of Disease
    B.   Chapter 3 Medical Asepsis
    C.   Chapter 4 Data Collection
    D.   Chapter 5 Vital Signs
    E.   Chapter 6 Assisting with the Physical Examination
    F.   Chapter 7 Bandages and Dressings
    G.   Chapter 8 Surgical Instruments and Supplies
    H.   Chapter 9 Office Surgery
    I.   Chapter 10 The Healing Process
    J.   Chapter 11 Pharmacology
    K.   Chapter 12 Administration of Medications
    L.   Chapter 13 Specimen Collection
    M.   Chapter 14 Laboratory Examinations
    N.   Chapter 15 Other Diagnostic Tests
    O.   Chapter 16 Treatment Modalities
    P.   Chapter 17 Emergencies
    Q.   Chapter 18 Health Maintenance

4.0   PERFORM CLINICAL DUTIES

4.1   Apply Principles of Aseptic Technique and Infection Control
    A.   Chapter 2 Agents of Disease
    B.   Chapter 3 Medical Asepsis
    C.   Chapter 6 Assisting with the Physical Examination
    D.   Chapter 8 Surgical Instruments and Supplies
    E.   Chapter 9 Office Surgery

4.2   Take Vital Signs
    A.   Chapter 5 Vital Signs

4.3   Recognize Emergencies
    A.   Chapter 15 Other Diagnostic Tests
    B.   Chapter 17 Emergencies

4.4   Perform First Aid and CPR
    A.   Chapter 1 Introduction to Clinical Medical Assisting
    B.   Chapter 7 Bandages and Dressings
    C.   Chapter 17 Emergencies

4.5   Prepare and Maintain Examination and Treatment Areas
    A.   Chapter 3 Medical Asepsis
    B.   Chapter 6 Assisting with the Physical Examination
    C.   Chapter 8 Surgical Instruments and Supplies
    D.   Chapter 9 Office Surgery
    E.   Chapter 10 The Healing Process
    F.   Chapter 13 Specimen Collection

B. Chapter 14 Laboratory Examinations
C. Chapter 15 Other Diagnostic Tests

4.12 Screen and Follow-up Patient Test Results
A. Chapter 5 Vital Signs
B. Chapter 14 Laboratory Examinations
C. Chapter 15 Other Diagnostic Tests

4.13 Prepare and Administer Medications as Directed by Physician
A. Chapter 11 Pharmacology
B. Chapter 12 Administration of Medications

4.14 Maintain Medication Records
A. Chapter 11 Pharmacology
B. Chapter 12 Administration of Medications

4.15 Respond to Medical Emergencies
A. Chapter 17 Emergencies

5.0 APPLY LEGAL CONCEPTS TO PRACTICE

5.1 Document Accurately
A. Chapter 1 Introduction to Clinical Medical Assisting
B. Chapter 4 Data Collection
C. Chapter 5 Vital Signs
D. Chapter 6 Assisting with the Physical Examination
E. Chapter 7 Bandages and Dressings
F. Chapter 9 Office Surgery
G. Chapter 10 The Healing Process
H. Chapter 11 Pharmacology
I. Chapter 12 Administration of Medications
J. Chapter 13 Specimen Collection
K. Chapter 14 Laboratory Examinations
L. Chapter 15 Other Diagnostic Tests
M. Chapter 16 Treatment Modalities
N. Chapter 17 Emergencies

5.2 Determine Needs for Documentation and Reporting
A. Chapter 4 Data Collection
B. Chapter 5 Vital Signs
C. Chapter 7 Bandages and Dressings
D. Chapter 10 The Healing Process
E. Chapter 12 Administration of Medications
F. Chapter 13 Specimen Collection
G. Chapter 14 Laboratory Examinations
H. Chapter 15 Other Diagnostic Tests
I. Chapter 16 Treatment Modalities
J. Chapter 17 Emergencies
K. Chapter 18 Health Maintenance

5.5 Dispose of Controlled Substances in Compliance with Government Regulations
    A.   Chapter 11 Pharmacology
    B.   Chapter 12 Administration of Medications

5.7 Monitor Legislation Related to Current Healthcare Issues and Practice
    A.   Chapter 1 Introduction to Clinical Medical Assisting
    B.   Chapter 14 Laboratory Examinations
    C.   Chapter 19 Professionalism

7.0 PROVIDE INSTRUCTION

7.2 Instruct Patients with Special Needs
    A.   Chapter 7 Bandages and Dressings
    B.   Chapter 9 Office Surgery
    C.   Chapter 10 The Healing Process
    D.   Chapter 12 Administration of Medications
    E.   Chapter 13 Specimen Collection
    F.   Chapter 15 Other Diagnostic Tests
    G.   Chapter 16 Treatment Modalities
    H.   Chapter 17 Emergencies
    I.   Chapter 18 Health Maintenance

7.3 Teach Patients Methods of Health Promotion and Disease Prevention
    A.   Chapter 2 Agents of Disease
    B.   Chapter 18 Health Maintenance

Index

Note: Page numbers in **bold** type reference to non-text material.